CULTURAL CONSIDERATIONS

LIFESPAN CONSIDERATIONS

ACTION STATS

St_____

DISORDER CLOSE-UPS

Mosby's
EXPERT
PHYSICAL
EXAM HANDBOOK
Rapid Inpatient and Outpatient Assessments

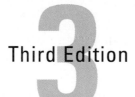

Third Edition

Frances D. Monahan, PhD, RN, ANEF
Professor of Nursing
SUNY Rockland Community College
Suffern, New York
and
Consulting Faculty
Excelsior College
Albany, New York

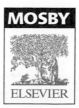

MOSBY

ELSEVIER

MOSBY
ELSEVIER

11830 Westline Industrial Drive
St. Louis, Missouri 63146

Mosby's Expert Physical Exam Handbook: ISBN: 978-0-323-05791-2
Rapid Inpatient and Outpatient Assessments

Notice

Knowledge and best practice in this field are constantly changing. As new research and experience broaden our knowledge, changes in practice, treatment and drug therapy may become necessary or appropriate. Readers are advised to check the most current information provided (i) on procedures featured or (ii) by the manufacturer of each product to be administered, to verify the recommended dose or formula, the method and duration of administration, and contraindications. It is the responsibility of the practitioner, relying on their own experience and knowledge of the patient, to make diagnoses, to determine dosages and the best treatment for each individual patient, and to take all appropriate safety precautions. To the fullest extent of the law, neither the Publisher nor the Author assumes any liability for any injury and/or damage to persons or property arising out of or related to any use of the material contained in this book.

The Publisher

Previous editions copyrighted 2005, 1997.

Library of Congress Cataloging in Publication Data
Monahan, Frances Donovan.
   Mosby's expert physical exam handbook: rapid inpatient and outpatient assessments/Frances D. Monahan.—3rd ed.
      p.; cm.
   Rev ed. of: Mosby's expert 10-minute physical examinations.
   Includes index.
   ISBN 978-0-323-05791-2 (pbk. : alk. paper) 1. Physical diagnosis—Handbooks, manuals, etc. 2. Nursing diagnosis—Handbooks, manuals, etc. I. Mosby, Inc. II. Mosby's expert 10-minute physical examinations. III. Title.
   [DNLM: 1. Physical Examination—Handbooks. 2. Nursing Assessment—Handbooks. WB 39 M734m 2009]
   RC76.E97 2009
   616.07′54—dc22   2008030802

Acquisitions Editor: Robin Carter
Developmental Editor: Deanna Davis
Publishing Services Manager: Deborah L. Vogel
Project Manager: Ann E. Rogers
Book Designer: Kimberly Denando

Working together to grow
libraries in developing countries

www.elsevier.com | www.bookaid.org | www.sabre.org

ELSEVIER   BOOK AID International   Sabre Foundation

Printed in United States of America
Last digit is the print number: 9 8 7 6 5 4 3 2 1

REVIEWERS

Jody F. Agins, MSN, RNP, BC-FNP/GNP
Executive Director
Seminars for Healthcare Education, Inc
and
Family & Geriatric Nurse Practitioner
Evercare
Tucson, Arizona

Erin Bagshaw, RN, MSN, C-ANP
Owner/Practice Director
Northwest Nurse Practitioner Associates
Washington, DC

Tim J. Bristol, RN, PhD
Director of Nursing
Crown College
St. Bonifacius, Minnesota

Mary Ann Siciliano McLaughlin, MSN, RN
Nurse Educator
Hospital of the University of Pennsylvania
Philadelphia, Pennsylvania

PREFACE

When you open this latest edition of *Mosby's Expert Physical Exam Handbook: Rapid Inpatient and Outpatient Assessments*, you'll see a physical examination book like no other. Packed with time-saving tips, this portable handbook will help you to organize your physical examination so that you can move through the examination quickly—and without missing critical findings. The book's organization allows you to rapidly find what you need, easily accessed in either a hospital or clinical setting. Physical exam content is organized by body region—for example, chest and back—rather than by body system, an approach that provides an excellent method for conducting a thorough examination. What's more, the book will help you realize when to shift gears and focus the examination on a critical sign or chief complaint.

HOW TO USE THIS BOOK

There are two ways to use this handbook and approach the physical examination. First, working methodically with a patient who is no immediate distress, you can cover all areas of the body, picking up any abnormal findings. You can pace yourself knowing you'll need to spend extra time examining the areas that reflect the patient's recovery from a specific condition. You'll find that Chapters 1 through 9 provide you with detailed knowledge of how to examine the major body regions. Chapter 10 then weaves together all aspects of a head-to-toe examination, and Chapter 11 highlights key information to document during the initial assessment and presents guidelines for documenting findings for more than 20 selected conditions.

If you have quickly identified a chief complaint from your patient, you'll want to begin a focused, rapid assessment that addresses the most pressing problem. That's why throughout this book you've been given techniques for isolating your patient's chief complaint (such as chest pain, dyspnea, and nausea), performing a focused assessment, and pinpointing its probable cause.

SPECIAL FEATURES

Several special features, signaled by quick-reference symbols within the text, help speed you to important assessment information.

Q *Disorder Close-Ups* focus on the most common disorders encountered by nurses today, listing their characteristic findings as well as complications. Disorders include angina pectoris, asthma, diabetes mellitus, hypertension, myocardial infarction, and many others.

Q *Action STATs* tell you exactly what to do if, during your examination, you discover that your patient is in a potentially life-threatening situation.

Q *Anatomy Reviews* present detailed illustrations of major body parts and organs.

Q *Normal Findings* summarize characteristic findings and acceptable variations based on age, sex, and condition of the patient.

Q *Interpreting Abnormal Findings* help you analyze abnormal findings and determine their causes.

Exam Tips feature time-saving pointers that make the examination faster and easier—and more accurate.

Lifespan Considerations help you individualize exams for patients of various ages and for those who are pregnant or lactating.

Cultural Considerations provide information on variations in findings and transcultural considerations.

The **step-by-step format** is easy to follow and covers all aspects of physical examination: inspection, palpation, percussion, and auscultation.

Chief complaints with **interview questions and guidelines** are provided for focused assessments.

How-to tips on individualizing the physical exam for patients with serious illnesses, pain, or handicaps provide specific approaches for special situations.

NEW TO THIS EDITION

To keep you on the right track, we've packed even more information and features into the third edition of *Mosby's Expert Physical Exam Handbook*.

Updated content throughout provides you with the latest information on assessment techniques, normal and abnormal findings, and the assessment of patients with specific diseases and disorders.

Expert Exam Checklists throughout the book review the most important steps to cover when examining patients.

Spanish-English Assessment Terms provide you with key assessment questions and findings.

The **dual-function table of contents** now provides body systems cross-referencing in addition to a body regions organization.

The **new companion Evolve website** offers easily accessible resources such as heart and lung audio clips, highly detailed and clear exam animations, and printable or PDA-downloadable versions of the Expert Exam Checklists. The website can be accessed, free with your purchase of this book, at http://evolve.elsevier.com/Mosby/expertexam/.

These added features have been selected, prepared, and reviewed with your time constraints and patient-care needs in mind. The new and improved *Mosby's Expert Physical Exam Handbook* is a reference tool that no nurse should be without.

CONTENTS

Health History and Physical Examination Review

An accurate, complete health history coupled with a general physical survey provides the foundation for a thorough, head-to-toe physical examination. Health history information helps focus your assessment on the patient's most important health problems. The health history interview provides an opportunity to assess your patient's understanding of his health problems or health maintenance needs and guides you as you devise a plan of care.

The following are keys to obtaining a reliable health history:

- Establish a rapport with your patient to promote cooperation.
- Make the patient comfortable both physically and psychologically.
  - Ensure privacy by drawing the curtains, closing the door, keeping your voice low, and asking others to leave the room if possible.
  - Make sure the room temperature is comfortable.
  - Find out if the patient has any immediate needs, for example, for a glass of water or use of the bathroom. Address those needs before proceeding with the interview.
- Use appropriate body language.
  - Sit down for the interview to avoid intimidating the patient and to indicate that you have time to spend meeting his or her needs.
  - Keep a *social distance,* staying several feet away from the patient, to set a proper tone for the interview.

CULTURAL CONSIDERATIONS

Certain cultural groups perceive personal space differently. For example, patients of Hispanic or Middle Eastern ancestry often feel more comfortable with less personal space (less than 4 feet between you and the patient) than those from other cultures. If your patient moves closer to create a more intimate space, try not to move away—a reaction that may offend the patient. On the other hand, patients of other cultural backgrounds, for example those of Native American, Vietnamese, Chinese, Korean, and West Indian heritage, may prefer that you maintain more distance during the interview.

- Keep focused on the patient to detect nonverbal clues to the patient's feelings and thoughts.
  - Maintain eye contact as much as possible.
  - Keep note taking to a minimum.

CULTURAL CONSIDERATIONS

Comfort with eye contact varies greatly among cultural groups. Patients who are of Asian, Arabic, Native American, or Hispanic heritage may avoid eye contact. Some cultural groups view steady eye contact as a form of aggression, whereas others avert their eyes as a sign of respect to authority.

- Communicate effectively.
  - Word questions wisely.
    - Use closed-ended questions for obtaining basic information, such as name and age.
    - Use open-ended questions to elicit details, such as when exploring the chief complaint.
    - Use nonjudgmental questions, not biased or leading questions (e.g., "Are you sexually active?" rather than "You are not sexually active, are you?")
  - Give the patient a chance to describe symptoms and concerns without interruption.
  - Listen closely to what the patient says, interrupting only to ask for clarification.
  - Avoid asking several consecutive questions that require yes-or-no answers because this can become confusing and also discourage the patient from providing additional information.

CULTURAL CONSIDERATIONS

If you and your patient speak different languages, enlist the help of an interpreter to get through the history and physical examination. Although it is often more convenient for a family member to translate, a professionally trained medical interpreter offers added benefits because he knows medical terminology, understands patient rights, and can provide culturally sensitive teaching and advice. If you use a family member to interpret, keep in mind that the patient might shield the family member from embarrassing or alarming information. Whomever you choose to translate, be sure to speak clearly and plainly (avoiding complicated terms), and pause every one or two sentences to allow for interpretation and responses.

OBTAINING THE HEALTH HISTORY: A SYSTEMATIC APPROACH

Use a systematic approach to the health history to save time and help organize your thoughts and questions. Before starting the interview, review the patient's available medical records to help identify areas that need further exploration.

Reviewing a patient's medical records is never a substitute for obtaining a health history directly from the patient.

Next, begin the interview and proceed through the following steps:

- Collect basic patient information.
- Determine the chief complaint.
- Obtain a history of the present illness.
- Obtain a past medical and surgical history.
- Obtain a family history.
- Obtain a social history.
- Conduct a review of body systems.
- Conclude the health history.

Safeguard the privacy of all medical records and information obtained during the history and physical examination in compliance with the regulations put forth by the Health Insurance Portability and Accountability Act (HIPAA) of 1996 (see Putting HIPAA into Practice).

PUTTING HIPAA INTO PRACTICE

The Health Insurance Portability and Accountability Act (HIPAA) national legislation was enacted to protect patients' privacy by safeguarding disclosure of health care information, such as medical records and medical information collected by or communicated to health care providers by oral, electronic, or paper routes, as well as any information related to the patient's health, health care, or payment history. This act aims to provide patients with better control over their personal health records and to give health care workers uniform standards of practice. Here is how you can comply with HIPAA standards when performing and documenting a health history and physical examination:

- When admitting a patient, provide him with a copy of his privacy rights.
- When taking a health history, keep your voice low and ask others to leave the room, if possible.
- Keep the results of the health history and physical examination, indeed all medical records, in a secure location. If charts are kept at the nurse's station, shield the names from the view of those passing by.
- If you are recording the health history and physical examination electronically, make sure the computer screen is not visible to visitors and others.
- Request and distribute the results of the health history and physical examination, as well as all other private information, on a need-to-know basis. This rule applies to information given in writing, by phone or fax, or electronically.
- Check your institution's policies and procedures, or check with an administrator to determine if you need patient authorization before sharing information.
- Remove any patient identifiers, such as name and social security number, from documents that you transmit by fax or e-mail.

COLLECTING BASIC PATIENT INFORMATION

Begin the health history by noting basic information, such as the source of the patient's referral, the source of patient information, and the reliability of the information provided.

To judge the reliability of the information provided, determine the patient's level of alertness and orientation. (You may not be able to judge reliability until later in the interview, when evaluating the patient's mental health status.) If you must gather information from a person other than the patient, find out how well that person knows the patient.

DETERMINING THE CHIEF COMPLAINT

Next, determine the chief complaint, which is the main reason the patient is seeking health care. Record the chief complaint in the patient's own words, using quotation marks (e.g., "I've had chest pain since early this morning"); then gather details about the symptom or symptoms (see Investigating the Chief Complaint).

INVESTIGATING THE CHIEF COMPLAINT

Ask your patient to describe the chief complaint, the main symptom or reason for seeking health care, as fully as possible. Further description may help you identify the underlying cause of the patient's problem. If the problem is life threatening, obtaining detailed information also promotes rapid intervention.

Dig for details
Obtain as many details as possible about the chief complaint. For instance, if the chief complaint is pain, ask whether the pain is sharp or dull, aching, burning, or shooting.

Find out what the patient was doing when his symptom began and how often the symptom occurs. Does he experience it during such activities as exercising, walking, doing housework, or showering? Does it occur during rest or awaken him from sleep?

Ask about onset, duration, and location
Determine the time of onset and the duration of the chief complaint. Ask when the patient first felt the symptom and how long it lasted; then ask about its location. Find out if the symptom is confined to one area or if it affects other areas as well. To help identify symptom location, ask the patient to point to the affected area.

Use terms the patient is familiar with. For example, instead of asking if the pain radiates, ask if the patient feels pain in any other part of the body.

Evaluate symptom severity
Next, explore the severity or degree of the chief complaint by asking the patient to quantify the symptom. Suppose, for example, your patient reports he has been coughing up blood. You will want to find out how often this happens and how much blood is involved. To elicit this information, ask the following (or similar) questions:
- "How many times have you coughed up blood?"
- "Was the sputum merely streaked with blood, or was a larger amount of blood present?"
- "How big was the bloody area? About the size of a nickel or more like the size of a half dollar?"
- "Did you cough into a tissue? If so, did the blood fill the tissue?"

continued

INVESTIGATING THE CHIEF COMPLAINT—cont'd

Ask about aggravating and relieving factors

Aggravating and relieving factors can provide insight into the cause of the chief complaint. Ask the patient if the symptom seems to get worse at certain times, for instance, with a change in seasons or temperature, when he consumes certain foods or beverages, or when he takes part in certain activities.

   Find out what measures, if any, bring relief. Does the symptom improve with rest? With medication? With heat or cold application?

Explore associated symptoms

Find out if the patient has other symptoms that could be associated with the chief complaint. These symptoms could provide clues to the underlying cause. For example, if chest pain is the chief complaint, ask if it is ever accompanied by nausea, shortness of breath, palpitations, or sweating.

If the patient has several complaints, ask which one is of most concern. After investigating the primary complaint, explore the others.

OBTAINING A HISTORY OF THE PRESENT ILLNESS
The history of the present illness usually provides additional information about the chief complaint. It may also help identify the underlying cause by placing the symptoms in the context of recent events.

Find out whether the patient has ever been evaluated or treated for the symptoms. If so, then determine the type of treatment and its outcome.

Ask the patient about his health status before symptoms began and before any treatment was received; then find out how much time elapsed between the treatment and the recurrence or worsening of the symptoms. Look for possible reasons for symptom recurrence. Has the patient complied with prescribed treatment—kept medical appointments and taken prescribed medication or maintained a restricted diet, if recommended, to treat the chief complaint? Has he recently changed his diet; started exercising; begun taking new medications, herbs, or dietary supplements; changed jobs; or made other lifestyle changes?

Finally, once you have gathered the history of the present illness, review it and read the main points back to the patient. Doing this will allow the patient to clarify any misconceptions and offer additional details, while helping you to confirm your understanding of the present illness. After completing this step, obtain the rest of the health history.

OBTAINING THE MEDICAL-SURGICAL HISTORY
A patient's past medical conditions and surgeries can affect current health status. A patient with long-standing diabetes mellitus, for example, may experience delayed wound healing. This is important information to bear in mind if the patient has been admitted for surgery. Medical and surgical history data also may provide insight into the patient's perception of his health and health education needs.

When obtaining the medical-surgical history, be sure to cover the major categories (see 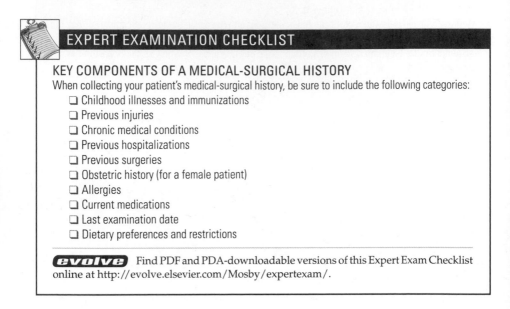 Key Components of a Medical-Surgical History).

EXPERT EXAMINATION CHECKLIST

KEY COMPONENTS OF A MEDICAL-SURGICAL HISTORY
When collecting your patient's medical-surgical history, be sure to include the following categories:
- ❏ Childhood illnesses and immunizations
- ❏ Previous injuries
- ❏ Chronic medical conditions
- ❏ Previous hospitalizations
- ❏ Previous surgeries
- ❏ Obstetric history (for a female patient)
- ❏ Allergies
- ❏ Current medications
- ❏ Last examination date
- ❏ Dietary preferences and restrictions

evolve Find PDF and PDA-downloadable versions of this Expert Exam Checklist online at http://evolve.elsevier.com/Mosby/expertexam/.

Childhood Illnesses and Immunizations
Ask your patient which common childhood illnesses he has had, such as measles, mumps, chickenpox, rubella, and whooping cough. In addition, ask about childhood immunizations. Adults who did not have the usual childhood diseases and have not been vaccinated against them are at increased risk for contracting them. This information may point to a possible cause of the patient's chief complaint and help to fine-tune the physical examination.

Also ask about recent immunizations, such as hepatitis B, pneumococcal, and influenza vaccines. Hepatitis B status is particularly important if the patient is being admitted to the hospital and is likely to receive blood transfusions.

Previous Injuries
Injuries and accidents may explain certain changes in a patient's physical condition and cognitive or motor function. They also may complicate a patient's current health problems and predispose him to certain secondary disorders. Therefore be sure to note the circumstances surrounding any previous injuries. If an injury occurred during an alcohol-related accident, explore the patient's current alcohol consumption habits. If the patient was injured in a fall, try to find out if the fall resulted from syncope, a possible indicator of an underlying illness.

Chronic Medical Conditions
Chronic medical conditions may affect the course of the present illness and help determine the physician's choice of treatments. Ask the patient if he has any chronic illness, such as diabetes mellitus, a thyroid disorder, anemia, hypertension, renal dysfunction, or heart disease.

Previous Hospitalizations

Ask the patient about previous hospitalizations. If the patient has been hospitalized, find out the reason or reasons for treatment, the length of stay, the treatment received, any associated complications, and the names of the hospital and health care providers for each hospitalization. If the patient is now being admitted again, be sure to explore his psychologic responses to the previous hospitalizations.

Previous Surgeries

Ask about all previous surgeries and medical procedures the patient has had. Determine their dates, where they were performed, and the length of the patient's recovery. Find out if the patient experienced postprocedure complications; if so, have the patient describe each complication. In addition, ask if the patient experienced excessive bleeding or adverse effects of anesthesia after the procedure and note whether blood transfusions were received.

Obstetric History

Obtain an obstetric history from all female patients. This history consists of the number of pregnancies (gravida), number of pregnancies carried to term (para), and number of miscarriages and elective abortions.

If the patient is of childbearing age, find out the date of her last menstrual period and ask if she may be pregnant. In addition, inquire about her current use of birth control.

For female patients who are perimenopausal or postmenopausal, ask about symptoms such as hot flashes, as well as the methods, if any, she uses or has used to relieve them. In addition, ask whether or not the patient is using or has used hormone replacement therapy.

Sexual History

A detailed sexual history is not always possible or necessary, but some information on sexual activity is essential. A few basic questions that should be asked, because they could provide important information about your patient's health condition, are as follows:
- Do you have more than one sexual partner?
- Do you ever have pain during intercourse?
- Do you have vaginal, anal, or oral sex?
- Have you ever had difficulty having sex because of physical or psychologic problems?

Allergies

Ask whether the patient is allergic to any medications, foods, environmental substances, or other conditions. Determine what happens when the patient comes in contact with the identified allergen; have the patient describe the symptoms in detail.

Try to differentiate true allergies from medication side effects by asking if the patient was taking medication when the allergy symptoms arose. Remember that usual allergic responses include anaphylaxis, shortness of breath, rash, pruritus, rhinorrhea, and watery eyes, whereas nausea and vomiting are typical medication-related side effects.

Clearly document reactions that you believe indicate true allergies, describing the patient's reaction in detail.

Current Medications

Medications may cause or contribute to a patient's current health problem. Ask the patient which medications, both prescription and over-the-counter, he currently takes. List the name of each medication, along with the dose, administration route, frequency, and duration of use (see Exploring the Patient's Medication Use).

EXPLORING THE PATIENT'S MEDICATION USE

When taking a patient's health history, ask to see any medication bottles he may have brought with him. Besides allowing you to take a more accurate medication history, inspecting the bottles can help you detect and correct dangerous medication errors. For example, you may discover that the patient is doubling up on a particular medication, taking it under both a generic name and a trade name (e.g., taking both propranolol and Inderal).

Verify medication names
Some patients may identify their medications only as "that blue pill" or "my water pill." If the bottles are available for inspection, note the exact drug name. Also check to see if any of the medications are outdated or show signs of improper storage.

Check for compliance
Find out if the patient complies with the prescribed drug regimen. Does he take the full dose as often as prescribed? Or does the patient sometimes skip doses or cut tablets in half to save money?

Other considerations
• Check for drug combinations that may lead to unwanted interactions.
• Ask if the patient has experienced any undesirable effects from a particular medication. If he has, ask what action, if any, the patient took. Did he call the doctor or simply stop taking the medication?

In addition, ask if the patient uses home remedies or alternative treatments, such as herbs or dietary supplements.

CULTURAL CONSIDERATIONS

Certain cultural groups, such as Chinese, Arab, and Hispanic cultures, view wellness in terms of balancing good and bad external forces. To maintain health and balance, these cultural groups often take a naturalistic approach to healing, using opposite forces to treat a condition. For example, hot conditions require cold foods, medications, and herbs. Not all cultural groups, however, use the same terms or define opposing forces in the same way. Chinese patients, for example, may use the terms *yin* for cold and *yang* for hot.

Last Examination Date

Find out when a physician last examined the patient. This information provides insight into how often the patient receives health care, as well as other aspects of the patient's health maintenance habits. In addition, ask if the patient has ever had a chest radiograph, tuberculin test, or electrocardiogram (ECG) and whether he gets routine dental care. Ask female patients if they get regular Pap smears and breast examinations.

Dietary Preferences and Restrictions

Ask your patient to describe a typical day's meals and snacks; then analyze his dietary report for nutritional value. Is the patient consuming too many high-fat foods or too few carbohydrates or proteins?

In addition, find out if the patient adheres to a special diet, such as vegetarian or kosher, or if his diet is restricted for health reasons, such as renal disease or celiac sprue. If a restricted diet has been prescribed, determine patient compliance.

OBTAINING THE FAMILY HISTORY

A complete family history can reveal whether the patient is at risk for a disorder or disease with a genetic or familial tendency. To obtain the family history, ask the patient about the health of parents, siblings, and grandparents (both maternal and paternal). Mention specific diseases by their names or symptoms to help the patient recall whether any family member has had them. Be sure to include such significant conditions as diabetes mellitus, hypertension, stroke, arthritis, pulmonary disease, cardiovascular disease, cancer, renal disease, mental illness, and alcoholism.

OBTAINING THE SOCIAL HISTORY

Social history data help place the patient within the context of his family and community. Because this part of the history requires you to ask about highly personal matters, be sure to convey a nonjudgmental attitude.

If you have not already determined the patient's age and marital status, start the social history by obtaining this information. Then explore educational level, occupation, financial status, religious beliefs, leisure activities, sleep patterns, home environment, support systems, and personal habits.

Marital Status and Social Support

Marital status is a possible indicator of the patient's support system. However, do not assume an unmarried patient lacks adequate support; investigate further by asking if a companion or close friend is available who can be contacted in case of an emergency. Also find out if the patient has children, either living at home or independently.

This might be a good time to investigate possible abuse. You can start by asking the patient if he feels safe at home or in his relationships and progress to more direct questions as appropriate.

Educational Level

Ask how many years of school the patient has completed, and find out if he can read and perform simple calculations. However, never make assumptions about a patient's intellectual abilities or understanding of his current condition based solely on his educational level.

Occupation

Occupational data may provide clues to work-related health hazards, such as asbestos exposure or chronic back pain caused by heavy lifting. Find out if the patient does manual labor or desk work, and determine if he works regularly, seasonally, or on a temporary or as-needed basis. Also ask if the patient's employer provides health insurance. If the patient is unemployed, find out if he is able to pay for food, medication, and health care.

Religious, Spiritual, and Cultural Beliefs

A patient's religious, spiritual, and cultural beliefs and customs may color his attitude toward health, illness, and medical treatment. For example, most Jehovah's Witnesses will not accept blood transfusions; consequently, major surgery may pose an increased risk for them.

The patient's belief system may also serve as a source of emotional support during illness. Ask if the patient belongs to a church, religious organization, or other spiritual group that could be a resource during or after illness or hospitalization.

Living Conditions

Have the patient describe his home. Does it have heat, running water, electricity, and telephone service? Is there a smoke detector? Does it have a carbon monoxide detector? Does the home have more than one story? If so, is the patient able to negotiate the stairs easily?

If you have not done so already, find out how many people the patient lives with. An overcrowded living environment may be responsible for the spread of certain infections.

Tobacco Use

Ask if the patient uses tobacco in any form: cigarettes, cigars, pipes, or chewing tobacco. If so, find out how long he has used tobacco and how much he uses daily. Document cigarette use in terms of pack-years (See Determining Pack-Years).

DETERMINING PACK-YEARS

If your patient smokes cigarettes, document the number of cigarettes smoked daily and the length of time the patient has been smoking. A concise way to report this information is by describing the patient's smoking history in terms of pack-years (the number of packs of cigarettes the patient smokes per day multiplied by the number of years he has been smoking). Following is an example of how to perform this calculation:

A patient has smoked two packs of cigarettes per day for 20 years. To determine the patient's pack-years, multiply two packs by 20 years; the result is 40 pack-years ($2 \times 20 = 40$).

Find out if the patient has ever quit smoking and, if so, when he quit and for how long. If he says he has quit smoking, ask when he last smoked. Some patients say they have quit when in reality, they have merely cut down on the number of cigarettes they smoke.

If the patient still smokes, ask if he would like to stop. Later, you can help him explore options for smoking cessation.

Alcohol Use

Excessive alcohol use can cause or contribute to many medical conditions; however, many health care providers hesitate to delve into this topic, perhaps fearing that questions about alcohol use might seem nosy or embarrassing. Nonetheless, because your goal is to obtain a thorough health history, you must investigate alcohol use. Keep in mind that the key to obtaining frank answers is to remain nonjudgmental.

Begin by asking if the patient drinks alcohol. If the answer is affirmative, ask when he last had a drink. Find out what kind of liquor the patient drinks and how many drinks he has on a typical day. If the patient's drinking seems excessive, ask if he thinks he has a drinking problem or if alcohol has ever interfered with his family life, occupation, or lifestyle.

Consider using the CAGE questionnaire to gather information about your patient's alcohol use (see Using the CAGE Questionnaire).

USING THE CAGE QUESTIONNAIRE

The CAGE questionnaire can help evaluate a patient's history of alcohol use. If he answers "yes" to any of the following questions, suspect that the patient may have a drinking problem:

C: Have you ever felt you should *Cut* down on your drinking?

A: Have people *Annoyed* you by criticizing your drinking?

G: Have you ever felt bad or *Guilty* about your drinking?

E: Have you ever had a drink first thing in the morning to steady your nerves or to get rid of a hangover *(Eye-opener)*?

Recreational Drug Use

Like tobacco and alcohol use, recreational drug use may lead to or compound certain health problems. Ask if the patient has ever used "street" drugs, such as cocaine, crack, amphetamine agents, LSD (lysergic acid diethylamide), or "downers." If so, determine frequency of use and the effect. Also ask whether the patient has ever injected illegal drugs; if so, ask if he has been tested for human immunodeficiency virus (HIV) or hepatitis.

CONDUCTING A REVIEW OF BODY SYSTEMS

After gathering the patient's social history, continue the health history interview by asking questions about each body system. The information you obtain from the review of systems may reinforce your initial impression of the patient's health problems. In addition, exploring each system in detail may prompt the patient to mention additional signs and symptoms, not just the most distressing one (see 🔲 Performing a Thorough Body-System Review).

EXPERT EXAMINATION CHECKLIST

PERFORMING A THOROUGH BODY-SYSTEM REVIEW

When performing a general review of body systems, be sure to ask the patient about the signs and symptoms listed below, noting anything unusual or abnormal, and addressing specific complaints.

Integumentary system
- ❏ Unusual hair loss or breakage
- ❏ Skin lesions or discoloration
- ❏ Unusual nail breakage or discoloration

Musculoskeletal system
- ❏ Joint pain or stiffness
- ❏ Tendon, ligament, or muscle pains or strains
- ❏ Bone aches or pains
- ❏ Muscle weakness

Head and neck
- ❏ Headaches
- ❏ Neck pain and stiffness
- ❏ Nasal discharge
- ❏ Nosebleeds
- ❏ Mouth lesions
- ❏ Sore throat
- ❏ Voice changes, such as hoarseness
- ❏ Dental problems

Eyes and ears
- ❏ Changes in vision, such as double or blurred vision
- ❏ Loss of vision
- ❏ Redness of eyes
- ❏ Eye drainage
- ❏ Eye pain
- ❏ Changes in hearing
- ❏ Loss of hearing
- ❏ Ear drainage
- ❏ Ear pain

Endocrine system
- ❏ Excessive thirst
- ❏ Excessive hunger
- ❏ Excessive urination
- ❏ Cold intolerance
- ❏ Heat intolerance
- ❏ Excessive sweating

Neurologic system
- ❏ Blackouts
- ❏ Seizures
- ❏ Loss of memory
- ❏ Mood swings
- ❏ Hallucinations
- ❏ Weakness
- ❏ Numbness
- ❏ Tremors
- ❏ Paralysis
- ❏ Loss of coordination

Cardiovascular system
- ❏ Chest pain
- ❏ Shortness of breath when lying flat
- ❏ Palpitations
- ❏ Edema
- ❏ Excessive urination at night
- ❏ Varicose veins
- ❏ Limb pain during exercise

Pulmonary system
- ❏ Shortness of breath
- ❏ Painful breathing
- ❏ Wheezing
- ❏ Sputum production
- ❏ Bloody sputum

Gastrointestinal system
- ❏ Changes in stool color, consistency, or frequency
- ❏ Heartburn
- ❏ Loss of appetite
- ❏ Food intolerances
- ❏ Painful swallowing
- ❏ Abdominal pain
- ❏ Blood in vomit or stool
- ❏ Nausea
- ❏ Constipation
- ❏ Diarrhea
- ❏ Fecal incontinence

continued

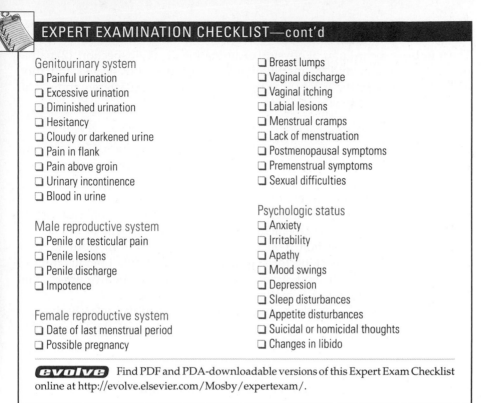

EXPERT EXAMINATION CHECKLIST—cont'd

Genitourinary system
- ❏ Painful urination
- ❏ Excessive urination
- ❏ Diminished urination
- ❏ Hesitancy
- ❏ Cloudy or darkened urine
- ❏ Pain in flank
- ❏ Pain above groin
- ❏ Urinary incontinence
- ❏ Blood in urine

Male reproductive system
- ❏ Penile or testicular pain
- ❏ Penile lesions
- ❏ Penile discharge
- ❏ Impotence

Female reproductive system
- ❏ Date of last menstrual period
- ❏ Possible pregnancy

- ❏ Breast lumps
- ❏ Vaginal discharge
- ❏ Vaginal itching
- ❏ Labial lesions
- ❏ Menstrual cramps
- ❏ Lack of menstruation
- ❏ Postmenopausal symptoms
- ❏ Premenstrual symptoms
- ❏ Sexual difficulties

Psychologic status
- ❏ Anxiety
- ❏ Irritability
- ❏ Apathy
- ❏ Mood swings
- ❏ Depression
- ❏ Sleep disturbances
- ❏ Appetite disturbances
- ❏ Suicidal or homicidal thoughts
- ❏ Changes in libido

evolve Find PDF and PDA-downloadable versions of this Expert Exam Checklist online at http://evolve.elsevier.com/Mosby/expertexam/.

As you conduct the review, maintain a systematic approach. Begin the review of systems by assessing the patient's overall health. Ask the patient to describe his present health status and how he feels overall. Be sure to note any general complaints, such as malaise, fatigue, or weakness, as well as problems with healing or unusual bleeding or bruising. Inquire about the patient's weight and the presence of possible indicators of systemic diseases, such as lymphoma, tuberculosis, and acquired immunodeficiency syndrome (AIDS). Next, focus on one body system at a time by asking questions relating to that system. (Later, when performing the physical examination, you will proceed from head to toe.)

CONCLUDING THE HEALTH HISTORY

After collecting health history data from your patient, take a few minutes to review your findings. Then, if necessary, ask more questions to clarify the patient's responses. For instance, if he gave conflicting or ambiguous information about a particular symptom, ask, "What do you think the problem is?" or "What concerns you most right now?"

Then thank the patient for his time and cooperation and explain that you will proceed with the physical examination.

PHYSICAL EXAMINATION TECHNIQUES

The four basic techniques of physical examination are (1) inspection, (2) palpation, (3) percussion, and (4) auscultation. Findings from physical examination are reliable only to the extent that these techniques are mastered and use of examination equipment is proficient.

INSPECTION

During inspection, the first step of the physical examination, observe your patient critically, evaluating what you see in light of your knowledge as a health care professional.

In an informal sense, inspection begins the moment you first encounter the patient. However, the formal inspection you conduct during the physical examination has two parts: (1) the general inspection and (2) the systematic inspection.

In the general inspection, you observe the patient from front to back and from each side, checking for symmetry of body parts, obvious injuries or abnormalities, and overall appearance. In the systematic inspection, you inspect each body region systematically from head to toe.

Accurate inspection requires adequate lighting, good exposure of the area to be inspected, and appropriate equipment, such as a penlight and possibly an ophthalmoscope and otoscope.

PALPATION

Palpation is used to elicit information about skin temperature, bodily pulsations and vibrations, internal masses, and tenderness or rigidity of organs and structures. Palpation can be light or deep and may involve the use of one or both hands (see Palpation Techniques).

PALPATION TECHNIQUES

Depending on the part of the body being examined or the particular characteristic you are assessing for, you may use light, deep, or bimanual palpation.

Light palpation
In this technique, you press gently on the patient's skin to a depth of no more than 1 cm, using one hand. Light palpation is best for assessing texture, temperature, moisture, pulsations, tenderness, vibrations, superficial masses, and papular lesions.

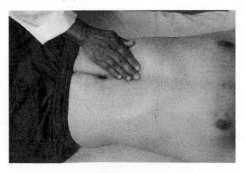

continued

PALPATION TECHNIQUES—cont'd

Deep palpation

In deep palpation, you press evenly on the patient's skin to a depth of approximately 4 cm. You may use one or both hands, keeping your fingers extended. Deep palpation is best for assessing abdominal structures, particularly the liver.

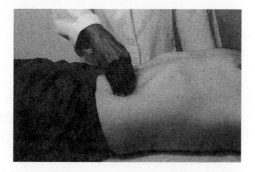

Bimanual palpation

This method involves the use of both hands to "trap" an organ and assess its texture and firmness. Expect to use this technique to assess the kidneys and female reproductive organs.

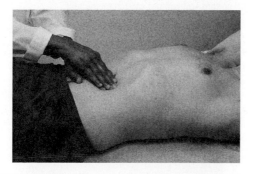

Photographs from Wilson SF, Giddens JF: *Health Assessment for Nursing Practice,* ed 2, St. Louis, 2001, Mosby.

Guidelines for obtaining the most accurate data from palpation are as follows:
- Use the part of the hand or hands best suited to the specific characteristic being assessed.
  - Finger pads for palpating texture, shape, and pulsations
  - Fingertips and nail tips for eliciting reflexes, such as the abdominal reflex
  - Forefinger and thumb for grasping tissue, hair, and nodules
  - Ball of the hand for detecting vibrations and thrills
  - Back of the hand for assessing temperature and moisture
  - Entire hand for testing strength and grip
- Palpate as the second step of the physical examination after inspection (except when assessing the abdomen).

When assessing the abdomen, always perform palpation after inspection and auscultation because palpation may increase the patient's intestinal activity, causing misleading auscultation findings, such as increased bowel sounds.

- Palpate areas of tenderness or pain last to enable changes from surrounding nonpainful tissue to be felt and to avoid patient tensing or withdrawal, which may interfere with palpation.

PERCUSSION

Perhaps the most challenging physical examination skill, percussion involves tapping or striking the patient's skin surface with the fingers or hands to elicit sounds, evaluate reflexes, uncover abnormal masses, and detect pain or tenderness. The tapping produces an audible vibration that helps to reveal the location, size, and density of the underlying structure. The three basic percussion techniques are (1) direct, (2) indirect, and (3) blunt percussion (see Comparing Percussion Techniques).

COMPARING PERCUSSION TECHNIQUES

To conduct a thorough physical examination, you must become proficient in the three percussion techniques: (1) direct, (2) indirect, and (3) blunt percussion. No matter what technique you use, your nails should be trimmed so that you will not scratch the patient.

Direct percussion
To perform direct percussion, tap directly on the patient's skin, using short, sharp strokes of your fist or the fingertips of your dominant hand. Make sure the tapping movement originates from your wrist, not your elbow. After tapping, immediately lift your wrist from the skin surface so that you do not muffle the sound. You can use this technique on any part of the body, including the back and the paranasal sinuses.

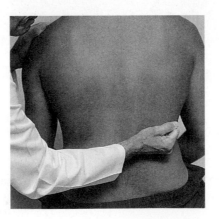

Indirect percussion
In this technique, used for most parts of the body, your nondominant hand serves as the striking surface. Place the middle finger of your nondominant hand firmly against the patient's skin surface;

continued

COMPARING PERCUSSION TECHNIQUES—cont'd

keep the other fingers of that hand fanned out slightly above the skin surface. Be sure to place only the pad of your finger against the skin. Next, with your dominant hand, strike the middle finger of your nondominant hand above or below the interphalangeal joint of your finger. Avoid striking directly on the joint because this can affect the sounds produced.

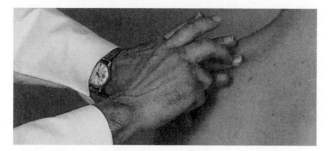

Blunt percussion

To perform blunt percussion, either strike the ulnar surface of your fist against the patient's skin surface or place your nondominant hand over the area and use it as a striking surface for your fist. Blunt percussion is useful for detecting pain or inflammation.

Before using this technique on a patient, practice it until you have learned to apply just enough force to elicit tenderness without hurting the patient.

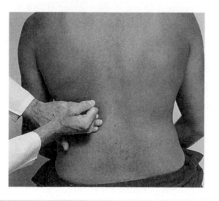

Photographs from Wilson SF, Giddens JF: *Health Assessment for Nursing Practice*, ed 2, St. Louis, 2001, Mosby.

Because the body's organs, structures, and cavities differ in density, they produce sounds that differ in loudness, pitch, and duration. The types of percussion sounds and the locations where each is heard are as follows:

- Tympany, a high-pitched, drum-like sound, is usually heard over the stomach.
- Resonance, a low-pitched, hollow sound, is usually heard over normal lung tissue.
- Hyperresonance, a loud, booming sound, is usually heard over a hyper-inflated lung, as in patients with emphysema.

- Dullness, a soft, high-pitched, thudding sound, is usually heard over dense organs, such as the liver.
- Flatness, a soft, high-pitched sound, is usually heard over bones, muscles, and tumors.

AUSCULTATION

Auscultation involves listening to sounds produced by internal body structures, usually the heart, lungs, blood vessels, and bowels. Generally auscultation follows inspection, palpation, and percussion. However, when examining the abdomen, you should auscultate *after* inspection and *before* palpation and percussion, because the effects of palpation and percussion may influence auscultation findings. To auscultate accurately, you must block out noises in the environment and sounds emanating from other organs. To help isolate sounds, close your eyes and concentrate on one auscultation sound at a time.

USING PHYSICAL EXAMINATION EQUIPMENT CORRECTLY

Incorrect use of physical examination equipment can result in erroneous findings. Guidelines to be followed for the accurate use of basic physical assessment equipment in day-to-day practice are as follows:
- When using a stethoscope:
  - Make certain the tubing is no more than 30 to 40 cm long and 4 mm in diameter. Longer and wider tubing may distort transmitted sounds.
  - Make sure the earpieces fit comfortably and snugly in your ear canal. Angle them toward your nose so that sounds are directed toward the tympanic membrane.
  - Hold the end piece between your second and third fingers, and avoid holding or rubbing the tubing to minimize extraneous noise.
  - Avoid placing the end piece of the stethoscope on the patient's gown or clothing. Friction between the fabric and stethoscope could produce false sounds.
  - Use the diaphragm of the stethoscope to detect high-pitched sounds, such as heart, lung, and bowel sounds, making sure you place it firmly on the skin surface. To detect soft, low-pitched sounds, such as heart murmurs and atrial and ventricular gallops, use the bell.
- When using an oral thermometer:
  - Always wait 15 minutes after your patient has consumed a cold or hot beverage and 2 to 3 minutes after he has smoked a cigarette before measuring oral temperature.
- When using a tympanic membrane thermometer:
  - Remove cerumen from the ear canal by irrigation or use of a softening agent, such as carbamide peroxide, and clean the probe window according to the manufacturer's instructions. If you fail to do this, the infrared sensor used to detect the temperature of blood flowing through the tympanic membrane may be blocked and a falsely low temperature reading may result.

- Straighten the adult patient's ear canal to insert the temperature probe, making sure to pull the external part of the ear (the pinna) upward and back.
- Insert the probe gently into the ear canal to avoid injuring or perforating the tympanic membrane. If you meet resistance, *stop*. Never force the probe into the canal.
- Advance the probe far enough into the ear canal to seal the opening to avoid an accurate reading.
- When using a sphygmomanometer:
  - Avoid using an arm on the same side of the body on which a radical mastectomy has been performed or when an arteriovenous (AV) shunt is present.
  - Use a cuff with a correct size inflatable rubber bladder. The bladder should be about 40% as wide as the patient's arm circumference and about 80% as long as his arm circumference. For most adult patients, expect to use a cuff that is 12 to 14 cm wide. Too narrow a cuff results in a falsely high reading; too wide a cuff results in a falsely low reading.
  - Support the limb at heart level. If the limb is unsupported or above the level of the heart, a falsely high reading will be obtained. If the limb is below heart level, the pressure will be falsely low.
  - Wrap the cuff smoothly and tightly; an uneven or too loose cuff causes a falsely high reading.
  - Deflate the cuff at a rate of 2 to 3 mm Hg/sec. If the cuff is deflated too slowly, the diastolic pressure may be falsely high. If the cuff is deflated too quickly, the systolic reading may be falsely low and the diastolic falsely high.
  - Wait 1 to 2 minutes before repeating the procedure; if redone immediately, systolic readings can be falsely high and diastolic falsely low.
  - After measuring blood pressure in one arm, measure it in the other. Be aware that blood pressure commonly differs by 5 to 10 mm Hg between arms.
- When using an automatic blood pressure cuff:
  - If the patient has an irregular heart rhythm, such as that which occurs with atrial fibrillation, the automatic blood pressure cuff may not produce accurate results. When in doubt, compare your reading with one obtained manually.
- When using an otoscope:
  - Tilt the patient's head slightly toward the side opposite the ear being examined to bring the eardrum into better view.
  - Pull the pinna up and back to straighten out the ear canal of an adult.
  - Keeping your hand alongside the patient's face to steady the otoscope, gently insert the speculum into the ear, then hold the otoscope against the patient's head, handle end in the upward position.
- When using an ophthalmoscope:
  - Darken the room before beginning the ophthalmoscopic examination.
  - Ask your patient to remove his eyeglasses. If you wear eyeglasses, remove them unless you are very nearsighted or astigmatic. (Contact lenses, on the other hand, can be worn during the examination.)

- Use your right hand and right eye to examine the patient's right eye. Use your left hand and left eye to examine his left eye.
- To help the patient hold his gaze steady, have him focus on a point on the opposite wall.
- Approach your patient from slightly off to one side, from a distance of about 15 inches. As you move toward the patient, place the thumb of your other hand on his eyebrow for guidance.

- Using a pulse oximeter:
  - Before placing the sensor probe, make sure the photodetectors in the probe are aligned. The pulse oximeter measures a patient's arterial oxygen saturation (SaO_2) by means of a cutaneous sensor probe that emits red and infrared light. The probe measures the light passing through the capillaries, detecting the relative amount of color absorbed by the arterial blood, and then calculates the SaO_2 value.
  - Place the probe at a site where capillaries are near the skin surface, such as a nail bed, an earlobe, or the bridge of the nose. If you choose the nail bed, remove any nail polish from the patient's finger to ensure the most accurate SaO_2 value. (To promote patient comfort, alternate probe sites periodically if the oximeter is being used for continuous measurements.)
  - Instruct the patient to stay still during the measurement because movement can cause inaccuracies in the reading.
  - Once the probe is in position, turn the pulse oximeter on and correlate your patient's radial pulse with the value on the digital display.

Examining Patients with Special Needs

A wide range of conditions, such as serious illness, sensory and cognitive impairments, anxiety, and hostility, can impede a thorough and accurate health history and physical examination. A patient with a cognitive impairment, for instance, may not understand your questions. An extremely anxious patient may be unable to focus on the interview.

Your assessment approach and techniques must be tailored for these patients, not only to save you time but also to obtain reliable findings while preserving the patient's dignity.

SERIOUSLY ILL PATIENTS

Patients suffering from acute illnesses or serious injuries, such as cerebrovascular accident or head trauma, may be unable to communicate or respond fully because of their medical condition, mechanical ventilation, or heavy sedation. If your seriously ill patient cannot supply a complete health history, obtain only the most important information: chief complaint, history of present illness, medications, and allergies. To prevent the patient from feeling rushed or physically taxed, explain that you will ask more questions later. Providing adequate time for the patient to feel comfortable will make it more likely that she will answer your questions fully.

ESTABLISHING A COMMUNICATION SYSTEM

A patient who is conscious but cannot speak (e.g., because of mechanical ventilation) may be able to respond nonverbally to simple questions. To obtain basic history information and assess the patient's level of pain and anxiety, establish gestures she can use to indicate her response to questions. For example, tell the patient to squeeze your hand once to indicate *no* and twice to indicate *yes*. Before recording any answers, test the patient to make sure that she understands and uses the gestures appropriately. For example, ask a simple question, such as "Is your name Mary?" Then make sure the patient responds correctly by squeezing your hand the proper number of times.

PROVIDING COMFORT MEASURES

Some seriously ill patients have trouble focusing on questions or instructions because of immobility, pain, discomfort, anxiety, or depression. Therefore, after establishing a communication system, evaluate your patient's ability to participate fully in the interview. Ask the patient how she is feeling. Note if she is able to talk at length despite discomfort or if she keeps her responses short to get back to coping with the discomfort.

Before you can start the health history interview, you must address the immediate source of the patient's discomfort. Respond to her needs by helping her to a more comfortable position or offering a cool beverage (if permitted). If the patient is in pain, administer the prescribed analgesic drugs and wait for the medication to take effect before proceeding with the interview.

You may also guide the patient through progressive muscle relaxation to ease pain and discomfort. For instance, you can instruct her to progressively tighten and then relax individual muscle groups until her whole body is relaxed. This exercise usually takes 10 to 30 minutes.

Some patients respond better to guided imagery. In this method, you gently instruct the patient to imagine she is in one of her favorite places. This should have a relaxing effect and enable you to proceed with the health history interview (see Interviewing a Seriously Ill Patient).

INTERVIEWING A SERIOUSLY ILL PATIENT

You will need to use your best interview skills when questioning a patient who is in marked pain or discomfort. To help the interview go more smoothly, follow these suggestions:

Get off to a good start

If your patient feels well enough to talk at length, start the history with open-ended questions. This will help the patient to feel more comfortable with you. Then use natural pauses in the conversation to ask closed-ended questions so that you can obtain more detailed information.

Maintain the flow of conversation so that the patient's attention stays focused on your questions, not on her discomfort or the surroundings. In addition, nod your head or make a brief remark to show the patient that you are listening closely to her responses.

Deal with the patient's fears

What if your patient asks you if she is going to die or be permanently disabled or disfigured? Usually your best response is to answer this type of question honestly. Remember that most patients do not ask such questions unless they are ready to hear the answer, whether it is good or bad.

However, before this situation arises, do some serious soul searching. Before you can deal with the patient's fears, you need to examine your own fears and attitudes toward illness, disability, disfigurement, and death. Can you talk openly about these topics without getting lost in your anxieties?

If you do not think you are up to the task, ask the patient if she would like to speak with a counselor, religious leader, or some other person who feels comfortable discussing these difficult matters.

continued

> ## INTERVIEWING A SERIOUSLY ILL PATIENT—cont'd
>
> Accept the patient's crying
> A patient who finds she is seriously ill may cry during the interview. Although this may make you uncomfortable, resist the urge to cut the crying short. Usually, the best approach is to do nothing. Do not move away from the patient or rush to say something you hope will make her feel better. Instead quietly offer a box of tissues or touch the patient on the arm to show that you are available and that you accept her feelings.
>
> If you feel uncomfortable with her crying, resist the urge to talk just to fill the time. If you must speak, offer a few sympathetic words about how hard it must be for the patient to go through such an ordeal. If you can accept the crying for what it is—coming to terms with painful emotions—you will help the patient to recognize that it is all right to feel the way she does.

PERFORMING AN ABBREVIATED ASSESSMENT

With an acutely ill patient, expect to condense the health history interview and physical examination so that you can address the most immediate and life-threatening problem. For example, if you suspect your patient is experiencing a myocardial infarction, perform a brief but focused assessment of the cardiovascular system and other affected body systems so you can rapidly intervene. Later, when the patient's condition has stabilized, you can complete the history and physical examination at a more leisurely pace.

MODIFYING THE PHYSICAL EXAMINATION

The order of the physical examination may need to be changed and parts may need to be omitted to meet the needs of patients with special needs. For example, a bedridden or immobile patient may be unable to participate in some parts of the physical examination, such as evaluation of gait or active range of motion.

If the patient cannot change her position easily, ask another nurse or caregiver to move the patient while you examine hard-to-reach areas. For instance, have a colleague hold the patient on her side so that you can freely examine her posterior.

EXAMINING A NONRESPONSIVE PATIENT

Never assume a nonresponsive patient cannot hear you.

If the patient is unconscious or comatose, speak to her as you conduct the examination. Provide explanations as if she were awake and conscious: "Now I'm going to listen to your heart." Remember that she may be able to hear what you are saying and may find your words soothing.

ANXIOUS PATIENTS

Many people feel anxious and intimidated in a medical setting. Mild anxiety can be helpful during the assessment because it focuses the patient's attention on answering questions and following instructions and provides the patient with the energy needed to complete the procedure.

For most patients, a reassuring manner is enough to reduce mild anxiety and promote cooperation. To convey empathy, tell the patient that you understand the stress she is feeling. For instance, you might say, "I know this experience can seem overwhelming. Take a deep breath and try to relax."

Do not make reassuring statements just to calm the patient if the statement may not be true (for example, "Everything will be okay"). False reassurance may jeopardize the patient's trust in you or other members of the health care team.

DEALING WITH MODERATELY TO SEVERELY ANXIOUS PATIENTS

A high anxiety level may interfere with a thorough history and physical examination. If your patient is moderately anxious, suggest breathing or relaxation exercises. Then, when she is more calm, start the interview with an open-ended question to invite her to begin talking and proceed as appropriate.

If the patient is extremely anxious, antianxiety medication may be needed before you can begin the assessment. In some cases you may even need to consider discussing with the physician the need for a psychiatric consultation.

MODIFYING THE PHYSICAL EXAMINATION

An anxious patient may fear that the physical examination will cause pain or embarrassment, or worse, reveal a serious illness. Therefore take special care to maintain patient privacy. Close the door and draw the curtain. Do not allow others to enter the room without the patient's permission.

During the examination, expose only the area of the body you are about to examine. Then promptly cover it when you are finished. As you examine the patient, state in advance what you are going to do so that the patient knows what to expect. For example, before auscultating the lungs you can say, "Now I'm going to listen to your lungs. You'll feel the end of my stethoscope on your back. It might feel a little cold." By doing this you will avoid startling the patient and can keep her involved in the examination process.

If you need extra time to perform a certain part of the examination, such as auscultating heart sounds, tell the patient you are going to spend a few minutes listening to her heart. Otherwise the patient might become anxious, fearing that the additional time you are spending listening to her heart means you have found something abnormal. After you have finished listening, say something reassuring like, "Your heartbeat is regular and strong." (However, if this is not true, do not give false reassurance.)

If you discover an abnormal finding, try to control your facial expressions and verbal response. Otherwise the patient may become alarmed.

WITHDRAWN PATIENTS

Most withdrawn patients are anxious but will become more communicative with a little encouragement. One way to encourage communication is to explain to the patient that you need to ask some questions about her health. Next, pose a few simple questions to elicit basic information, such as the patient's full name, address, and telephone number, to give the patient an idea of what to expect during the rest of the interview. Once the patient becomes more comfortable, you can follow up with open-ended questions.

If the patient remains uncommunicative during the interview, you may be able to draw her out by listening to concerns, clearing up misconceptions, or providing assistance. Ask if she is troubled by something, and then offer assistance in dealing with her concern.

Suppose, for instance, the patient expresses a concern about a pet left unattended during her hospital stay. To relieve the patient of her worry and establish rapport, provide access to a telephone (or offer to make a call) so that the patient can arrange for someone check on the pet. With this situation handled, the patient will be more likely to cooperate during the assessment.

You may also consider using touch to help draw a patient out (see Using Touch Appropriately).

USING TOUCH APPROPRIATELY

When used in a genuine way (rather than in a forced or scripted manner), touching can be helpful in dealing with a withdrawn patient. Holding the patient's hand or putting your hand on the patient's arm or shoulder can send the message that you are in the moment with her. Touching also serves to help connect the patient's inner world with the outside world.

Try to exercise good judgment when you are about to touch a patient. Not all patients are comfortable being touched; some patients may misinterpret your intentions and become upset.

A person's cultural background may also influence views on when touching is acceptable and when it is an invasion of personal space.

COPING WITH SILENCE
Expect frequent silences when interviewing a withdrawn patient. However, keep in mind that a silent period does not mean that your interview skills are inadequate or that you should take these pauses personally. Instead, learn to become comfortable with them so that you can resist the urge to jump in and "rescue" the patient.

When used appropriately, silent pauses can help elicit information. For instance, they can help the patient remember facts, organize thoughts, or think over important details. They also give the patient a chance to process painful emotions associated with her medical condition or personal life.

MODIFYING THE PHYSICAL EXAMINATION
The withdrawn patient is usually anxious, so modify your physical examination as you would for an anxious patient by ensuring privacy, telling the patient in advance what you are going to do, and controlling your facial expressions and verbal responses.

OVERLY TALKATIVE PATIENTS

Like withdrawn patients, many overly talkative patients are highly anxious. Typically the overly talkative patient channels anxiety through speech, fearing that unless she relates every detail of her condition she will not be diagnosed correctly. Your primary task with this type of patient is to maintain control while addressing her need to reduce anxiety.

ALLOWING A "FREE SPEECH" PERIOD

As the interview begins, give the patient an opportunity to talk without interruption. During this "free speech" period, make sure that every now and then you nod or say a few words to indicate that you are listening. As the patient talks, observe her and listen closely to what she is saying. By doing this, you can gain valuable insight into the patient's thought processes, emotional state, coping mechanisms, and interaction style.

Note the patient's speech pattern and characteristics. Is her speech pressured (rapid or urgent)? If so, this may indicate bipolar disorder. Is her speech incoherent, circumstantial, or tangential (veering off the subject)? These patterns suggest a possible thought disorder, such as schizophrenia. Does the content of her speech contradict her affect (i.e., does she look sad but say she feels happy?). In addition, observe nonverbal messages, such as body language and gestures. Are they consistent with what the patient is saying?

TAKING CONTROL OF THE INTERVIEW

After listening to the patient for a short time, wait for a natural break in the conversation. Then say you have some specific questions that will require short answers and proceed with closed-ended questions to elicit the information you need to complete your assessment.

If the patient's answers veer from the topic, gently interrupt to clarify information or steer the conversation back to the topic. For example, if the patient goes into excessive detail about events that occurred years ago, you might say, "It sounds like a lot happened to you in 1978. However, before you go on, could you tell me about any other surgeries you've had?" Most overly talkative patients will tolerate interruptions if they believe the other party is truly listening to them.

You might also want to ask the overly talkative patient to fill out questionnaires and other forms. This can help channel her energy into something productive while giving her the sense of participating in her own care. It might also save you some time. Remember, though, that such forms are not a substitute for formal history taking.

MODIFYING THE PHYSICAL EXAMINATION

During the examination, allow the patient to continue talking, provided it does not interfere with your ability to concentrate on findings or listen to sounds. If, for example, you need to listen to breath sounds, ask her not to speak because you do not want to miss important sounds; however, emphasize that you will gladly listen to her after you have finished this part of the examination.

HOSTILE PATIENTS

How you react to a hostile patient can be crucial to conducting a successful health history and physical examination. Often hostility and anger are expressions of fear. When this is the case, expect the patient to watch you closely to observe how you handle her emotions. If you can deal with them effectively, the patient may realize that her emotions aren't so overwhelming that she can't handle them.

Don't take a patient's expression of anger personally. To a hostile patient, you may symbolize everything she is upset about at the moment—the health care facility, the medical profession, or even her illness. The patient may vent her anger at you because you are a convenient target.

DEFUSING ANGER

Before you start the interview, give the patient a chance to express her feelings. Simply by listening, you may be able to defuse her anger and frustration. Show the patient that you can tolerate her feelings as long as the situation does not escalate into abuse.

Be genuine, acknowledging those things that you would find frustrating if you were the patient. Empathize with how difficult it must be for her to be hospitalized, to receive treatment for an acute illness, or to live with a chronic condition.

If the patient yells, do not yell back. Doing so could cause the situation to escalate into a confrontation. Instead, recognize that she is yelling because she feels the need to be heard. Listen in a noncritical manner, providing the sounding board she is seeking.

Avoid taking sides either for or against the patient. Arguing with her would probably prove pointless because most hostile patients are not willing to listen to other people's arguments. Only after you have established rapport through supportive listening should you consider providing information that might change her mind.

As your patient calms down, redirect her attention to her primary goal: feeling better, getting well, or going home. Affirm your commitment to helping the patient reach this goal and to providing her with the best possible care. Help the patient to use her determination and energy to focus on her recovery and the will to live.

DEALING WITH ABUSE AND VIOLENCE
Never tolerate abuse.

If a patient becomes verbally abusive, firmly explain that you will continue the interview later, when she can express her thoughts in a respectful manner. Set boundaries and be consistent in maintaining them.

Make sure you are familiar with your facility's policies and procedures regarding violent patients. Keep in mind that past behavior is the best predictor of future behavior. If you know a patient has a history of violent outbursts, take extra precautions when dealing with her. Notify another staff member that you will be interviewing a potentially dangerous patient and ask that staff member to check on you periodically (see Managing a Hostile Patient).

MANAGING A HOSTILE PATIENT

When coping with a hostile patient, let the phrase CALM DOWN be your guide. Each letter of this mnemonic stands for one of the eight steps to follow when trying to keep the situation under control.

C: *Check* to see that everyone is safe.

A: *Agree* with the patient's affect, not her opinion. Let her know you understand her feelings without necessarily agreeing with her opinion.

L: *Listen* to the patient, hearing out her concerns.

M: Redirect the patient to your common goal: getting her the best *medical* care possible.

D: *Do not debate* with your patient.

O: *Old* (past) behavior is the best predictor of future behavior. If your patient has shown violence toward caregivers in the past, assume she may do so again.

W: *Walk away* from the patient if you feel threatened or abused.

N: Listen carefully and try to determine the patient's underlying *need*. What is the patient really trying to tell you?

If you suspect a patient is about to become violent, position yourself between the patient and the door, making sure that the door stays open. If she does become violent, or you feel she poses a risk to herself or others, leave the room and alert security. Ask the physician to order a sedative and restraints. After a violent episode, be sure to document your interventions and the patient's response.

MODIFYING THE PHYSICAL EXAMINATION

You may need to provide the hostile patient with additional explanations and privacy measures before you can start the physical examination. Before you touch the patient, ask permission so that she will not react violently or accuse you of battery.

If you are worried about being alone with the patient behind a closed door, ask a colleague to be present during the examination. As you examine the patient, stay alert for clues that the patient is becoming more hostile or losing control (e.g., rapid breathing, gritting of the teeth, avoiding eye contact). If you notice these signs, stop the examination and tell the patient that you will resume later when she is calmer. If necessary, ask for help from others for your protection.

COGNITIVELY IMPAIRED PATIENTS

Most patients with mild cognitive impairments can function adequately in daily life and can speak for themselves. This means you will probably be able to obtain at least some health history information directly from the patient. However, some patients with mild cognitive impairments may not understand the complexities of their condition and may have emotional outbursts if they become confused or overstimulated. A few may even show psychotic symptoms.

Of course, patients with more severe cognitive impairments may be unable to provide any health history information. In that case you will need to interview a family member or other caregiver (see Taking a Patient History From a Family Member or Caregiver).

TAKING A PATIENT HISTORY FROM A FAMILY MEMBER OR CAREGIVER

If your patient cannot speak (e.g., if she is severely ill, comatose, or has a severe cognitive impairment), you will probably need to obtain health history information from a family member or caregiver. Try to follow these important guidelines:

Ensure a conducive environment
Conduct the interview in a quiet, private, comfortable area away from the patient's room, if possible. Otherwise, the patient's presence may distract the family member or caregiver from concentrating on your questions.

After introducing yourself and explaining that you need to take the patient's health history, ask the family member or caregiver if she needs anything. Offer coffee, water, or another beverage, and ask how the caregiver is holding up. Reassure her that the patient is receiving proper attention, even though the two of you have left the patient's room. If the person is upset, allow her to express her thoughts and feelings. Offer reassurance and empathize with the difficulty of her circumstances.

Obtain basic information
Start the interview by asking simple, direct questions to obtain the patient's name, age, and telephone number. Find out the nature of the relationship between the person you are interviewing and the patient. If the person is a family member, is she a close relative? If she is a friend or caregiver, how long has she known the patient? How often does she normally see the patient? Is the relationship informal or more distant? This will help you judge if the data the person provides are reliable, especially information about the patient's health habits and other sensitive areas.

INTERVIEWING THE PATIENT WITH A MILD IMPAIRMENT
Before starting the health history interview, eliminate distractions. The mildly impaired patient may not cope well with the stress or stimulation of being in an unfamiliar environment. Turn off any television or radio, and close the door to the interview room if a lot of activity is occurring in the hall.

Direct your questions to the patient even if a family member or caregiver is present. Because it is faster and easier, there is often a tendency to bypass the patient and interview the third party. Guard against this because it can destroy any chance of building rapport with the patient. If, after interviewing the patient, you need more information, ask the patient for permission to speak with the family member or caregiver.

Additional guidelines that help in obtaining a health history from a mildly impaired patient are as follows:
• Tailor your language to your patient's verbal abilities. Avoid jargon and technical terms, use concrete language whenever possible, and ask only one question at a time.

- Do not talk down to the patient. Doing so could work against your efforts to establish rapport.
- If the patient reports a symptom, such as pain, ask her to rate its intensity on a scale of 1 to 10. This not only will help you assess the severity of the symptom but also could prove useful for later comparison once treatment begins.

INTERVIEWING THE PATIENT WITH A MORE SEVERE IMPAIRMENT

Try to obtain this patient's health history from a family member or caregiver. Be sure to include questions about the patient's ability to perform activities of daily living, such as dressing, toileting, personal hygiene, and managing money for small purchases. Besides indicating the patient's functioning level, the answers to these questions can give you a sense of the patient's ability to learn about her health care.

MODIFYING THE PHYSICAL EXAMINATION

Like the health history interview, the physical examination of a patient with a cognitive impairment will proceed more smoothly if you have established rapport. Other measures to help promote a successful examination are as follows:

- Arrange for a family member or caregiver to be present, if possible, to help calm and reassure the patient.
- If necessary, change the sequence of examination steps so that you start with less intrusive areas, such as the hands, skin, and hair. Once you have shown the patient you are not going to hurt her, proceed to more intrusive areas.
- If you think a certain part of the examination will be painful or uncomfortable, tell the patient in advance; however, choose your words carefully to avoid frightening the patient. "This might sting a little" is less frightening than "This might hurt."

HEARING-IMPAIRED PATIENTS

Dealing with hearing-impaired patients can present a number of challenges. If your patient communicates mainly in sign language, sign if you are able or try to find an interpreter. If you must rely on an interpreter, explain the importance of not summarizing what the patient is saying; otherwise you might miss important details or clues about the patient's thought process.

If the patient can read lips, face her, speak slowly, and articulate your words clearly; where appropriate, add gestures or pantomime. If the patient relies largely on visual cues and wears eyeglasses, make sure she is wearing them and that the room is adequately lit.

If the patient has some hearing, determine whether her hearing loss is unilateral or bilateral. If it is unilateral, position yourself near her good ear when speaking. If the patient has hearing aids, ask her to use them during the interview. Remember that older patients with presbycusis lose the ability to hear high-pitched sounds such as consonants, so it is important that you lower your voice and speak distinctly; do not speak more loudly and raise the pitch of your voice.

COMMUNICATING ON PAPER

If the patient has adequate reading and writing skills, you can gather some health history information by having her fill out questionnaires and other pre-printed forms during the interview or afterward. Another option would be to write down questions and have the patient write down her answers.

Remember, however, that if you leave preprinted forms for the patient to complete on her own, you will not be able to ask immediate follow-up questions to the responses the patient supplies. This could prevent you from obtaining a complete history.

MODIFYING THE PHYSICAL EXAMINATION

You may need to give specific instructions to a hearing-impaired patient during the examination. For example, you may have to ask her to change her position. If so, provide written instructions, pictures, or diagrams whenever possible.

VISUALLY IMPAIRED PATIENTS

Most visually impaired patients can respond to questions without difficulty. When you first approach the patient, introduce yourself and describe the purpose and format of the interview. Be sure to use a normal tone of voice, speak at a moderate speed, and enunciate words clearly. If the visually impaired patient also uses a hearing aid, ask her to wear it during the interview.

ORIENTING THE PATIENT

To reassure the patient and orient her to your location, use subtle gestures, such as resting your hand on her arm. If the patient has not been previously oriented to the room, take a few minutes to describe where everything is so that she can get a sense of the surroundings. Whenever possible, use other aids to supplement oral instructions, such as materials on audio CD or in Braille.

MODIFYING THE PHYSICAL EXAMINATION

Move slowly and deliberately during the examination, providing explanations and directions as you proceed. Tell the patient what you are about to do before you do it. Explain where you are going to touch the patient and why.

OLDER ADULTS

From your first contact with an older adult, be sure to convey respect. Never address an older adult by a first name unless the patient asks you to do so.

Early in the health history interview, determine if the patient has any sensory impairments. Some older adults with declining visual or hearing ability do not wear eyeglasses or hearing aids because of cost. Others refuse because they want to maintain a sense of independence and dignity. Unfortunately, this only compounds the sensory impairment. What's more, poor vision or hearing can lead to or worsen confusion when an older adult is in unfamiliar surroundings.

Older adults are likely to have a longer health history than are younger patients. Try to allow more time for the health history interview so that you will not need to rush through the interview or gloss over aspects of the patient's history that she feels are important.

CHECKING FOR MEMORY DEFICITS

Memory normally declines somewhat with age. Usually, age-related memory loss involves spontaneous recall of information about recent events. Thus the older adult may have trouble recalling what she had for dinner the previous night but have no difficulty remembering the name of her high school.

Be sure to consider the possible impact of memory problems when assessing the patient's ability to perform activities of daily living. For example, does the patient sometimes forget that she is cooking something on the stove? Does she occasionally forget where she is, even in her own neighborhood? To obtain such information, you may need to interview a close friend or family member (see Assessing a Patient's Psychosocial Status).

ASSESSING A PATIENT'S PSYCHOSOCIAL STATUS

Stay alert for signs that an older adult is experiencing personal or social difficulties. Such signs include poor hygiene and grooming, as well as indications of abuse, neglect, or malnutrition. If you uncover these signs, you will need to investigate the causes and be prepared to contact a social worker, if appropriate.

When assessing for depression and other psychologic disorders, keep in mind that although depression is more common among older adults, its symptoms may be less severe in this age-group. What is more, they may mimic normal signs of aging.

Make sure that you check for subtle indicators of depression, such as disruptions in a patient's sleep patterns (trouble falling asleep or waking up early in the morning), changes in eating habits (eating too little or too much), and changes in personal interests (loss of enjoyment derived from hobbies that the patient used to enjoy).

If during the health history interview you suspect that the patient has a significant memory problem, interrupt the interview to assess her mental status and level of consciousness. (For more information on assessing level of consciousness, see Chapter 3.) Later, interview a friend or family member to obtain complete health data.

DEALING WITH AN INCOMPETENT PATIENT

Competency can be an issue with patients of all ages and with a variety of conditions. Older adults with age-related dementia are one such group of patients. Competency is a legal issue, and your facility will need to take certain steps to protect the patient's welfare and civil liberties. If you suspect your patient is incompetent or unable to make decisions for herself, contact her physician and your nurse manager to determine who will make decisions about the patient's care.

Consult with your nurse manager about the need to document specific patient deficits, such as lack of judgment, as well as how to involve your facility's risk-management team in the patient's care. In addition, talk to the physician about obtaining a psychiatric consultation for the patient.

MODIFYING THE PHYSICAL EXAMINATION

Proceed more slowly when examining an older adult to allow for a slower response to your instructions or an increased number of symptoms to investigate. In addition, keep in mind that the patient may be unable to assume certain positions because of decreased flexibility.

During the examination, do not confuse normal signs of aging with signs of disease. Age brings on many bodily alterations, including changes in fat distribution, skin elasticity, and posture. Age can also reduce a person's pain perception, so take special care to be gentle. This is particularly important if you suspect the patient may have osteoporosis. Blunt percussion, for instance, may be contraindicated in this patient.

Also consider whether any medications the patient is taking could affect your physical findings. For example, if the patient is taking a beta-blocker, expect her heart rate to be slower than normal.

OBESE PATIENTS

When obtaining a health history from an obese patient, be sensitive to the patient's feelings, especially when asking about weight and eating habits. Most obese people are painfully aware that they are overweight; some have tried to lose weight numerous times. In addition, many know of the health risks associated with obesity and feel guilty about endangering their health.

CHECKING FOR OBESITY-RELATED HEALTH PROBLEMS

Obesity in itself is good cause for a thorough investigation of the patient's health status. Ask about a history of obesity-related disorders such as diabetes mellitus and hypertension. Also find out if the patient's serum cholesterol and triglyceride levels have been checked recently. If they have and the results were elevated, find out if the patient is currently being treated for these conditions.

Review the patient's dietary habits and discuss any past attempts at weight loss. Try to determine whether the obesity is long standing or more recent. If it is recent, ask if the patient knows what prompted the weight gain. For instance, did she recently begin taking a medication that promotes weight gain, such as a corticosteroid agent?

In addition, investigate whether the patient is depressed, bored, or less mobile as a result of an injury or a disorder. Ask about recent pregnancies and changes in menstrual patterns.

MODIFYING THE PHYSICAL EXAMINATION

Be sensitive to the patient's need for privacy and discretion. If an examination gown is not large enough to fully cover the patient's body, let her wear her own clothing, when appropriate.

Be sure to use the proper examination equipment, such as a large blood pressure cuff, to ensure accurate findings. In body areas that may be hard for the obese patient to reach, such as skin folds, feet, and toenails, carefully examine the skin for signs of disease or poor hygiene.

Be aware that you may have difficulty performing certain examination steps with an obese patient, including eliciting deep tendon reflexes and palpating peripheral pulses and abdominal organs. To palpate, you may need to use both hands (bimanual palpation) to trap or hook an organ.

PREGNANT PATIENTS

You may care for a pregnant patient when she seeks health care for another problem. Therefore you will need to be prepared to alter the health history and physical examination for the patient's special needs. Because her pregnancy may not be obvious, always ask a female patient of childbearing age if she is pregnant. When in doubt, check with the physician about ordering a pregnancy test.

GETTING THE DETAILS

In addition to other components of the health history, you will need to ask specific questions about the progression of the patient's pregnancy, including duration of gestation, delivery due date, presence of contractions, and any complications, such as hypertension. In addition, find out if this is the patient's first pregnancy or if she has had previous pregnancies, abortions (spontaneous and induced), or deliveries.

While obtaining the patient's nutritional history, ask about her typical daily diet and any food intolerances, as you would ask any patient. However, also ask about food cravings. If the patient craves nonnutritive substances (pica), such as dirt, find out what she has eaten and how much. Also, ask if she's taking nutritional supplements, such as prenatal vitamins. If possible, determine the patient's prenatal weight, and calculate her weight gain during pregnancy.

Be sure to ask about smoking, alcohol intake, and recreational drug use. If there's evidence of the use of any of these substances, warn her about the potential effects on the fetus and consider a referral to a social worker or counselor.

Finally, try to get a handle on the patient's social and emotional state. If you have not asked earlier, determine whether your patient is married or in a safe, stable relationship. If the patient is single and unattached, explore options for support during the pregnancy and after the delivery. Also try to gauge her reaction (positive or negative) to the pregnancy. Keep in mind that ambivalence and anxiety are common emotions, especially early in the pregnancy.

MODIFYING THE PHYSICAL EXAMINATION

As you would with any patient, be sure to provide the pregnant patient with warmth, privacy, and comfort during the physical examination. Make sure that the examination gown is large enough to cover an advanced pregnancy, or allow the patient to wear her own clothing. If needed, bring a large-sized blood pressure cuff to the bedside, as well as an ultrasound stethoscope or fetoscope and measuring tape, if you perform a fetal examination.

Before starting the examination, ask the patient if she needs to void; increased glomerular blood flow and uterine pressure on the bladder can cause urinary frequency in the first and third trimester. As you proceed with the examination, pay special attention to her positioning. Whenever possible, keep the patient in the seated position or in the left-sided supine position, with the head of the bed elevated. Avoid having the patient lie flat on her back for very long because the enlarged uterus places pressure on the descending aorta and inferior vena cava, compromising blood flow to and from the lower extremities. If the blood flow is severely compromised, it can lead to supine hypotension, marked by a feeling of faintness (vena cava syndrome). When the patient needs to lie on her back (e.g., when you are examining her abdomen), place a pillow beneath her bent knees to relax her abdominal muscles. Because the enlarged uterus can keep the diaphragm from descending fully and prevent complete lung expansion, keep the patient's head elevated to help ease her breathing.

When you examine a pregnant patient, be prepared for the normal, physiologic changes that pregnancy produces. Signs and symptoms present in a healthy, pregnant female might otherwise cause alarm if found in a nonpregnant patient (see ▥ How Pregnancy Affects Findings on the Physical Examination).

LIFESPAN CONSIDERATIONS

HOW PREGNANCY AFFECTS FINDINGS ON THE PHYSICAL EXAMINATION

Body Region	Expected Changes	Possible Cause
Head and neck	• Irregularly shaped, brown patches on the face (chloasma), darkening of scars and moles, spider nevi	• Increased melanocyte activity
	• Increased facial hair, loss or thinning of scalp hair, oily scalp	• Increased androgen and corticotropic hormone formation
	• Gingival hyperplasia	• Increased gingival vascularity caused by hormonal changes
	• Symmetrically enlarged thyroid gland	• Increased thyroid gland vascularity, new thyroid follicle formation, hyperplasia of glandular tissue
	• Nasal congestion	• Increased vascularity and swelling of nasal mucosa
Eyes and ears	• Blurred vision when wearing contact lenses	• Increased lysosome content in tears
	• Darkening of eyelids	• Increased melanocyte activity
	• Feeling of fullness in ears	• Increased vascularity of auditory canal and tympanic membrane

continued

LIFESPAN CONSIDERATIONS—cont'd

Body Region	Expected Changes	Possible Cause
Chest and back	• Point of maximal impulse (PMI) displaced upward and to left, shallow respirations with increased rate, reduced respiratory excursion	• Upward displacement of diaphragm
	• Soft, blowing systolic murmurs, S_3 heart sound	• Increased blood volume and velocity
	• Darkening of areolae and nipples	• Increased melanocyte activity
	• Breast hypertrophy and tenderness, superficial venous pattern	• Increased breast glandular tissue and vascularity
Upper extremities and abdominal region	• Palmar erythema	• Cause unknown
	• Midline, brownish-black streak (linea nigra)	• Increased melanocyte activity
	• Purple or red striae	• Stretching of skin caused by uterine, fetal growth
	• Hypoactive bowel sounds, nausea, vomiting, dyspepsia, constipation	• Intestinal smooth-muscle relaxation
	• Abdominal tenseness or firmness during palpation	• Uterine contractions caused by palpation (commonly third trimester)
	• Hemorrhoids	• Increased regional blood flow
Lower extremities	• Edema, varicosities	• Increased lower extremity venous pressure, caused by pressure on enlarged uterus

First Encounter: A General Survey of the Patient

From the moment you meet your patient during admission to the hospital, on your first encounter during your shift, or at the start of a clinic visit, you should begin to form a sound clinical impression of the patient's physical and psychologic well-being. You build on that impression step by step as you conduct the general survey and head to toe physical examination.

ASSESSING GENERAL PRESENTATION

A patient's general presentation can provide important clues to health and well-being. To assess general presentation, observe the patient's facial expression, evaluate self-care, and note any unusual odors.

FACIAL EXPRESSION

A person's facial expression usually reveals the emotions he is experiencing at the time, such as fear, happiness, or anxiety. As you first encounter a patient, check his expression for signs of distress. If the patient is distressed, it may affect the way you conduct the examination. For example, if he is grimacing in pain, you will need to respond to the need for relief before proceeding. Continue to assess facial expression for clues to discomfort as you perform each examination step. Watch for grimacing, gritting teeth, or flushing. In addition, observe for pallor and diaphoresis, which suggest hypotension from severe discomfort that triggers a vasovagal reaction.

Try to determine if the patient's facial expression is consistent with what he is saying or appropriate for the conversation. For instance, does the patient look tense, even though he is telling you he feels fine? If so, he may be reluctant to tell you that something is bothering him. On the other hand, if the patient complains of excruciating pain but has a relaxed or happy facial expression, then he could be malingering.

CULTURAL CONSIDERATIONS

Cultural factors can play a role in facial expressiveness and the extent of eye contact a patient makes. A patient who comes from a culture that values stoicism may try to hide any sign of pain on his face. Also, be aware that in some cultures, avoiding eye contact does not indicate lack of interest or distrust. Rather, it is a sign of respect or deference to authority.

SELF-CARE

Components of self-care include personal hygiene and grooming. Signs of poor hygiene and grooming may be obvious as you approach the patient. You can assess hygiene further by noting whether the patient's hair, nails, and skin are clean. To assess grooming, note whether the patient has combed his hair and fastened his clothing properly, as well as whether or not the patient is dressed appropriately.

Poor hygiene and grooming may reflect illness or malaise, lack of social support or financial resources, or impaired thought processes related to depression or other mental disorder.

CULTURAL CONSIDERATIONS

Different cultures have different customs and standards regarding hygiene. For example, in some cultures the use of deodorant and the shaving of axillary hair is rare.

UNUSUAL ODORS

Unusual body odors may result from a variety of physical illnesses. Fruity breath, for example, may indicate diabetic ketoacidosis. Other body odors may simply reflect variations in hygienic and grooming practices. If you detect an unusual odor, try to determine if the underlying cause calls for prompt attention (see Identifying Unusual Odors).

IDENTIFYING UNUSUAL ODORS

Odor	Probable Causes
Fruity breath	• Diabetic ketoacidosis
Halitosis	• Dental decay • Throat infection
Putrid breath or body odor	• Infection (e.g., lung abscess, wound infection) • Malignancy
Fishy vaginal odor	• Vaginal infection
Urine or ammonia-like odor	• Dehydration • Incontinence • Urinary tract infection
Fecal breath or body odor	• Bowel obstruction (with fecal breath odor) • Incontinence • Poor hygiene

ASSESSING VITAL SIGNS

Obtaining your patient's vital signs early in the assessment enables you to immediately detect certain life-threatening problems, such as profound hypotension or tachycardia.

TEMPERATURE

Core body temperature is the most reliable standard for temperature measurement and can be measured with a tympanic thermometer. If the patient is in a critical care area and has a pulmonary artery catheter or an indwelling urinary catheter that records temperature, measurement can be made using the thermistor port of the catheter.

NORMAL FINDINGS

- Body temperature ranging from 96.8° to 99.5° F (36° to 37.5° C), depending on type of measurement and time of day (see Normal Temperature Variations)

NORMAL FINDINGS

NORMAL TEMPERATURE VARIATIONS
- Oral temperature: 96.8° to 99.5° F (36° to 37.5° C)
- Rectal temperature: 97.3° to 100.2° F (36.3° to 37.9° C)
- Tympanic (core) temperature: 97.2° to 100° F (36.2° to 37.8° C)

Fluctuating temperatures
Body temperature tends to fluctuate throughout the day, peaking in the late afternoon and reaching its low point at about 3 to 4 AM. Body temperature also varies over the life span, decreasing with age. This is why older adults are more vulnerable to hypothermia and less capable of mounting a febrile response.

ABNORMAL FINDINGS

- Temperature higher than normal range (This requires investigation for possible causes of the fever, such as infection, tissue trauma, infarction, malignancy, blood disorder, medication reaction, or immune disorder.)
- Core body temperature exceeding 105° F (40.5° C), indicating a medical emergency called *hyperpyrexia*, which can lead to death unless the temperature is promptly reduced (Clinical effects of hyperpyrexia include neurologic symptoms [e.g., seizures or changes in mental status] and direct thermal injury to muscle tissue. Such injury may lead to rhabdomyolysis [breakdown of muscle tissue into myoglobin], which in turn may lead to renal failure. Other possible consequences of thermal tissue injury include disseminated intravascular coagulation, hypoxemia, and hypotension. In adults, hyperpyrexia rarely results from an infection. More often, heatstroke or damage to the hypothalamus causes it.)

- Rapid and potentially fatal temperature elevation characterized by muscle rigidity, indicating a rare hereditary phenomenon called *malignant hyperthermia* (This may follow administration of inhaled anesthetic agents or muscle relaxants. Malignant hyperthermia may cause tachycardia, tachypnea, muscle rigidity, cyanosis, and skin mottling. To avert death, treat it rapidly. Treatment may include a direct-acting muscle relaxant [e.g., dantrolene], discontinuation of the offending agent, and fever reduction through the use of cooling blankets.)
- Core body temperature less than 95°F (35°C), indicating hypothermia (This may result from prolonged exposure to cold, starvation, hypothyroidism, or hypoglycemia. Alcohol intoxication and sepsis worsen hypothermia by impairing vasoconstriction [the mechanism by which blood vessels constrict], reducing blood flow to peripheral organs and preserving body heat necessary for the vital organs. Hypothermia is life threatening and calls for rapid intervention [see Assessing the Severity of Hypothermia].)

ASSESSING THE SEVERITY OF HYPOTHERMIA

Hypothermia may be mild, moderate, or severe.

Mild hypothermia
Defined as a body temperature between 90° and 95°F (32.2° to 35°C), mild hypothermia causes shivering, piloerection (gooseflesh), cool skin, pallor, and cyanotic nail beds with slow capillary refill.

Moderate hypothermia
A body temperature between 82.4° and 90°F (28° and 32.2°C) causes loss of the ability to shiver, diminished deep tendon reflexes, and cardiac arrhythmias (e.g., atrial fibrillation). Although moderate hypothermia typically causes a decreased cardiac output and a slow heart rate, the person usually can maintain a normal blood pressure.

Severe hypothermia
A body temperature less than 82.4°F (28°C) causes decreased blood pressure, ventricular arrhythmias, progressive bradycardia, and coma. If the temperature falls below 64°F (18°C), the heart may stop beating and brain wave activity may cease. Death ensues unless normal body temperature is restored.

PULSE

Assessing the pulse rate and rhythm provides information about heart function. The pulse amplitude (weak, strong, or bounding) is indicative of the circulating blood volume, strength of left ventricular contractions, and blood vessel tone. Pulse contour or configuration reflects the amount and force of blood ejected into the aorta.

Key guidelines for accurate pulse assessment when a pulse is hard to palpate or irregular are as follows:

- Palpate the carotid or femoral pulse if the radial pulse is very weak or thready.
- If the pulse is irregular, determine if the irregularity has a regular pattern or no detectable pattern.
- Confirm an irregular pulse rate by auscultating an apical heart rate (in case some of the heart's impulses are not reaching the radial pulse).
- Record any pulse deficit (difference between apical and radial pulse rates).

NORMAL FINDINGS

- Pulse rate between 60 and 100 beats per minute
- Regular rhythm
- Strong amplitude
- Contour with a smooth upstroke and downstroke
- Variations in pulse rate and amplitude within normal limits (For example, pulse rates less than 60 beats per minute are common in athletes and in people taking beta-adrenergic blockers. In addition, any condition that stimulates the sympathetic nervous system, such as exercise, stress, fear, caffeine ingestion, or medications like pseudoephedrine, may increase the pulse rate and amplitude.)

ABNORMAL FINDINGS

- Weak, thready pulse, possibly indicating decreased pulse pressure, reduced stroke volume (e.g., from heart failure, hypovolemia, or aortic stenosis), and increased peripheral vascular resistance (PVR)
- Bounding pulse, which is easy to palpate and typically has a sharp upstroke followed by a quick downstroke (The pulsations may seem to throb against your finger, then quickly collapse or retreat [called *water-hammer* or *Corrigan's pulse*]. Conditions that may cause a bounding pulse include bradycardia; hypervolemia; severe hypertension; disorders that increase circulating catecholamine agents [e.g., pheochromocytoma, hyperthyroidism]; disorders that increase stroke volume, reduce PVR, or do both [e.g., anemia, aortic regurgitation, hyperthyroidism, arteriovenous fistula, patent ductus arteriosus]; and decreased blood vessel compliance [see Identifying Pulse Abnormalities].)

IDENTIFYING PULSE ABNORMALITIES

Pulse Abnormality	Characteristics	Probable Causes
Pulsus alternans	• Weak beats alternating with strong beats • Regular rhythm	• Left ventricular failure
Pulsus bigeminus (bigeminal pulse)	• Two beats occurring in rapid succession, followed by a pause during which no pulse is felt	• Cardiac arrhythmias, such as premature ventricular contractions

continued

IDENTIFYING PULSE ABNORMALITIES—cont'd

Pulse Abnormality	Characteristics	Probable Causes
	• Irregular rhythm • Premature beat with smaller amplitude than normal sinus contraction	
Pulsus paradoxus	• Pulse amplitude that decreases with inspiration and increases with expiration	• Conditions that impede left ventricular outflow during inspiration, such as constrictive pericarditis, cardiac tamponade, end-stage heart failure, and severe chronic obstructive pulmonary disease
Pulsus tardus	• Slow pulse rate • Gradual upstroke; prolonged, blunted downstroke	• Severe aortic stenosis

RESPIRATIONS

Changes in the rate, depth, or character of a patient's respirations may suggest neurologic, respiratory, or cardiovascular compromise. If respirations are abnormal, always investigate for associated symptoms to help uncover the underlying cause.

NORMAL FINDINGS

- Breathing quiet and effortless
- Rate between 12 and 20 breaths per minute
- Regular rhythm
- Slight thoracic movement and pronounced abdominal movement when the patient is supine; more obvious thoracic movement if sitting up

ABNORMAL FINDINGS

- Respiratory rate exceeding 20 breaths per minute (tachypnea) may indicate restrictive lung disease, pleuritic chest pain, an elevated diaphragm, fever, metabolic acidosis, or salicylate poisoning. Breathing may be shallow as well. (For information on other abnormal respiratory patterns, see Chapter 6.)

BLOOD PRESSURE

Blood pressure measurement provides information about cardiac output, circulation, hydration, and arterial elasticity. Extremely high or low blood pressure may be life threatening, requiring rapid assessment and quick intervention (see Hypertension).

DISORDER CLOSE-UP

HYPERTENSION

A common disorder often of unknown cause, hypertension is marked by an intermittent or sustained rise in systolic or diastolic blood pressure. Most physicians diagnose and treat hypertension when a patient has three consecutive blood pressure readings of 140/90 mm Hg or higher. The threshold for treating a patient with diabetes mellitus or chronic renal failure is lower. For these patients, treatment begins when the blood pressure reaches 130/80 mm Hg. Patients with blood pressure readings of 120/80 to 139/89 mm Hg are considered prehypertensive.

Typically, hypertension causes no symptoms and is detected incidentally during routine screening or evaluation for another problem. If it seems to have no underlying cause, the disorder is called *primary (or essential) hypertension.* When the condition does have a detectable cause, as when the patient has an adrenal disorder, it is called *secondary hypertension.* If the patient's diastolic pressure rises when he stands up, the patient probably has primary hypertension. If it drops when he stands up, he probably has secondary hypertension.

Blood pressure rises in response to increased blood volume, heart rate, and stroke volume, or because of arteriolar vasoconstriction, which increases peripheral vascular resistance (PVR). Eventually the result of hypertension can be seen in the patient's blood vessels. In the arterioles, alternating areas of dilation and constriction develop, leading to vascular injury and increased intraarterial pressure.

Characteristic findings

Health history and physical examination findings vary, depending on the extent and severity of the disorder. Use the following information to help distinguish between expected and unexpected findings.

Health history

- Family history of hypertension
- African heritage
- Stress
- Obesity or sedentary lifestyle
- Diet high in sodium or saturated fat
- Tobacco use
- Oral contraceptive use
- History of diabetes mellitus, arteriosclerotic disease, or renovascular disease
- Pheochromocytoma
- Cushing's syndrome
- Primary aldosteronism
- Renal failure
- Coarctation of the aorta
- Thyroid or parathyroid disease
- Sleep apnea
- Morning headache in the occipital region
- Fatigue, dizziness, or weakness
- Blurred vision
- Epistaxis
- Chest pain
- Dyspnea

Inspection

- Peripheral edema (in late stages, with heart failure)
- Retinal hemorrhages, exudates, and papilledema (in late stages, with hypertensive retinopathy)

Palpation

- Pulsating mass in the abdomen (suggests aneurysm, which can result from hypertension)
- Enlarged kidneys (suggests polycystic disease, which can cause hypertension)

Auscultation

- Abdominal bruit
- Femoral bruit
- Elevated systolic or diastolic pressure (or both)
- Prehypertension: Systolic pressure 120 to 139 mm Hg, diastolic 80 to 89 mm Hg
- Stage 1 hypertension: Systolic pressure 140 to 159 mm Hg, diastolic 90 to 99 mm Hg
- Stage 2 hypertension: Systolic pressure greater than or equal to 160 mm Hg, diastolic pressure greater than or equal to 100 mm Hg

continued

DISORDER CLOSE-UP—cont'd

Complications
- Cerebrovascular accident
- Coronary artery disease
- Angina
- Myocardial infarction
- Heart failure

- Arrhythmias
- Sudden cardiac death
- Renal failure
- Hypertensive encephalopathy
- Blindness

Blood pressure taken in three positions, with the patient lying down, sitting, and standing up, helps detect orthostatic hypotension, which is a drop of 20 mm Hg or more in systolic pressure when the patient rises from a sitting or lying position (see Checking for Orthostatic Hypotension).

EXAMINATION TIP

CHECKING FOR ORTHOSTATIC HYPOTENSION

If your patient appears dehydrated, complains of light-headedness or fainting, or is taking antihypertensive medication, be sure to check for orthostatic hypotension (a decrease in blood pressure when rising from a sitting or reclining [lying down] position).

Take three readings
First, measure blood pressure when the patient is lying down. Then, after waiting 1 to 5 minutes, have the patient sit up (with the blood pressure cuff still around the arm) and take the blood pressure again. Finally, after waiting 1 to 5 minutes, have the patient stand (with the cuff still in place) and obtain a third measurement. Also auscultate the patient's heart rate in these three positions.

Interpret the readings properly
Consider orthostatic hypotension if the patient's sitting or standing systolic pressure is 20 mm Hg (or more) lower than the recumbent pressure and the pulse rises by 10 to 20 beats per minute, especially if the patient says he feels light-headed when rising to a vertical position.

NORMAL FINDINGS

- Systolic pressure between 90 and 119 mm Hg in an adult
- Diastolic pressure between 60 and 80 mm Hg in an adult
- Systolic pressure that drops only slightly (less than 20 mm Hg) when the patient rises from a sitting to a standing position
- Diastolic pressure that rises only slightly when the patient rises from a sitting to a standing position
- Pulse pressure (the difference between systolic and diastolic pressures) between 30 and 40 mm Hg
- Pressure that follows a typical diurnal pattern, peaking at midmorning and falling progressively throughout the day to reach its lowest point at 3 to 4 AM
- Blood pressure that rises slightly as the patient ages (Diastolic pressure increases up to about age 60; systolic pressure also increases [from stiffening of the arterial and aortic walls], as does pulse pressure.)

ABNORMAL FINDINGS

- Below normal blood pressure, indicating hypotension (Generally, this involves a systolic pressure less than 90 mm Hg or a diastolic pressure less than 60 mm Hg. However, a patient with pressures higher than this range may still be hypotensive if readings are considerably lower than the patient's baseline. Possible causes include heart failure, dehydration, endocrine disorders [e.g., Addison's disease or hypothyroidism], neurogenic shock, vena cava obstruction, cardiac tamponade, adrenal hypofunction, and a vasovagal reaction.)

- Pulse increase of 10 beats per minute and light-headedness or syncope when the patient is standing, indicating orthostatic hypotension (Possible causes include decreased autonomic tone [as seen in older adults and diabetics], decreased vasomotor tone, and medications such as diuretics, alpha-blockers, and tricyclic antidepressants.)

- Blood pressure ranging from 120/80 to 139/89 mm Hg obtained on at least three occasions, indicating prehypertension (Although not always treated with medication [unless the patient has diabetes mellitus or renal disease], patients with prehypertension should be instructed to implement lifestyle changes, such as weight loss and a low-sodium diet.)

- Blood pressure 140/90 mm Hg or higher obtained on at least three occasions, indicating hypertension (Be aware that pain, emotional stress, and use of medications such as cyclosporine may cause blood pressure to rise. [For more information on hypertension, see Chapter 7.] If an older patient's systolic blood pressure is greater than 140 mm Hg, but the diastolic reading is less than 90 mm Hg, consider isolated systolic hypertension, a variation commonly seen with aging [see Recognizing Systolic Hypertension in an Older Adult].)

LIFESPAN CONSIDERATIONS

RECOGNIZING SYSTOLIC HYPERTENSION IN AN OLDER ADULT

Until the age of 50 years, both systolic and diastolic pressures tend to rise. After this age, diastolic pressure tends to level off in most people. If systolic pressure continues to rise, then isolated systolic hypertension (systolic pressure greater than or equal to 140 mm Hg, with a diastolic pressure less than 90 mm Hg) and a widening in pulse pressure results. A loss of elasticity in the large arteries caused by atherosclerosis contributes to the development of isolated systolic hypertension.

Previously, isolated systolic hypertension was not treated because researchers believed it to be part of the normal aging process. Now it has been shown that isolated systolic hypertension increases the risk of stroke and cardiovascular disease in older adults, even when the diastolic pressure is normal; hence it should be treated. Track your older patient's blood pressure with each visit to detect isolated systolic hypertension, and monitor the effects of treatment. Include orthostatic blood pressure measurements, because impaired baroreceptor reflex mechanisms may occur in an older patient, especially if he has isolated systolic hypertension.

- Widened pulse pressure, or a difference of more than 40 mm Hg between the systolic and diastolic pressures (This may result from aortic insufficiency or thyrotoxicosis.)

- Narrowed pulse pressure, or a difference of less than 30 mm Hg between systolic and diastolic pressures (This may result from tachycardia, severe aortic stenosis, constrictive pericarditis, cardiac tamponade, pericardial effusion, or ascites.)

EVALUATING BODY BUILD AND POSTURE

Continue your initial assessment by evaluating the patient's body build and posture. Be sure to check the symmetry of the shoulders, scapulae, and iliac crests. In addition, inspect the alignment and curvature of the spinal column. This part of the assessment also includes measuring the patient's height and weight.

HEIGHT AND WEIGHT

Measure your patient's height and weight without his shoes. If the patient is hospitalized, try to weigh him every day on the same scale, at the same time, and in the same clothing to ensure an accurate comparison. Record both English and metric values for each measurement.

If a chair or bed scale is used, subtract the weight of sheets, padding, and any other items with which the patient must be measured. If height cannot be measured, rely on the patient's report of his height.

Determining if a Patient Is Overweight

Next, refer to a body mass index (BMI) chart to determine if the patient's weight is appropriate for his age and height (see Assessing Body Mass Index). BMI is weight in kilograms divided by height in meters squared. The chart shows BMIs for various heights and weights and determines whether the patient is a healthy weight, overweight, or obese. Individuals with a BMI greater than 25 are over their ideal body weights and considered at increased risk for obesity-related disorders.

If your patient has gained or lost weight recently, determine the percentage of weight change by using the following steps:

- If the patient has lost weight, subtract the current body weight from the previous weight (e.g., his weight from 6 months ago). If the patient has gained weight, subtract the previous weight from the current weight.
- Multiply the result by 100.
- Divide the result you obtained in the previous step by the patient's previous weight. This is the percentage of recent weight change.

The following example is calculated for a patient now weighing 185 lb who weighed 162 lb 6 months ago. As the result shows, his recent weight gain represents 14.2% of his previous weight.

$$\frac{(185 - 162) \times 100}{162} \div 162 = 14.2$$

Consider any change exceeding 10% of the patient's usual weight as significant, and be sure to document it.

ASSESSING BODY MASS INDEX

Body mass index (BMI) is a value that reflects body weight adjusted for height. For individuals 20 years or older, BMI is categorized as underweight (less than 18.5), normal (18.5 to 24.9), overweight (25.0 to 29.9), or obese (greater than 30). The following chart displays corresponding inches and pounds for individuals with BMIs ranging from 19 to 35.

Weight in Pounds

Height (feet and inches)	19	20	21	22	23	24	25	26	27	28	29	30	31	32	33	34	35
4'10" (58")	91	96	100	105	110	115	119	124	129	134	138	143	148	153	158	162	167
4'11" (59")	94	99	104	109	114	119	124	128	133	138	143	148	153	158	163	168	173
5' (60")	97	102	107	112	118	123	128	133	138	143	148	153	158	163	168	174	179
5'1" (61")	100	106	111	116	122	127	132	137	143	148	153	158	164	169	174	180	185
5'2" (62")	104	109	115	120	126	131	136	142	147	153	158	164	169	175	180	186	191
5'3" (63")	107	113	118	124	130	135	141	146	152	158	163	169	175	180	186	192	197
5'4" (64")	110	116	122	128	134	140	145	151	157	163	169	174	180	186	192	197	204
5'5" (65")	114	120	126	132	138	144	150	156	162	168	174	180	186	192	198	204	210
5'6" (66")	118	124	130	136	142	148	155	161	167	173	179	186	192	198	204	210	216
5'7" (67")	121	127	134	140	146	153	159	166	172	178	185	191	198	204	211	217	223
5'8" (68")	125	131	138	144	151	158	164	171	177	184	190	197	203	210	216	223	230
5'9" (69")	128	135	142	149	155	162	169	176	182	189	196	203	209	216	223	230	236
5'10" (70")	132	139	146	153	160	167	174	181	188	195	202	209	216	222	229	236	243
5'11" (71")	136	143	150	157	165	172	179	186	193	200	208	215	222	229	236	243	250
6' (72")	140	147	154	162	169	177	184	191	199	206	213	221	228	235	242	250	258
6'1" (73")	144	151	159	166	174	182	189	197	204	212	219	227	235	242	250	257	265
6'2" (74")	148	155	163	171	179	186	194	202	210	218	225	233	241	249	256	264	272
6'3" (75")	152	160	168	176	184	192	200	208	216	224	232	240	248	256	264	272	279
BMI	**19**	**20**	**21**	**22**	**23**	**24**	**25**	**26**	**27**	**28**	**29**	**30**	**31**	**32**	**33**	**34**	**35**

From NIH/National Heart, Lung, and Blood Institute (NHLBI): *Evidence report of clinical guidelines on the identification, evaluation, and treatment of overweight and obesity in adults*, Bethesda, Md, 1998, National Institutes of Health.

NORMAL FINDINGS

- Shoulders, scapulae, and iliac crests symmetrical bilaterally
- Spinal column midline, with aligned spinal processes, when patient is bent forward
- Spinal curvature concave in lumbar region and convex in thoracic region with patient standing
- BMI within normal range for weight and height

LIFESPAN CONSIDERATIONS

AGE-RELATED CHANGES WITHIN NORMAL LIMITS

With age, a person's posture changes and height decreases as the intervertebral disks shrink, the bony structures between the disks become shorter, and full knee and hip extension becomes more difficult. In addition, the lower abdomen typically protrudes from weakened abdominal muscles and redistribution of fat to the hips and lower abdomen. Spinal column alterations may lead to kyphosis.

ABNORMAL FINDINGS

- Accentuated lateral curvature of the spine when the patient bends forward, indicating structural scoliosis (The shoulders appear uneven, and the rib cage seems to bulge to one side. This form of scoliosis is associated with thoracic deformity and vertebral rotation.)
- BMI outside normal range for weight and height

ASSESSING BODY MOVEMENTS AND GAIT

Body movements and gait can provide clues to such disorders as Parkinson's disease and other neuromuscular or neurologic conditions. Assessing these features helps to gauge the patient's functional status and progress, and it alerts you to the need for possible intervention. For example, a patient with a gait disturbance that predisposes him to falls may require safety interventions or physical therapy for gait or balance retraining.

Observe your patient's body movements both at rest and in motion, paying special attention to movements of the arms, legs, and head. Check for involuntary movements, such as tremors or tics.

TESTING FOR INVOLUNTARY MOVEMENTS

You may be able to detect involuntary movements simply by observing as the patient moves about the room or performs simple activities. Alternatively, you can ask the patient to hold the arms forward and flex the wrists upward with fingers spread as you watch for abnormal involuntary movements.

Another way to check for involuntary movements is to perform *point-to-point testing*. Used mainly to assess coordination, this test also may reveal tremors. Ask the patient to place an index finger on his nose and then touch your finger as you hold it 12 inches to 14 inches directly in front of his nose.

Have the patient continue to alternately touch his nose and your finger several times while you watch closely for tremors.

NORMAL FINDINGS

- Body movements smooth, easily controlled, and coordinated
- Patient able to hold the arms forward with little difficulty or extraneous movement
- Point-to-point testing smooth, with reasonably accurate movements (The patient should touch his nose and your finger without missing the target or trembling.)

ABNORMAL FINDINGS

- Tremors, tics, and dystonic movements, possibly indicating neurologic, neuromuscular, endocrine, or psychologic disorder (If you note tremors, tics, or other involuntary movements, document their location, rate, rhythm, and amplitude. In addition, note whether they are related to particular postures, activities, or emotions.)

OBSERVING A PERSON'S GAIT

Analyzing a patient's manner or style of walking may help you detect various neurologic disorders. Observing the gait of a patient who has suffered a neurologic or musculoskeletal injury or amputation can also help you assess recovery and rehabilitation.

To analyze a patient's gait, ask him to walk a straight line for several feet and then turn and walk back toward you. Observe the patient's walking rhythm, cadence, and speed, as well as his posture, balance, leg movements, and arm swing (see Identifying Ataxic Gaits).

Observe gait during both the stance and swing phases of walking. The stance phase occurs when one leg and one foot bear most of the patient's weight; it includes double stance, when both feet are in contact with the ground. Most gait abnormalities occur during the stance phase. The swing phase occurs when one foot is raised above the walking surface and the opposite leg and foot bear all of the patient's weight.

During a complete two-step cycle, the stance phase accounts for 60% of total gait time (a quarter of this time in double stance, when both feet are in contact with the ground); the swing phase accounts for the remaining 40%.

When assessing a person's gait, be sure to rule out painful or restrictive foot conditions, such as corns and calluses, which can affect the way someone walks.

NORMAL FINDINGS

- Patient holding the body and head erect, maintaining balance easily, swinging the arms at the sides, and turning smoothly, with the shoulders and hips remaining level with each stride (The patient's center of gravity moves up and down about 2 inches, and the pelvis and trunk shift laterally about 1 inch. The patient's feet are held about 2 to 4 inches apart, and his step averages 15 inches.)

LIFESPAN CONSIDERATIONS

AGE-RELATED CHANGES WITHIN NORMAL LIMITS

A person's gait slows, and balance and grace diminish with age. Reduced muscle strength, especially in the quadriceps, results in short, shuffling steps. Older men typically have a wide-based, short-stepped gait; older women typically have a narrow-based, waddling gait.

ABNORMAL FINDINGS

- Short-stanced, limping gait (antalgic gait), which is often associated with pain originating from the feet or knees
- Waddling gait characterized by exaggerated alternation of lateral trunk movements and increased hip elevation (gluteal gait) (Possible causes include gluteal medius paralysis, progressive muscular dystrophy, bilateral hip dislocations from joint infections, spastic paralysis, and polio.)
- Wide-based, unsteady, uncoordinated gait (ataxic gait)
- Slow, stiff gait in which the thighs cross each other at each step; it appears as if the patient is walking through water (scissors gait) (This may result from bilateral spastic paresis of the legs.)
- Slow gait, with the patient taking short accelerating steps, possibly indicating festinating gait (generally associated with Parkinson's disease) (Other features include a decreased arm swing, stiff turning, stooped posture, forward lurching of the head and neck, slight flexion of the hips and knees, and arm flexion at the elbows and wrists.)

EXAMINATION TIP

IDENTIFYING ATAXIC GAITS

When evaluating your patient's gait, check for signs of ataxia, a condition marked by impaired ability to coordinate body movements. Depending on the cause of ataxia, the patient may display either a sensory ataxic gait or a cerebellar ataxic gait.

Sensory ataxic gait

In this uncoordinated gait, the patient may watch the ground for guidance while walking and may throw the feet forward and outward, toes and heels striking the ground in tandem. This gait is usually caused by loss of position sense, resulting from such conditions as peripheral neuropathy (possibly caused by diabetes mellitus) or posterior spinal column damage.

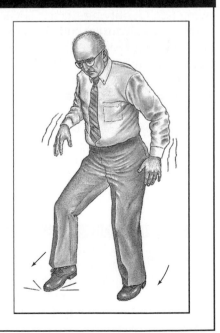

continued

EXAMINATION TIP—cont'd

Cerebellar ataxic gait
This wide-based, staggering gait is characterized by difficulty turning. The patient seems
to waver and has difficulty standing steadily
with eyes open or closed. Possible causes
include cerebellar disease, vestibular disease,
and alcohol intoxication.

Illustrations from Seidel HM, Ball JW, Dains
JE, Benedict GW: *Mosby's guide to physical
examination,* ed 5, St Louis, 2003 Mosby.

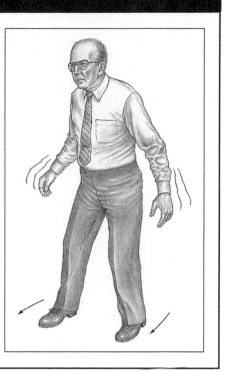

ASSESSING BALANCE, COORDINATION, AND POSITION SENSE

Balance is the ability to maintain the body's equilibrium. Coordination refers to
the harmonious functioning of various muscle groups to perform purposeful
actions. Position sense is the ability to perceive head, arm, and leg movements
and orient oneself without visual cues.

Balance, coordination, and position sense require the smooth integration
of the various parts of the nervous system. Use your clinical judgment to
determine whether your patient is able to perform tests that involve standing,
walking, or performing other maneuvers that require him to leave the bed or
expend energy. For example, you would defer most of these tests for a patient
who is recovering from surgery or a myocardial infarction until that patient is
stable or no longer in an acute care setting.

TESTING BALANCE AND COORDINATION

To test balance, have the patient perform Romberg's test by standing with
the feet together and eyes closed. Observe the patient for 45 to 60 seconds,
watching for signs that indicate loss of balance (see Evaluating Balance and
Coordination).

EVALUATING BALANCE AND COORDINATION

To assess your patient's balance and coordination, ask him to perform the following maneuvers. Throughout these tests, stand nearby to support the patient in case he starts to lose his balance. (Note: An older, weak, or disabled patient may be unable to perform some of these maneuvers.)

Romberg's test

In this test of balance, the patient stands with the feet together and then closes the eyes. Watch for swaying or loss of balance.

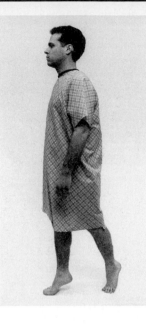

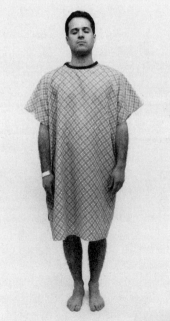

Hopping in place

To test proximal and distal muscle strength in the legs, instruct the patient to hop in place for 10 seconds on each foot. Ask a weak, frail, or older adult patient to stand up from a sitting position without using the arms. This also tests proximal muscles and hip extensors.

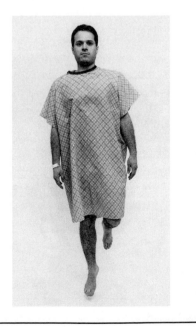

Walking on heels and toes

To evaluate balance and strength of the foot extensor and flexor muscles, instruct your patient to walk several feet on the heels and then turn around and walk toward you on the toes.

NORMAL FINDINGS

• Romberg's test showing that the patient can stand with the feet together without losing balance (Although the patient may sway slightly when the eyes are closed, he should not fall.)

ABNORMAL FINDINGS

• Marked swaying or loss of balance during Romberg's test, possibly indicating a cerebellar or vestibular (inner ear) problem

EVALUATING POSITION SENSE
Assess your patient's position sense by performing tests that evaluate symmetrical positioning, the ability to identify toe direction, and pronator drift.

Symmetrical Positioning
Have your patient close his eyes. Then move the patient's arm or leg into a specific position and ask him to place the other arm or leg in the same position. Determine how closely the patient duplicates the position in which you placed his arm or leg.

Identifying Toe Direction
Grasp the patient's great toe by the sides. Ask him to close his eyes; then move the toe up or down, and ask the patient to identify the direction in which it was moved. (Before performing this test, clarify which direction you are calling up and which you are calling down.)

Pronator Drift
Have the patient stand and extend the arms forward with the palms up. Then instruct the patient to close his eyes and maintain this position for 20 to 30 seconds.

Nylen-Bárány Test
To assess vestibular function, ask your patient to sit on the side of the bed and then recline to a lying position. As the patient reclines, have him turn his head toward you while keeping the eyes open.

NORMAL FINDINGS

• Symmetrical positioning test showing that the patient can duplicate the position in which you moved a leg or arm
• Toe direction test showing that the patient can accurately identify the position of a toe after you have moved it
• Pronator drift test showing that the patient can keep the arms extended without one of them drifting
• Nylen-Bárány's maneuver showing that the patient does not feel dizzy or make extraneous eye movements while moving into a reclining position

ABNORMAL FINDINGS

- Inability to accurately duplicate the position of the arm or leg, indicating poor position sense, possibly stemming from such conditions as posterior spinal column disease or a peripheral nerve root lesion
- Inability to identify the direction of toe movement, indicating poor position sense, possibly stemming from such conditions as posterior spinal column disease or a peripheral nerve root lesion
- Slow downward drift of the arm and supination of the hand during the pronator drift test, possibly indicating mild hemiparesis (paralysis of one side of the body) (The patient may rely on visual cues to maintain correct arm position. Hemiparesis may result from a lesion in the contralateral cerebral hemisphere or the corticospinal tract.)
- Reporting a sensation of revolving in space or of the surroundings revolving (vertigo) during Nylen-Bárány test, possibly indicating an inner ear problem
- Involuntary, rhythmic eye movements (nystagmus) when moving from a seated to a recumbent position, possibly indicating an inner ear problem

ASSESSING LEVEL OF CONSCIOUSNESS

From the first exchange, you should be able to assess your patient's level of consciousness (LOC) simply by calling the patient by name in a normal tone of voice and observing the response. The patient should turn the head when hearing your voice and should respond appropriately, indicating alertness.

If the patient does not respond, call his name again while gently touching the patient or shaking the shoulder. If no response occurs, you may need to apply strong stimulation, such as nail bed pressure. (Keep in mind, though, that a simple hearing impairment may explain a patient's lack of response to verbal stimulation.)

If you must use stimulation, be sure to document the amount and type of stimulation used, as well as your patient's response. That way, other caregivers can use the same type of pressure to reliably assess changes in the patient's LOC.

To document LOC, you can use the Glasgow Coma Scale, especially if the patient has been critically injured (see Using the Glasgow Coma Scale). On the other hand, you may prefer to document the patient's state of arousal using one of the following terms:

- *Alert.* The patient is awake and responds appropriately when addressed in a normal tone of voice.
- *Lethargic.* The patient awakens and responds briefly to a loud voice or gentle shaking but then falls back to sleep.
- *Obtunded.* The patient opens the eyes only when vigorously shaken or stimulated but does not fully awaken. Response may be slow and confused.
- *Stuporous.* The patient can be aroused only with strong stimulation (e.g., nail bed pressure) and lapses quickly back into an unresponsive state.
- *Comatose.* The patient cannot be aroused even with strong stimulation.

Remember that various facilities may define these terms differently. To avoid confusion, check your facility's policy on documenting LOC.

USING THE GLASGOW COMA SCALE

Once used mainly to evaluate patients' prognoses and recovery from head injuries, the Glasgow Coma Scale (GCS) is now widely used to evaluate level of consciousness (LOC). To use the GCS, score your patient's response to motor, verbal, and eye stimulation according to the numbers and responses listed; then total the score. When reporting the results, break down the total score into its components, such as M5, V3, E3 = GCS 11. A patient who scores 15 points, the maximum, is fully awake, alert, and oriented. A patient who scores 3 points is deeply comatose.

Motor response	6	Follows commands
	5	Localizes pain on stimulus
	4	Withdraws from painful stimulus
	3	Shows abnormal flexion in response to pain
	2	Shows abnormal extension in response to pain
	1	No responses
Verbal response	5	Oriented
	4	Confused
	3	Inappropriate words
	2	Unintelligible sounds
	1	No responses
Eye opening	4	Spontaneous
	3	Opens eyes on verbal command
	2	Opens eyes on painful stimulus
	1	No responses
Total		

ASSESSING SKIN, HAIR, AND NAILS

Careful assessment of the skin, hair, and nails (known as the *integumentary system*) usually provides a clear sense of a patient's overall health. Similarly, changes in the skin, hair, and nails are typically the first indications of declining health. Therefore, when assessing the skin, hair, and nails, you need to look for subtle changes in color, texture, moisture, and temperature, as well as unusual markings or areas of injury.

SKIN

The body's largest organ, the skin, often serves as a mirror reflecting underlying illnesses, such as those of the liver, kidney, or heart (see Structures of the Skin, Hair, and Nails).

A thorough skin assessment requires removal of some or all of the patient's clothing. Before you start the examination, make sure the room is well lit, comfortably warm, and private. For greater efficiency, you may reserve much of the skin examination for later, when you assess the different parts of the patient's body. For example, you can assess the skin on the legs when examining the lower extremities.

ANATOMY REVIEW

STRUCTURES OF THE SKIN, HAIR, AND NAILS

The top illustration shows a cross-section of skin and hair structures. The bottom illustration shows the structures of the nail and surrounding tissue.

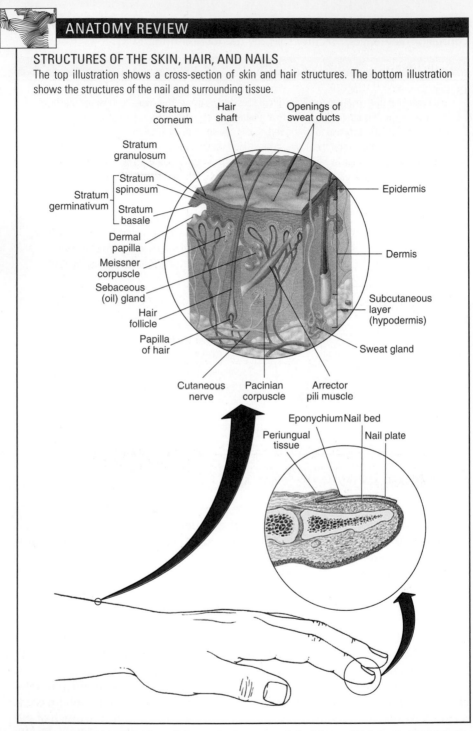

Top illustration from Thibodeau G, Patton K: *Anatomy and physiology,* ed 5, St Louis, 2003, Mosby; bottom illustration modified from Thompson JM, McFarland GK, Hirsch JE, et al: *Mosby's clinical nursing,* ed 5, St Louis, 2002, Mosby.

Inspection

Start the examination by inspecting all exposed areas of the patient's skin. Pay particular attention to areas associated with the patient's chief complaint and other symptoms. Check skin pigmentation and complexion, and note areas of skin breakdown, lesions, and bruising.

Inspect the pigmentation and general color of the patient's skin, checking for mottling, cyanosis, or jaundice.

CULTURAL CONSIDERATIONS

To check for cyanosis in a dark-skinned patient, look for an ashen color in the conjunctivae, oral mucosa, or nail beds. Jaundice, on the other hand, is best observed in the soles of the feet and palmar surfaces of the hands. However, remember that color irregularities may be difficult to determine in a dark-skinned patient.

Also note pigment abnormalities, freckles, birthmarks, and moles. Ask the patient if he has noticed any changes in the color, shape, or size of a mole.

If the patient appears sunburned or tan, ask if he uses sunscreen, especially if taking a medication that makes his skin photosensitive, such as ciprofloxacin, methoxsalen, or a tetracycline.

If the patient is chronically ill or hospitalized, look closely for signs of skin breakdown.

CULTURAL CONSIDERATIONS

Patients with dark skin may manifest pressure changes differently than patients with lighter skin. In a darker-skinned patient, look for gray or yellowish-brown discoloration at the site of pressure, which can turn purple before returning to its baseline color.

In areas that have served as recent insertion sites for intravenous (IV) lines or catheters, look for signs of infiltration of medication or IV fluid, infection (manifested by pus or erythema), phlebitis, and tape burns. In addition, check for skin breakdown at all pressure points, such as the ears, scalp, scapulae, shoulders, iliac crests, sacrum, malleoli, and heels.

Always look beneath dressings, prostheses, and restraints.

Inspect any area that may be excoriated or infected from heavy perspiration, lack of exposure to air, obesity, or incontinence. Typically, these areas include the skin beneath the breasts, in the axillae, between the thighs, and in the gluteal folds.

Finally, check the skin for lesions, rashes, wounds, and bruising. Note the location, size, color, and other physical characteristics (e.g., distribution, type of border, presence of drainage) as appropriate.

LIFESPAN CONSIDERATIONS

In an older adult, normal changes that occur with aging include wrinkled, thinned, pale, or translucent skin. You might also observe purple macular lesions that resemble bruises, called *actinic purpura*, bright-red lesions called *cherry angiomas*, or brownish-gray macular lesions (known as *liver spots*) called *actinic lentigines*.

Palpation

For optimal patient comfort, warm your hands before beginning palpation. If you think the patient may have an infection that can be transmitted through the skin, don gloves before touching lesions.

Palpate skin temperature using the back of your hand, which is more sensitive to temperature. To help detect a temperature abnormality, simultaneously compare the patient's skin temperature to your own, using both hands. To check for localized temperature changes, compare body parts on both sides of the body. For example, move your hand rapidly from the left leg to the right leg to compare their temperatures.

To check skin turgor (resiliency or elasticity), gently pinch the patient's skin between your thumb and forefinger. Then release it. In an older or dehydrated patient, you should test skin turgor on the forehead, sternal area, or beneath the clavicle areas where the skin normally is more taut.

LIFESPAN CONSIDERATIONS

Expect skin turgor changes in the older adult that reveal loosened, thinning skin on the back of the hands, forearms, and other areas.

Using the tips and pads of your fingers, palpate for areas of increased roughness or smoothness. Also check the skin for suppleness or tautness, thickness, and strength.

Palpate for dry areas. To avoid confusing the patient's skin moisture with your own, use the backs of your hands and fingers. If you are wearing gloves, you can defer this part of the examination because gloves will interfere with moisture assessment.

If inspection reveals a skin lesion, gently palpate the borders of the lesion to see if the area is raised (papular) or flat (macular). Because the lesion may be infectious, either wear gloves or avoid direct palpation.

NORMAL FINDINGS

- Skin color varying with race but appearing even over the entire body

CULTURAL CONSIDERATIONS

Dark-skinned people have lighter skin on the palms, the soles of the feet, and the nail beds. In addition, in areas that get regular sun exposure, expect darker skin and greater pigmentation.

ABNORMAL FINDINGS

- Skin abnormalities reflecting a wide range of conditions (see Recognizing Skin Abnormalities)

INTERPRETING ABNORMAL FINDINGS

RECOGNIZING SKIN ABNORMALITIES

An abnormal skin finding may suggest that the patient has a particular disease or disorder. Use the following table to correlate skin abnormalities with possible causes.

Abnormality	Probable Causes
Patchy pigmentation	• Vitiligo • Tinea versicolor
Absence of pigmentation	• Albinism
Jaundice	• Hepatic disease
Cyanosis	• Hypoxemia
Mottling	• Blood flow disturbance (e.g., from hypotension, if generalized, or a blood clot, if localized)
Flushing	• Fever • Embarrassment • Too-rapid infusion of certain drugs (e.g., vancomycin) • Medications or supplemental vitamins (e.g., niacin)
Pallor	• Anemia • Hypotension
Erythema	• Polycythemia • If localized: infection, burn, or infiltration of intravenous (IV) medication
Skin breakdown	• Pressure ulcer • Infection
Macule (flat lesion)	• Allergic reaction • Pigmentation change • Systemic lupus erythematosus (butterfly rash)
Papule (raised lesion)	• Hives • Acne
Scaling patches	• Psoriasis • Seborrheic dermatitis
Bruising	• Clotting disorder • Anticoagulant therapy • Trauma

continued

INTERPRETING ABNORMAL FINDINGS—cont'd

Abnormality	Probable Causes
Change in appearance of mole	• Melanoma
Hot, dry skin	• Fever
Cool, moist skin	• Circulatory compromise • Hypotension
Decreased turgor	• Dehydration
Oily skin	• Hyperthyroidism
Dry, thin skin	• Hypothyroidism

HAIR

Like changes in the skin, changes in a patient's hair may reflect underlying illness; therefore you will need to examine the patient's hair carefully. Be sure to assess both types of hair: terminal and vellus. Terminal hair is long, coarse in texture, and found on the scalp, eyebrows, axillae, and pubic areas. Vellus hair is short, fine in texture, and lighter than terminal hair; it covers most areas of the skin except the palms and soles.

For efficiency, you can assess the patient's hair at the same time you assess the skin. Provide adequate lighting for inspection and, to prevent piloerection (gooseflesh), ensure warmth. If you suspect the patient's hair and scalp are infested with lice, wear protective gear, such as gloves.

Begin your assessment of the hair by inspecting the terminal hair on the patient's scalp, noting its color, distribution, and quantity. If you see areas of hair loss or thinning, determine if the hair shafts are broken or burned off or if the hair is completely absent.

LIFESPAN CONSIDERATIONS

Hair quantity and thickness tends to diminish with age. Fewer functioning melanocytes in the hair shafts result in loss of hair color.

Grasp the hair between your thumb and forefinger, noting its moisture, texture, and whether the hair falls out as you gently grasp it. Next, part the hair and inspect the scalp, noting any wounds, lesions, dryness or oiliness, scaling, infection, or signs of infestation.

Then inspect the fine vellus hairs on the patient's face, chest, back, arms, legs, and abdomen. Note the color, distribution, and quantity. Check for areas of hair loss or unusually dense or coarse hair, especially on the face of a female patient.

Finally, inspect the coarse, terminal hairs in the axillae and pubic areas, noting color, texture, and distribution. Remember, the pubic hair normally forms an upright triangle in male patients and an inverted triangle in female patients.

NORMAL FINDINGS

- Hair distributed evenly over the scalp and body, except in male patients with male-pattern thinning or baldness (Thin, fine, lighter-colored [vellus] hair covers all areas of the body except the palms and soles. Terminal hair is coarser, darker, and thicker than vellus hair.)
- Hair color usually ranging from light blond to black (Hair color is consistent throughout the scalp, except in patients who use hair coloring or have graying hair.)
- Hair fine or coarse, straight or curly
- Scalp free of injuries, lesions, excessive dryness or oiliness, scaling, infection, or signs of infestation

ABNORMAL FINDINGS

- Decreased hair growth, possibly indicating hypopituitarism (Patchy baldness with breakage of the hair shaft at the scalp surface indicates alopecia areata, a disease of unknown origin. Hair loss associated with scalp scarring and destroyed hair follicles typifies scarring alopecia. Incomplete hair loss or thinning may result from wearing tightly bound hairstyles [traction alopecia], or from habitual hair pulling [trichotillomania]. These disorders also cause scalp inflammation. Hirsutism [excessive body hair] may result from hormonal dysfunction [e.g., Cushing's syndrome], hereditary factors, porphyria, or certain medications.)
- Altered hair color, possibly indicating malnutrition (Sometimes graying is associated with pernicious anemia. Nerve injury may cause patchy graying.)
- Dry, brittle hair, possibly indicating malnutrition or hypothyroidism (Increased silkiness and fineness of the hair may be associated with hyperthyroidism.)
- Scaling eruptions of the scalp, possibly indicating psoriasis or seborrheic dermatitis (Excoriation of the scalp, eyelids, and pubic area with small, nit-like flakes along the hair shaft indicates infestation with *Pediculus humanus corporis* [lice]. Infection of one or more hair follicles results in folliculitis or carbuncles [clusters of staphylococcal boils or abscesses beneath the skin].)

NAILS

Because nails are extensions of the epidermis, disease may affect their shape, color, texture, and condition. In addition, capillaries visible under the nail plate may reflect color changes associated with altered circulation and oxygenation.

For efficiency, you can assess the patient's nails when examining the upper and lower extremities. Before examining the nails, make sure the room temperature is comfortable; extremes in temperature can affect nail bed color. In addition, check for nail polish, artificial nails, and nail wraps, which can interfere with your assessment. If you must check the nail bed for signs of circulatory or oxygenation problems, have the patient immerse artificial nails or nail wraps in an acetone solution to loosen or dissolve them.

You can inspect and palpate the nails simultaneously. To begin, inspect the nail surface, noting its shape, color, and opacity. Feel the nail surface to determine smoothness and areas of unevenness. Check for horizontal or longitudinal ridges, opaque white spots, and small, splinter hemorrhages visible through the nail bed. Inspect the curvature to detect clubbing or spooning. (see Assessing for Finger Clubbing).

EXAMINATION TIP

ASSESSING FOR FINGER CLUBBING

You can use the Schamroth technique to identify clubbing of the fingers and nail beds, an abnormality resulting from chronic hypoxemia. Ask your patient to place the first phalanges of both index fingers together, as shown. Check the space between the two nail tips (normally, small and diamond shaped). With clubbed fingers, no space is seen between the two nail tips, and the transverse diameter of the nail is wider than the distal phalanx. This is because the angle between the nail and the point at which the nail enters the skin is convex, exceeding 180 degrees.

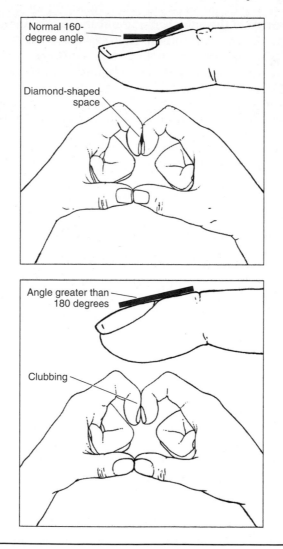

Normal 160-degree angle

Diamond-shaped space

Angle greater than 180 degrees

Clubbing

Next, gently squeeze the nail between your thumb and forefinger to determine how well the nail plate adheres to the nail bed, as well as to assess the firmness of the nail bed. In addition, note how long the nail bed takes to recover from blanching (capillary refill).

Finally, inspect and palpate the periungual tissue. Note any erythema, edema, induration, or tenderness.

NORMAL FINDINGS

- Nail plate smooth, round, fairly translucent, and firmly attached to the nail bed (The nails should have slightly convex curvature, with an angle of about 160 degrees between the nail and the skin at the nail base. The nail surface should feel smooth, even, and hard, with smooth, rounded edges.)

CULTURAL CONSIDERATIONS

Some dark-skinned patients normally have pigmented spots or bands on their nail plates.

LIFESPAN CONSIDERATIONS

Older adults often have thickened, yellowish nails, with longitudinal furrows, especially on the toes.

- Nail bed pinkish and firm on palpation (Capillary refill should take less than 4 seconds.)
- Cuticles smooth, flat, and unbroken

ABNORMAL FINDINGS

- Brittle, thinning, or peeling nail plates, suggesting nutritional or circulatory deficiencies (Occasionally the nail plate is congenitally absent.)
- Cracks or fissures in the nails, possibly indicating undernutrition
- Thickened nails, which may result from trauma, decreased circulation, or fungal infection
- White nail plates, suggesting hypoalbuminemia
- Pale nail plates, possibly indicating anemia
- Greenish-black nail plates, suggesting a fungal or bacterial infection (e.g., *Pseudomonas* spp.)
- Yellow nail plates, suggesting psoriasis or respiratory disease (Yellowing can also stem from cigarette smoking or use of nail polish.)
- Spoon-shaped nails, possibly reflecting iron deficiency
- Poor adhesion of the nail plate to the nail bed or pitting of the nail plates, suggesting psoriasis
- Rough, jagged, or bitten nails, possibly indicating poor hygiene or habits
- An abnormal curvature or a nail base angle of 180 degrees or greater, indicating clubbing, a sign of cardiopulmonary disease

- Splinter hemorrhages of the nail bed, possibly resulting from endocarditis, psoriasis, or trauma
- A white band suddenly appearing in the nail bed of a light-skinned person, suggesting melanoma
- Transverse white lines (Mees' lines) or grooves (Beau's lines), possibly after certain systemic illnesses (However, white lines occasionally result from clinically insignificant nail trauma as well.)
- Pallor of the nail bed, suggesting anemia
- Bluish mottling or cyanosis, indicating hypoxemia or compromised peripheral circulation
- Capillary refill greater than 4 seconds, indicating compromised circulation
- Broken, bitten, erythemic, or swollen cuticles, possibly indicating paronychia, an acute or chronic infection of the tissue around the nails

EVALUATING NUTRITIONAL STATUS

Nutritional status can affect a person's growth and development, wound healing, resistance to infection, and recovery from illness or surgery. The nurse is often the first staff member to consider a nutritional problem or to recognize that a patient's nutritional needs have changed. This means you are in a position to rapidly intervene to correct actual or potential nutritional deficiencies.

Before formally evaluating your patient's nutritional status, review the health history for possible risk factors for nutritional deficiencies. Look for recent weight changes, special dietary needs, changes in bowel elimination patterns (e.g., diarrhea), a history of chronic illness (e.g., chronic obstructive pulmonary disease), or a history of poor wound healing. In addition, review any prescription medications the patient is taking; some drugs can cause appetite changes. Note the presence of psychosocial factors that can affect nutritional status, such as low income, depression, alcoholism, or a history of anorexia or bulimia.

If possible, review the patient's 24-hour dietary recall and determine if he's consuming the proper number of servings from each of the six food groups: breads and grains, fruits, vegetables, dairy, meat or meat substitutes, and fats.

NUTRITIONAL IMBALANCES

Nutritional imbalances fall into one of two general categories: undernutrition and overnutrition. If your patient has an actual or potential nutritional imbalance, he will need to undergo a thorough examination, including anthropometric assessment. Anthropometric assessment includes height, weight, and skinfold measurement.

Undernutrition

If your patient is undernourished or at risk for undernutrition, try to identify the cause. Usually, undernutrition is associated with poor nutritional intake, altered nutrient digestion or absorption, increased nutrient excretion, inability to process nutrients, or increased nutritional demand.

Conditions that cause poor nutritional intake include appetite loss from nausea, dysphagia, and psychosocial problems such as depression, anorexia nervosa, bulimia, and alcoholism. Altered nutrient digestion or absorption can result from conditions such as diarrhea and pancreatitis, as well as procedures such as gastrectomy and small bowel resection.

Increased nutrient excretion can be caused by dialysis, diarrhea, and hemorrhage. Conditions that impair nutrient processing include alcoholism, congenital metabolic disorders (e.g., celiac sprue), and liver disease. Nutritional demands may increase from fever, sepsis, and surgery.

Overnutrition and Obesity

One of the largest health concerns facing the United States, obesity, is defined as a BMI that is greater than 30 (a BMI between 25.0 and 29.9 ranks as overweight). An obese, or overnourished, person typically consumes more calories than he expends, but that does not necessarily mean the person is getting adequate nutrition. For example, a patient who takes corticosteroid agents may be overweight and yet experience protein breakdown, a condition that may call for protein supplementation.

Sometimes, obesity stems from a medical condition, such as Cushing's syndrome (cortisol overproduction) or Klinefelter's syndrome (a chromosomal disorder). In addition, certain medications such as tricyclic antidepressant drugs (e.g., amitriptyline) and corticosteroid agents (e.g., prednisone) can predispose a person to weight gain. What is more, an obese patient is prone to related health problems, such as diabetes mellitus, cardiovascular disease, and osteoarthritis.

What to Do

If your assessment reveals that your patient is at risk for undernutrition or overnutrition, plan to refer him to a registered dietitian who can develop a diet plan that will address his nutritional needs.

4 Examining the Head and Neck

Once the health history and general assessment are complete, the head-to-toe physical examination begins. Throughout this examination keep pertinent points of your patient's health history and chief complaints foremost in your mind.

Begin the physical examination with the patient's head and neck. This region includes the skull, nose, mouth, throat, and neck to the clavicle. The examination also involves assessment of several cranial nerves that control various sensory functions, including taste and smell. Assessment of the eyes and ears, although mentioned occasionally in this chapter, appears in detail in Chapter 5.

The head is the part of the human body that interacts most (and at the highest level of complexity) with the environment. Partly because of this, the head is the site of a number of common ailments, including headaches, sinus congestion, neck pain, nosebleeds, sore throats, and injuries.

In general, the chief complaints related to the head can and often do result from simple, temporary medical problems. However, virtually all of these complaints can also stem from serious, even life-threatening disorders. That is why assessing this area of the body completely and accurately is so important. Before beginning, be sure you're familiar with the important structures and functions you will be assessing (see Structures of the Head and Neck).

STRUCTURES OF THE HEAD AND NECK

The skull
Composed of flat, irregular bones tightly joined by sutures, the skull houses and protects the brain. It also positions and protects the eyes, ears, and teeth. The skull's major bony structures are shown in the following illustrations:

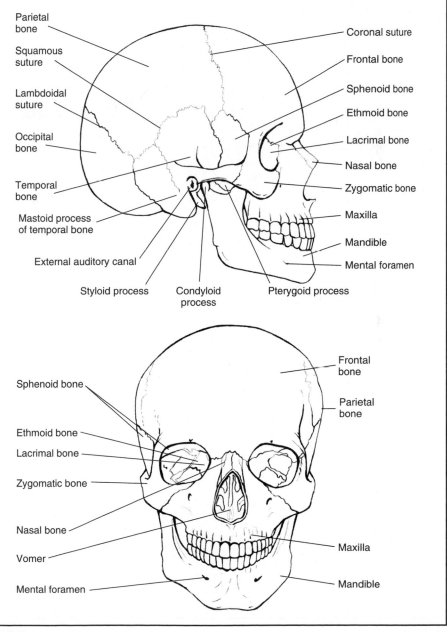

continued

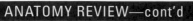

ANATOMY REVIEW—cont'd

Muscles

The neck is divided into two triangles by the sternocleidomastoid muscle. The mandible and the sternocleidomastoid muscle, which meet at the body's midline, form the boundaries of the anterior triangle. Midline structures of the neck are located in the anterior triangle. The trapezius muscle, the sternocleidomastoid muscle, and the clavicle form the boundaries of the posterior triangle. Major muscles of the head and neck are shown in the following illustrations:

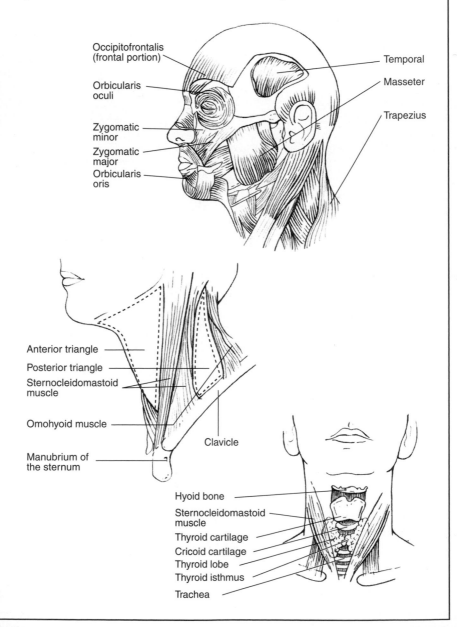

continued

ANATOMY REVIEW—cont'd

Internal structures

A wide variety of internal structures support the functions of the senses, respiratory system, digestive system, endocrine system, and lymphatic system.

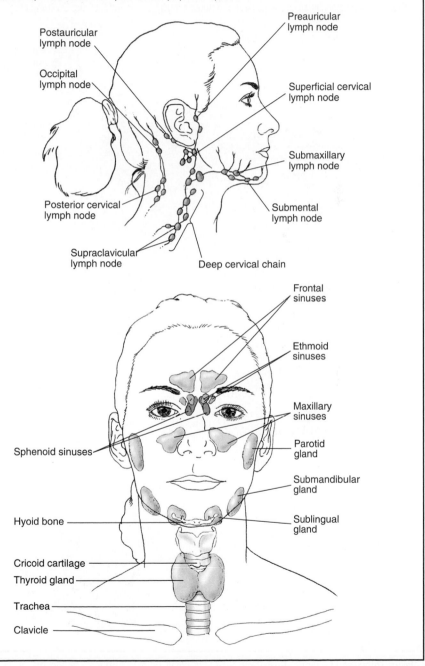

continued

ANATOMY REVIEW—cont'd

The mouth

Bordered superiorly by the hard and soft palates, inferiorly by the tongue, laterally by the pillars of the soft palate and tonsils, and anteriorly by the lips, the mouth serves as entryway to the digestive and respiratory systems. Major oral structures are shown in the following illustrations:

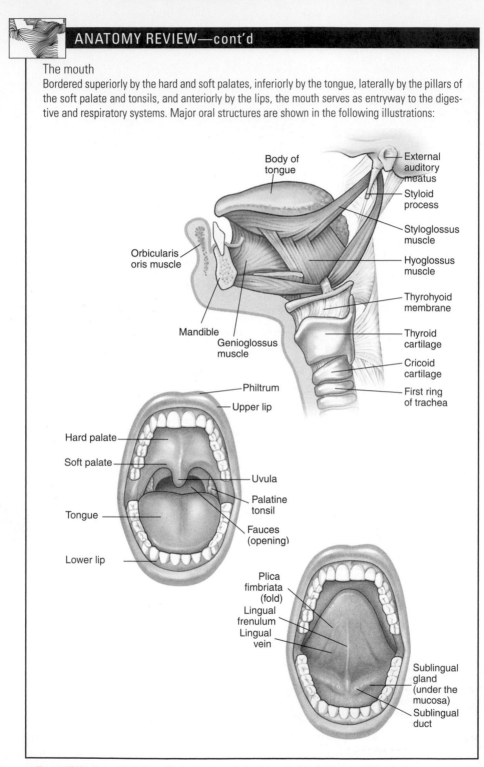

From Thibodeau G, Patton K: *Anatomy and physiology,* ed 5, St Louis, 2003, Mosby.

The brain exerts fine control over many of the characteristics you will be assessing. Therefore the brain is another structure with which you should be familiar if you want to bring your best talents to bear in the assessment (see Parts of the Brain).

ANATOMY REVIEW

PARTS OF THE BRAIN

Seat of the central nervous system, the brain is composed of three major parts: (1) cerebrum, (2) cerebellum, and (3) brain stem. Beneath the cerebrum and on top of the brain stem lie the structures of the diencephalon, including the thalamus and hypothalamus. The brain stem controls vital involuntary functions, such as breathing.

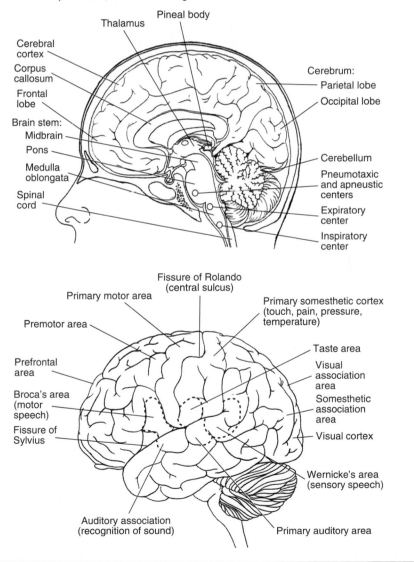

continued

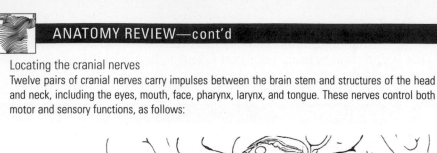

ANATOMY REVIEW—cont'd

Locating the cranial nerves

Twelve pairs of cranial nerves carry impulses between the brain stem and structures of the head and neck, including the eyes, mouth, face, pharynx, larynx, and tongue. These nerves control both motor and sensory functions, as follows:

Nerve		Function
I	Olfactory	Sensory
II	Optic	Sensory
III	Oculomotor	Motor
IV	Trochlear	Motor
V	Trigeminal	Mixed
VI	Abducens	Motor
VII	Facial	Mixed
VIII	Acoustic	Sensory
IX	Glossopharyngeal	Mixed
X	Vagus	Mixed
XI	Spinal accessory	Motor
XII	Hypoglossal	Motor

EXAMINATION STEPS AND FINDINGS

Before beginning your examination, be sure to assemble the necessary equipment, including examination gloves, a bright light source (e.g., penlight), an otoscope with a wide speculum (if available), a cotton-tipped applicator, a tongue blade, a sterile pin or other sharp object, several samples of familiar scents and tastes, and a stethoscope.

INSPECTION

In most cases you will start your examination at the top of the patient's head and proceed systematically downward toward the neck, performing inspection and palpation simultaneously to maximize your efficiency (see Key Examination Steps for the Head and Neck).

EXPERT EXAMINATION CHECKLIST

KEY EXAMINATION STEPS FOR THE HEAD AND NECK

Use this checklist to make sure you cover the most important steps when examining the head and neck.

☐ Inspect the scalp and face, noting any lesions, sores, and scars.

☐ Inspect the mucous membranes in the nose and mouth.

☐ Inspect the position and movement of the tongue, uvula, and soft palate.

☐ Check the gag reflex.

continued

EXPERT EXAMINATION CHECKLIST—cont'd

❏ Assess the patient's ability to recognize familiar tastes.

❏ Assess the patient's ability to recognize familiar odors.

❏ Assess the patient's ability to discern sharp and dull sensations on the face.

❏ Observe the patient's face for symmetry of structure and movement.

❏ Inspect the patient's neck for distention of the jugular vein.

❏ Estimate central venous pressure.

❏ Palpate for lymph node swelling.

❏ Palpate the thyroid gland.

❏ Inspect and palpate the position and movement of the trachea.

❏ Auscultate for carotid bruit and venous hum.

❏ Assess the symmetry and strength of the jaw, neck, and shoulder muscles.

evolve Find PDF and PDA-downloadable versions of this Expert Exam Checklist online at http://evolve.elsevier.com/Mosby/expertexam/.

Skull and Scalp

Begin by asking your patient to sit comfortably upright so you can easily examine the top of the head. Working step by step, inspect the patient's hair, noting its quantity, distribution, texture, and any evidence of hair loss. If the patient has hair loss, describe its pattern.

Part the patient's hair and inspect the scalp. Look for scales, redness, open lesions, scabbed areas, or nits (lice eggs). In addition, look for lumps. Observe the general size and shape of the patient's skull. Make note of any deformities, swelling, or masses. Finally, perform a general assessment of the ears, noting their position and size in relation to the patient's head.

Face

Observe the patient's face for symmetry. Watch for any involuntary movements or tics. Then test cranial nerve (CN) VII, the facial nerve, by asking the patient to perform a series of movements to demonstrate the use of facial muscles (see Understanding Cranial Nerves, pp. 75-76).

Ask the patient to raise the eyebrows, frown, smile, show the teeth, puff the cheeks, and close the eyes tightly. Later, when you are examining the patient's mouth, you can test for sense of taste.

Complete your examination of the patient's face by observing the facial skin. Note its color, pigmentation, texture, and the distribution of any hair. Document the size, shape, and configuration of any lesions.

Eyes

Perform a general inspection of the eyes, eyelids, eyebrows, and eyelashes. Note any asymmetry or obvious abnormalities. Inspect the skin beneath and around the eyebrows and eyelashes for erythema, scaling, or drainage. Note the distribution of the eyelashes and whether they are thick or sparse. Check the eyebrows as well. Keep in mind that many female patients (and some male patients) remove all or part of their eyebrows for cosmetic reasons. Inspect the patient's periorbital area for edema, erythema, and lesions (see Chapter 5 for a full assessment of the eyes and ears).

Nose

Inspect the patient's nose for symmetry, deformity, and inflammation. If the patient currently has or recently has had a nasogastric tube or nasal oxygen therapy, inspect the skin around the nares for signs of breakdown.

Ask the patient to tip the head back. Using an otoscope with a wide speculum, gently insert the speculum through one nostril and into the vestibule. Observe the mucosa for erythema, swelling, and drainage. Then inspect the nasal septum for bleeding, perforation, and deviation. Repeat the process for the other nostril.

If you notice any nasal drainage, be sure to document its color, amount, and consistency. If your patient has a possible or confirmed basilar skull fracture and you notice a clear, thin, nasal discharge, use a glucose-testing strip to see if it contains high levels of glucose, possibly indicating the presence of cerebrospinal fluid (CSF). Blood-tinged drainage that forms droplets with bloody centers and clear halos may also indicate the presence of CSF.

To assess the function of CN I (the olfactory nerve), ask your patient to identify familiar scents such as soap, coffee, chocolate, and vanilla. Before performing this part of the physical examination, however, first confirm the patency of the patient's nasal passages by obstructing one nostril and asking the patient to inhale through the other. If one side is obstructed, use the other nostril to assess olfactory function. With the patient's eyes closed, pass a fragrance under one nostril and ask your patient to identify the scent. Repeat this process with the other nostril and the remaining scents. Note the patient's responses. Omit this test if you have already observed inflamed nasal mucosa or nasal discharge because it could worsen the irritation.

Mouth

Inspect the patient's lips for color, moisture, and lesions. To examine the inside of her mouth, first ask your patient to remove any dentures; then use a penlight to examine the condition of the oral mucosa, noting any lesions or infected areas. Ask the patient to open her mouth widely; use a tongue blade to expose the mucosa on both sides of the mouth. Note the color, pigmentation, and overall condition of the interior structures. Inspect the color and shape of the hard palate. Look at the gingiva and teeth for swelling, bleeding, retraction, and discoloration. Identify any abnormalities in the position or shape of the teeth.

Next, observe the patient's tongue for symmetry, position, size, color, and texture. Ask her to touch the tongue to the roof of the mouth while you inspect its underside for lesions or other abnormalities. Inspect the lingual frenulum at the floor of the mouth. Look for the submandibular ducts, located on either side of the base of the frenulum.

Use your penlight and tongue blade to inspect the floor of the mouth and the underside of the tongue (where malignancies may occur) for white or red spots. If you find any ulcerations or nodules, palpate them with a gloved hand for tenderness and consistency. Inspect the soft palate, uvula, tonsils, and posterior pharynx. Look for symmetry of structures, color, and signs of exudate, edema, or ulceration. Note whether the patient still has her tonsils and whether they are enlarged.

LIFESPAN CONSIDERATIONS

Tonsils generally shrink after the age of 5 years. In some adults, the tonsils are not visible because they shrink back into the folds of the palatine arches.

Now test the function of CNs IX, X, and XII (glossopharyngeal, vagus, and hypoglossal). These nerves work together to control movements of the pharynx, larynx, soft palate, and tongue. If you have heard your patient speak and cough, you have already partially assessed these cranial nerves. Ask your patient to stick her tongue out and move it up, down, and sideways. Watch for awkward movements or deviations to one side or the other. To test the sensory function of CN VII, place sugar, salt, and lemon solutions on the anterior two thirds of the tongue and ask your patient to identify the tastes. To test the sensory function of CN IX, place those same recognizable tastes on the posterior third of the patient's tongue and ask her to identify them.

Next, using the tongue blade to depress the tongue and a penlight to illuminate the oral cavity, ask the patient to yawn or say "ah" and observe the movement of the soft palate, uvula, and posterior pharynx for symmetry. Finally, with the tongue still depressed with a tongue blade, use a clean cotton-tipped swab to touch either side of the pharynx to stimulate the gag reflex.

UNDERSTANDING CRANIAL NERVES

Use this table to assess cranial nerves and their functions and to help identify abnormalities.

Cranial Nerve	Function	Origin	Structures Innervated	Assessment
I Olfactory	Sensory	Olfactory bulbs below frontal lobes	Olfactory mucous membranes	Ability to identify familiar odors
II Optic	Sensory		Retina of the eye	Visual acuity Visual fields

continued

UNDERSTANDING CRANIAL NERVES—cont'd

Cranial Nerve	Function	Origin	Structures Innervated	Assessment
III Oculomotor	Motor	Midbrain	Medial, superior, and inferior rectus muscles of the eye	Extraocular movement Pupillary reaction to light and accommodation
IV Trochlear	Motor	Midbrain	Superior oblique muscle of the eye	Extraocular movement
V Trigeminal	Mixed	Pons	Sensory: pain, touch, and temperature sensations in the forehead, cheeks, jaw and chin, corneal reflex Motor: muscles of mastication	Sensation in the forehead, cheeks, jaw, and chin Mastication
VI Abducens	Motor	Pons	Lateral rectus muscle of the eye	Extraocular movements
VII Facial	Mixed	Pons	Sensory: anterior two thirds of the tongue Motor: muscles of the face, forehead, and eye	Taste for anterior two thirds of the tongue Movement of the facial muscles
VIII Acoustic	Sensory	Pons	Cochlea: organ of Corti Vestibule and semicircular canals	Hearing acuity Balance
IX Glossopharyngeal	Mixed	Medulla	Sensory: posterior third of the tongue Motor: muscles of the pharynx	Taste for posterior one third of the tongue Movement of the pharynx Gag reflex
X Vagus	Mixed	Medulla	Sensory: skin of external ear and mucous membranes Motor: muscles of larynx, pharynx, esophagus, and thoracic and abdominal viscera	Swallowing Movement of the pharynx Gag reflex
XI Spinal Accessory	Motor	Medulla	Sternocleidomastoid and trapezius muscles	Movement and strength of neck and shoulder
XII Hypoglossal	Motor	Medulla	Tongue	Movement and strength of tongue

Neck

Inspect the neck for symmetry, masses, scars, pulsations, or swelling. If the patient has no history of neck or spine trauma, ask her to drop the chin to the chest and then slowly roll the head in a full circle. Observe any limitations in movement or discomfort with movement. Note the position of the patient's trachea and whether it is deviated to one side or the other. Identify the thyroid gland. If your patient is thin, the thyroid's isthmus (the part that joins the two lobes) may be visible. However, the isthmus may be difficult or impossible to find if the patient's neck is short and thick.

NORMAL FINDINGS

- Head round and symmetrical (The scalp appears clean, with unbroken skin. The ears should be symmetrically shaped, in proportion to the face, and vertically positioned to line up with the eyes.)
- Facial expressions, such as smiles and frowns, leaving symmetrical wrinkles on the forehead (The cheeks should appear symmetrical when puffed with air.)
- Facial skin smooth, unbroken, and clean
- Eyes clear, bright, and symmetrical (The eyelids close completely. The eyebrows and eyelashes should be evenly distributed, with unbroken skin at the base.)
- Nasal mucosa moist, pink, and slightly darker than the oral mucosa (The nasal septum should be midline and intact.)
- Nasal passages patent bilaterally (The patient should be able to identify scents correctly in both nostrils, indicating normal function of CN I.)
- Lips soft, pink, and intact
- Oral mucosa smooth, moist, pink, and intact, without inflammation or lesions (Fordyce's spots [sebaceous glands], characterized by small yellowish spots on the buccal mucosa, are normal in adults.)
- Gingiva smooth and shiny (In light-skinned people, the gingiva is pale red. In dark-skinned people, it is commonly a patchy brown.)
- Margins around teeth sharp, and crevices between the gingiva and teeth shallow (The patient should have 32 teeth, each seated firmly in a bony socket.)
- Tongue pink and slightly rough, with a midline depression (Its underside should be smoother and pinker than the top; the sublingual fold should be pink and moist. The tongue should be midline, fill the floor of the mouth, and move freely from side to side.)
- Patient able to distinguish between sweet, sour, salty, and bitter tastes, indicating normal function for CN VII and CN IX
- Soft palate rising, uvula moving forward, and posterior pharynx moving inward (like a curtain closing) when your patient says "ah"
- Gag reflex when your patient's posterior pharynx touched
- Trachea at midline of patient's neck

ABNORMAL FINDINGS

- Scaling skin and erythema around the eyelashes and eyebrows from seborrheic dermatitis

- Red and swollen nasal mucosa, indicating rhinitis (With allergic rhinitis, the mucosa is swollen, but color varies from gray to dull red or blue.)
- Nasal polyps, characterized by mobile, gelatinous, gray lesions in the middle meatus of the septum
- Septal deviation, causing nasal obstruction, possibly congenital or caused by injury
- Reduction or loss of sense of smell (anosmia), possibly caused by frontal bone or sinus trauma, disorders of the base of the frontal lobe (e.g., tumors), or decreased blood flow from atherosclerosis (It can also result from sinus infection, nasal congestion, smoking, or cocaine use and can alter a patient's ability to recognize tastes.)
- Blisters caused by the herpes simplex virus (Clusters of vesicular blisters develop around the lips and mucous membranes. As the blisters break, a crust forms.)
- A thickened plaque, ulcer, or warty growth of the lower lip that does not heal, possibly indicating a carcinoma
- Painful, small, round or oval white ulcers surrounded by a halo of reddened mucosa (Known as *aphthous ulcers* or *canker sores*, these ulcers usually recur. Their cause is unknown.)
- White plaquelike exudate on the tongue and oral mucosa, resulting from moniliasis or thrush
- Gingival hypertrophy (swelling of the gingiva), possibly caused by pregnancy, leukemia, or medications such as phenytoin and cyclosporine
- Gingivitis (inflamed gingiva), characterized by erythema and swelling of the margins of the gingiva (The gingiva becomes fragile and bleeds easily. This condition typically results from poor oral or dental hygiene. If the disease progresses, gum margins recede and erode, causing teeth to loosen—a condition known as *periodontitis.*)
- A smooth, red tongue with loss of papillae, suggesting a deficiency of cyanocobalamin (vitamin B_{12}), niacin (vitamin B_3), or iron
- A swollen tongue, swollen face, rhinitis, and urticaria, possibly indicating anaphylaxis, a life-threatening allergic reaction (See ◹ Responding to Anaphylaxis.)
- Mildly red, slightly swollen pillars, and prominent lymphoid patches on the posterior wall of the pharynx, caused by viral pharyngitis (Severe redness, swelling, and patchy exudate may result from streptococcal pharyngitis.)
- Loss of gag reflex and a hoarse or nasal-sounding voice from dysfunction of CN X (Because CN X also controls involuntary functions, the patient's heart rate and respiratory patterns also may be affected. Loss of the gag reflex and dysphagia reveal dysfunction of CN IX.)
- Facial weakness (If the weakness affects the entire side of your patient's face, the problem most likely stems from damage to CN VII, as seen in Bell's palsy. If, however, your patient can wrinkle the forehead while one side of the lower part of her face remains weak or immobile, the problem most

likely stems from upper motor neuron damage from a cerebrovascular accident [CVA] or tumor.)

- Impaired sense of taste from damage to CN VII and CN IX, caused by chemotherapy, radiation of the head and neck, or aging (It may be a sign of myasthenia gravis or amyotrophic lateral sclerosis [ALS] if accompanied by anesthesia of the tongue and palate, difficulty swallowing, increased salivation, and difficulty speaking.)
- Soft palate that fails to rise, along with deviation of the uvula to one side (This may occur with paralysis of CN X.)

ACTION STAT

RESPONDING TO ANAPHYLAXIS

A life-threatening allergic reaction, anaphylaxis results from the body's overwhelming immunologic response to an allergen found in food, medication, blood products, insect venom, or chemicals (e.g., contrast medium used in medical testing).

On first exposure to the antigen, the body becomes sensitized to it. Then, on second exposure, the allergic person's humoral immune system activates immunoglobulin (Ig)E, IgG, and IgM, prompting the release of chemical mediators, including histamine and complement, from mast cells.

Once released, these chemical mediators cause a massive systemic reaction marked by laryngeal edema and vasodilation. If allowed to progress, anaphylaxis leads rapidly to respiratory arrest, profound hypotension, and death. For any patient experiencing anaphylaxis, your response must be swift and sure. It could easily mean the difference between life and death.

What to look for

Signs and symptoms of an anaphylactic reaction can appear within seconds. Look for the following:

- Flushing of the skin
- Urticaria
- Pruritus
- Hoarseness and stridor
- Coughing and wheezing
- Extreme shortness of breath
- Angioedema, or swelling of the eyelids, lips, tongue, hands, and feet
- Copious watery nasal secretions
- Nasal congestion and sneezing
- Nausea, vomiting, and abdominal pain from edema of the gastrointestinal tract
- Signs of shock, including hypotension, tachycardia, and a weak, thready pulse

What to do immediately

Anaphylaxis requires rapid intervention. Have someone notify a physician immediately, then do the following:

- If the anaphylactic reaction is caused by a blood transfusion or intravenous (IV) medication, stop the infusion immediately and change the IV tubing down to the hub of the catheter. Then start an infusion of normal saline through new IV tubing.
- Ensure a patent airway by positioning the patient's head and neck in slight hyperextension.
- Administer supplemental oxygen.
- Insert an oral or nasal airway if the patient is unconscious.
- Prepare for endotracheal intubation or tracheotomy if the airway cannot be restored.
- Administer epinephrine (1:1000 aqueous solution) immediately, as prescribed, to counteract the effects of chemical mediators and reduce bronchospasm. The usual dosage is 0.1 to 0.5 ml every 10 to 15 minutes subcutaneously (SC) or intramuscularly

continued

ACTION STAT—cont'd

(IM) until your patient responds. As an alternative, 1.0 to 2.5 ml IV (1:10,000 concentration) can be given every 5 to 15 minutes.
- When giving epinephrine SC or IM, massage the injection site to promote faster absorption.
- After giving epinephrine, expect to give the histamine-1 (H_1) antagonist diphenhydramine 1 to 2 mg/kg IV or IM. In addition, plan to give a histamine-2 (H_2) antagonist, such as ranitidine, 1.0 to 1.5 mg/kg IV or IM (to a maximum dose of 150 mg). These drugs prevent further release of histamine from mast cells.
- Maintain circulatory volume and blood pressure with IV fluids.

What to do next
Once your patient has been stabilized, identify and remove the allergen to prevent further reaction and respond as follows:

- If the reaction was to an insect bite, remove the stinger by gently scraping it out of the skin.
- If the reaction was caused by food, induce vomiting to prevent further absorption.
- Administer other medications as prescribed. Examples are a corticosteroid agent, such as methylprednisolone 1 to 2 mg/kg to prevent a late-phase reaction and an inhaled β_2-agonist, such as albuterol, to treat bronchospasm or wheezing.
- Monitor vital signs carefully after the event.
- Monitor respiratory effort and oxygenation.
- Comfort and reassure your patient.
- Teach the patient to avoid the suspected allergen.
- Instruct the patient to carry an anaphylaxis kit, and demonstrate how to use it.
- Encourage the patient to wear a medical information alert that lists the allergy.

PALPATION

To maximize efficiency, perform palpation during your inspection of the structures. Be sure to protect yourself from infection by wearing examination gloves when examining the mouth or other areas where transmission of microorganisms may occur.

Head and Neck

Begin by palpating the head and neck. Feel for the contour, symmetry, and size of the skull. Use your gloved hands to palpate lumps or lesions that you have observed, testing for tenderness, mobility, and consistency. Note their size and shape.

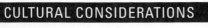

CULTURAL CONSIDERATIONS

If your patient is of Asian descent, make sure you ask permission before touching the patient's head; some Asians believe the soul exists in the head.

Next, test muscle strength in the neck and shoulders by asking the patient to shrug the shoulders against the resistance of your hands. Then have the patient turn the head side to side, also against the resistance of your hands.

Face

CN V (the trigeminal nerve) controls the strength of the temporal and masseter muscles and sensations around the face. To assess its function, first palpate the temporal muscle by placing your middle and index fingers on your patient's temples and asking her to clench the teeth. Compare the strength of contraction of each side. Then move your middle and index finger to the mastoid process and again ask your patient to clench the teeth.

To assess the sensory component of CN V, ask your patient to close the eyes. Using the stick end of a clean cotton-tipped swab, press the patient's forehead, cheeks, and jaw (but make sure you do not press too hard). Ask the patient to identify whether the stimulus is sharp or dull. Occasionally, substitute the soft, cotton-covered end of the swab to test your patient's reliability.

Palpate the temporal pulses, located near the temples on either side of the face. Be sure to compare sides. Note the strength, amplitude, and rhythm of the pulsations.

Next palpate the frontal and maxillary sinuses for tenderness. To palpate the frontal sinus, place your thumb on the upper inner aspect of the orbit and press gently but firmly upward, noting any increase in pain or tenderness. To assess the maxillary sinus, place your thumb under the zygomatic bone and gently press upward, also noting any increase in pain or tenderness. Avoid placing pressure directly on the eyes to prevent injury.

Mouth

Palpate the upper and lower lips with a gloved hand to evaluate muscle tone, lumps, or areas of tenderness. To palpate the tongue, grasp it with a 4 × 4-inch gauze pad and move it from side to side to inspect and palpate the lateral borders for lesions or tenderness.

Trachea

In addition to inspecting the trachea's position, you can also palpate it to see if it is displaced or moving. Place your thumbs on either side of the trachea and feel the space between it and the sternocleidomastoid muscle. Is it equal? Then, with your patient's neck extended, place your index fingers and thumbs on the sides of the trachea, below the thyroid's isthmus. Feel for the presence of tracheal movement or tugging.

Thyroid Gland

Examine the thyroid gland for size, texture, and pulsation (see Palpating the Thyroid Gland).

PALPATING THE THYROID GLAND

The thyroid gland has two lobes connected by a central isthmus, giving it a butterfly appearance. In most people, a normal or slightly enlarged thyroid cannot be palpated, although you can feel the isthmus rise as the patient swallows.

Palpating the thyroid gland is an advanced procedure you should perform with caution. It can release thyroid hormone into the circulation, possibly sparking a thyroid storm if the patient has hyperthyroidism. Do not palpate the thyroid if it is visibly enlarged.

The thyroid gland can be palpated by a posterior or anterior approach. Many nurses find the posterior approach to be the easier of the two.

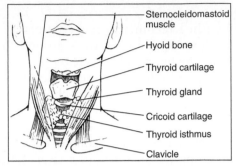

Midline structures of the neck

Sternocleidomastoid muscle
Hyoid bone
Thyroid cartilage
Thyroid gland
Cricoid cartilage
Thyroid isthmus
Clavicle

Posterior Approach

With your patient sitting upright, approach her from behind. Ask her to lower the chin slightly and relax the neck muscles. Then start by locating the thyroid isthmus, placing your thumbs against the back of the patient's neck and resting the tips of your forefingers over the lower half of the trachea. You will feel the isthmus rise in the patient's neck as she swallows.

To palpate the right lobe, have your patient keep the chin down and flex her neck slightly to the right. Use your left hand to displace the trachea to the right. Palpate the right lobe with your right hand as your patient swallows. Then assess the left lobe with your left hand while using your right hand to displace the trachea to the left.

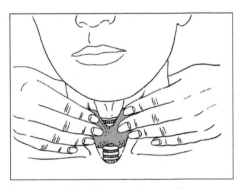

Palpating the right lobe by posterior approach

Anterior Approach

Approach your patient from the front and slightly to one side. Ask her to relax the neck muscles. To palpate the thyroid isthmus, use your index and middle fingers to palpate the cricoid cartilage as your patient swallows.

To palpate the lobes, grasp and palpate each one by placing your fingers on either side of the sternocleidomastoid muscles. Alternatively, you can displace the trachea toward your examining hand as with a posterior approach, thus moving the thyroid lobe to your fingertips.

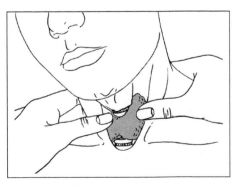

Palpating the right lobe by anterior approach

Lymph Nodes

For best results when examining the lymph nodes of the head and neck, ask your patient to relax her muscles and bend the neck slightly forward or toward the side that you are palpating. Use the pads of your index and middle fingers to gently move the skin over the tissue where the nodes are located. If you palpate an enlarged gland, note its size, consistency (hard or soft), mobility, tenderness, temperature, and location. Ask the patient if the enlarged node is tender. In addition, assess the areas adjacent to the lymph node for signs of infection or malignancy.

Systematically palpate the lymph nodes on both sides of the patient's neck. Be sure to include the following:

- Preauricular (in front of the ear)
- Postauricular (at the mastoid process)
- Occipital (at the base of the skull)
- Tonsillar (at the base of the mandible)
- Submaxillary (halfway between the angle and tip of the mandible)
- Submental (in the midline behind the tip of the mandible)
- Superficial cervical (just over the sternomastoid)
- Posterior cervical chain (just at the anterior edge of the trapezius)
- Deep cervical chain (deep in the sternomastoid)
- Supraclavicular (deep in the angle formed by the clavicle and sternomastoid)

As you palpate the lymph nodes, compare findings on the right and left sides for symmetry. Compare size, shape, borders, mobility, consistency, and tenderness.

Vascular Structures

When examining the neck, palpate the carotid artery's pulsations and evaluate the jugular veins for distention, which is a possible sign of overhydration or heart failure. For best results, ask your patient to lie down with the head elevated on a pillow. Elevate the head of the bed slightly to maximize visibility of the jugular veins. Keep the patient's neck in a neutral position, neither flexed nor extended. Use tangential lighting, and be sure to ask the patient to remove any clothing that might interfere with your examination. If the patient has difficulty changing positions, you can delay evaluating vascular structures until the patient is supine for a later part of the examination.

Palpate the carotid pulsations on either side of the neck one at a time. Use the pads of your fingertips to feel along the side of the trachea, midway between the angle of the jaw and the clavicles. Apply gentle pressure, noting the contour, rate, and rhythm of the pulsations. If you feel a thrill, be sure to note it. In addition, auscultate the carotid artery for bruits.

Distinguish between the internal and external jugular veins, which usually are not visible unless your patient is reclining at an angle of at least 45 degrees. The external jugular veins lie posterior to the internal jugular veins and appear just above the clavicles. The internal ones will pulsate in response to pressure changes in the right atrium as your patient reclines. You can distinguish internal jugular pulsations from those of the carotid artery because internal jugular pulsations are rarely palpable (only visible), and the level of pulsation usually diminishes with inspiration. In addition, when your patient is upright, the pulsations disappear.

To measure jugular venous pressure, follow these steps:

- Identify the highest point at which you can see the internal jugular vein's pulsations, and identify the sternal angle.
- Hold a centimeter ruler in a vertical position, with the bottom placed at the patient's sternal angle.
- Hold another ruler in a horizontal position so that one end rests at the highest jugular vein pulsation and the other intersects with the vertical ruler.
- Note the vertical distance on the centimeter ruler, where it intersects with the horizontal ruler; this equals the patient's jugular venous pressure. Normally it does not exceed 4 cm.
- Document the angle at which the head of the patient's bed is elevated.
- Estimate central venous pressure (right atrial pressure) by adding 4 cm to the patient's jugular venous pressure reading (because the right atrium lies about 4 cm below the sternal angle).

NORMAL FINDINGS

- Skull contour smooth and symmetrical
- Patient able to distinguish between sharp and dull stimuli bilaterally in all three distributions of CN V
- Temporomandibular joint (TMJ) smooth (Joint movement produces no pain or crepitation.)
- Frontal and maxillary sinuses nontender when palpated
- Lips smooth and nontender, with good muscle tone; tongue surface nontender and without palpable lesions
- Trachea straight and midline, without movement or tugging
- Thyroid thin, smooth, and mobile (The isthmus is the only portion of the thyroid that is usually palpable, although you may feel one or both lobes in some patients.)
- Lymph nodes nonpalpable or small, soft, round, and mobile; should not be tender
- Carotid pulse regular, full, and smooth
- Jugular venous pressure 3 cm or less above the sternal angle (at 45 degrees), reflecting a central venous pressure of approximately 7 cm (The pulsations of the internal jugular vein should be barely visible above the clavicles.)
- Neck and shoulders overcome resistance equally well, indicating intact function of CN XI (the spinal accessory nerve)

ABNORMAL FINDINGS

- Asymmetrical skull, with bulging or protrusions, possibly indicating injury or tumor
- Patient unable to distinguish sharp stimuli in one or all distributions of CN V, possibly indicating injury
- Sharp, bulletlike facial pain in the distribution of CN V, from trigeminal neuralgia (This pain is more common in female patients than in male patients and usually affects the right side of the face.)

- Limited jaw movement; crepitation or clicking heard on jaw movement; pain on jaw movement, possibly indicating TMJ dysfunction
- Tender frontal and maxillary sinuses, indicating fluid pressure, inflammation, or infection
- Lesions or tenderness involving the lips or tongue, indicating injury, infection, or malignancy
- Tracheal deviation, indicating a mediastinal shift
- Tracheal tugging in a downward direction in synchrony with the pulse, indicating an abdominal aortic aneurysm
- Diffusely enlarged thyroid gland. (The surface may feel lobulated [bumpy or lumpy], but no discrete nodules are palpable. Thyroid enlargement can be associated with hyperthyroidism, hypothyroidism, endemic goiter [normal levels of thyroid hormones], or thyroiditis [see Q Hyperthyroidism].)

DISORDER CLOSE-UP

HYPERTHYROIDISM

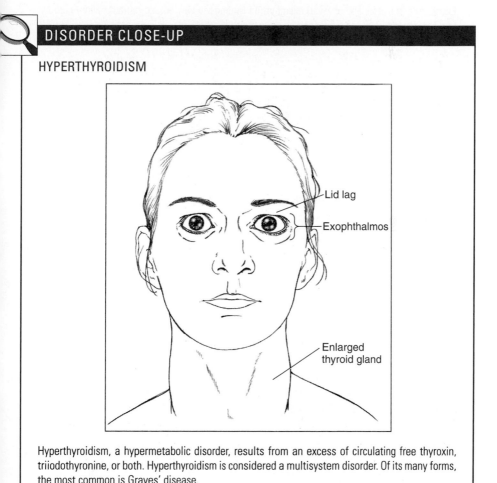

Hyperthyroidism, a hypermetabolic disorder, results from an excess of circulating free thyroxin, triiodothyronine, or both. Hyperthyroidism is considered a multisystem disorder. Of its many forms, the most common is Graves' disease.

continued

Pathophysiology

As secretion of thyroid hormones increases, the thyroid gland enlarges and becomes more vascular and thyroid function increases. As excessive thyroid hormones are secreted, systemic adrenergic activity magnifies, causing epinephrine overproduction and hypermetabolism. The result is a sustained hypermetabolic state with increased oxygen consumption, along with heightened sensitivity and stimulation of the sympathetic nervous system.

Hyperthyroidism also causes fluid accumulation in the fat pads behind the eyeball and inflammatory edema of the extraocular muscles. As a result, the eyeballs protrude and the extraocular muscles may become inflamed and fibrotic (see illustration). The skin may take on an orange-peel texture from hyperpigmentation and nonpitting edema of the pretibial area, ankles, and feet.

Characteristic findings

Expect health history and physical examination findings to vary among patients with hyperthyroidism, depending on the extent and severity of the disease. Use the information that follows to help distinguish between typical findings and complications.

Health history

- Family history of Graves' disease
- Heat intolerance accompanied by excessive sweating
- Weight loss despite increased appetite
- Diarrhea
- Tremors
- Palpitations
- Dyspnea on exertion and possibly at rest
- Pruritus
- Menstrual irregularities in female patients; impotence in male patients
- Emotional lability and nervousness
- Difficulty concentrating
- Insomnia

Inspection

- Anxious and restless appearance
- Tremors of the fingers and tongue
- Shaky handwriting
- Clumsiness
- Emotional instability
- Mood swings
- Flushed skin
- Soft, fine hair with premature graying and hair loss
- Fragile nails with distal nail separating from nail bed
- Raised, hyperpigmented, and well-demarcated pretibial edema on dorsa of legs and feet
- Plaquelike or nodular lesions
- Generalized or localized muscle atrophy
- Soft-tissue swelling, with underlying bone changes in areas of new bone formation
- Periorbital edema

continued

DISORDER CLOSE-UP—cont'd

- Infrequent blinking
- Staring and eyelid lag
- Exophthalmos
- Ocular muscle weakness, with impaired upward gaze, convergence, and strabismus

Palpation
- Asymmetrical, enlarged, and smooth or lobular thyroid gland
- Rubbery, soft, or firm thyroid gland
- Thrill over thyroid gland
- Moist, warm, smooth skin
- Bounding pulse
- Hyperreflexia

Auscultation
- Bruit over thyroid gland
- Supraventricular tachycardia and atrial fibrillation (especially in older adult patients)
- Systolic murmur at left sternal border (occasionally)
- Increased bowel sounds

Vital signs
- Tachycardia
- Bounding pulse
- Widened pulse pressure

Complications
- Thyrotoxicosis
- Arrhythmias, especially atrial fibrillation
- Cardiac insufficiency and decompensation
- Muscle weakness and atrophy
- Paralysis
- Osteoporosis
- Skin hyperpigmentation
- Corneal ulcers
- Impaired fertility
- Gynecomastia

- Enlarged thyroid with two or more identifiable nodules, known as *multinodular goiter,* suggesting metabolic disease, such as thyrotoxicosis
- Tender, palpable lymph nodes, indicating a recent infection (In an acute infection, the nodes feel large and well defined. In a chronic infection, node borders are less defined. Firmly enlarged, nontender, immobile lymph nodes may indicate malignancy. If three or more node groups are involved, the patient has generalized lymphadenopathy, possibly indicating an autoimmune disease or neoplasm.)

> **LIFESPAN CONSIDERATIONS**
>
> Palpable, nontender submandibular glands can be normal in an older patient. In addition, cervical lymph nodes are often palpable in late childhood and throughout adolescence.

- Jugular vein distention related to elevated central venous pressure (The internal jugular pulsations may be visible well above the clavicles, as high as the mandible or the tragus. It may indicate heart failure, fluid overload, constrictive pericarditis, or obstruction of the superior vena cava.)

> **LIFESPAN CONSIDERATIONS**
>
> If you suspect increased intracranial pressure (ICP) in a child, percuss the patient's skull with one finger behind the junction of the frontal, temporal, and parietal bones to try to elicit Macewen's sign. If you hear a sound that is more resonant than normal and resembles a cracking pot, consider increased ICP after fontanel closure.

- Bounding carotid pulse related to a hyperdynamic state, such as fever or thyroid storm
- Weak carotid pulse from decreased stroke volume, indicating left ventricular heart failure or profound hypotension
- Unilateral weakness or paralysis of muscles in the neck and shoulders, indicating a disorder of CN XI

PERCUSSION

When examining the head and neck, you will percuss only the frontal and maxillary paranasal sinuses. Using your index or middle finger as the plexor, gently tap the area above the eyebrow (frontal sinuses). To percuss the maxillary sinuses, tap your middle or index finger on both sides of the nose in line with the pupil.

NORMAL FINDINGS

- Resonance on percussion, indicating sinuses are filled with air
- No discomfort or tenderness on percussion

ABNORMAL FINDINGS

- Dullness or flatness on percussion of the maxillary and frontal sinuses, indicating fluid
- Pain and pressure on percussion in the maxillary and frontal sinuses, possibly indicating bacterial, viral, or allergic sinusitis

AUSCULTATION

When auscultating blood vessels in the head and neck for abnormal sounds, be sure to include the temporal and carotid arteries, as well as the jugular vein. First, place the bell of the stethoscope over the temporal artery, just lateral to the outer canthus of the eye. Listen for several seconds. Repeat this procedure on the opposite temporal artery.

To listen to the carotid arteries, gently place the bell of your stethoscope over each artery and ask your patient to hold her breath so that the sound of the respirations does not interfere with the examination. Do not press too hard, or you will occlude the artery.

Bruits are most readily heard at the lateral end of the clavicle and the posterior margin of the sternocleidomastoid muscle. If you need extra time to listen, let your patient take deep breaths between listening. Also be sure to listen to both sides of the neck.

To listen for venous hums, move the bell of your stethoscope to the medial end of the clavicle and the anterior border of the sternocleidomastoid muscle. With your patient's head turned away from the area of auscultation, press firmly on the end piece and listen for a continuous low-pitched sound during ventricular diastole. If you ask your patient to bear down, the sound will soften.

If the thyroid gland feels enlarged, auscultate it for a bruit as well. Using the bell of your stethoscope, listen over the lateral lobes of the thyroid gland while your patient holds her breath. To differentiate a bruit from a venous hum, gently occlude the jugular vein on the side you are auscultating. A venous hum will disappear when you compress the vein.

NORMAL FINDINGS

- No audible sounds when auscultating the temporal and carotid arteries (other than normal heart sounds commonly heard in the neck)
- Venous hum in pregnant female patients
- No audible sounds when auscultating the thyroid

ABNORMAL FINDINGS

- Soft, low-pitched, rushing sound heard during the cardiac cycle, indicating a bruit in the temporal or carotid artery (The bruit may signify narrowing of the artery or radiation of a systolic murmur from the aortic valve area, as heard in aortic stenosis.)
- Venous hum heard in the presence of anemia, thyrotoxicosis, or intracranial arteriovenous malformation
- Bruit in the thyroid gland caused by accelerated blood flow through an enlarged gland and found with hyperthyroidism

To close your examination of the head and neck, take a few minutes to summarize your findings (see ▉ What to Expect When Examining the Head and Neck).

NORMAL FINDINGS

WHAT TO EXPECT WHEN EXAMINING THE HEAD AND NECK

Use this review to confirm normal findings when examining the head and neck.

- Head round and symmetrical
- Scalp pink in color, without scales, and covered with hair; hair distributed evenly, without excess oil
- Facial features symmetrical; eyes open evenly and are equally displaced from the midline of the face
- Nasolabial folds symmetrical
- Skin of the face and neck pink, smooth, and firm in tone
- Nasal mucosa flat and somewhat redder than oral mucosa; nasal septum lies at midline of nose
- Lips moist, without cracks or fissures
- Gums with a red, stippled surface; margins around teeth sharp; teeth firm in sockets
- Internal jugular vein pulsations regular and vary with inspiration and expiration; not visible when patient sits upright; patient has no jugular distention
- Skin of head and neck warm and dry, without masses or tenderness
- Frontal and maxillary sinuses free of pain
- Trachea straight and at midline of the neck; thyroid gland moves freely when patient swallows; isthmus free of nodes

- Lymph nodes in neck nonpalpable, nontender, and not swollen; if palpable, nodes are soft, round, and freely mobile
- Carotid artery pulsation regular, full, and smooth
- Resonance on percussion of sinuses
- No audible sounds over carotid and temporal arteries, other than normal heart sounds generally heard in neck
- Venous hum over jugular vein in pregnancy

Cranial nerve function

- Patient able to identify various odors (CN I)
- Temporal and masseter muscles equal in strength bilaterally; patient able to differentiate between sharp versus dull in all three distributions of CN V
- Facial movements symmetrical (CN VII)
- Movements of pharynx, larynx, and palate symmetrical; gag reflex intact; patient's voice clear and easily audible (CN IX and X)
- Shoulder and neck muscles equal in strength and contraction bilaterally (CN XI)
- Tongue at midline of mouth, with full, rounded appearance and smooth movement (CN XII)

EXPLORING CHIEF COMPLAINTS

Most of your head and neck examinations will revolve around a chief complaint made by a patient seeking medical care. Information about common chief complaints, instructions on how to focus your assessments when examining patients with those complaints, and possible causes follow.

HEADACHES

If your patient complains of headaches, investigate further by asking the following questions:

- Is the pain on one side of your head or on both sides? Is it diffuse or localized?
- Is the pain so severe that it interrupts your activities of daily living, or can you carry on despite the pain?

- Would you describe the headache as viselike or stabbing? Are you nauseated and vomiting? Are you dizzy or experiencing visual changes or weakness?
- Do the headaches begin suddenly or gradually? Are they preceded by an aura or characteristic sensation, such as flashing lights?
- When did you first notice the headaches? How often do they occur? How long do they last? Have they become more severe over time?
- What seems to bring the headaches on (noise, lights, coughing or sneezing, sexual intercourse, fatigue, certain foods, or menstruation)?
- What relieves them (sleep, analgesics, or avoiding certain foods, alcohol, or cigarettes)?
- Have you experienced any changes in your sleep pattern? Do you awaken early without cause?

Focusing Your Assessment

When examining a patient who complains of headaches, focus your assessment as follows:

- Check the patient's vital signs because fever and hypertension can cause headache.
- Palpate the head and neck for tenderness or muscle tightness—signs of tension headaches.
- Assess for bruising, swelling, neck stiffness, otorrhea, and rhinorrhea— signs of trauma.
- Assess level of consciousness (LOC). Check for photophobia and pupil reaction to assess for migraines or hemorrhage.
- Auscultate for bruits in the temporal and carotid arteries—signs of temporal arteritis and carotid stenosis.
- If the headache is acute and very painful, check for nuchal rigidity and positive Kernig's sign or Brudzinski's sign—signs of meningeal irritation (see Assessing for Signs of Meningeal Irritation).
- Check muscle strength and reflexes for symmetry. Paresthesias may occur with migraines, hemorrhage, or tumors.
- Palpate and percuss the sinuses for tenderness.

Possible Causes

- *Muscular pain or tension.* This benign headache is characterized by aching, bandlike pain around the head and neck. Often, mild analgesic agents or muscle relaxant drugs can relieve tension headaches (see 🔲 Determining Causes of Headache).

ASSESSING FOR SIGNS OF MENINGEAL IRRITATION

If your patient with fever also complains of a stiff neck, check for signs of meningeal irritation, which can point to meningitis. Check for these cardinal signs of meningeal irritation: Kernig's and Brudzinski's signs, and nuchal rigidity.

Kernig's sign
With the patient supine, flex the patient's leg at the hip to a 90-degree angle. With the leg in this position, try to straighten the knee. If you feel resistance or the patient has severe lower back pain, Kernig's sign is present.

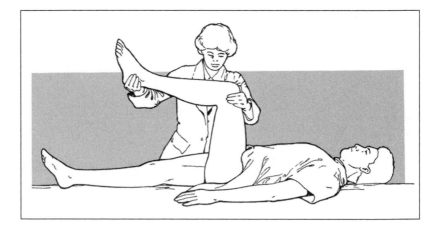

Nuchal rigidity and Brudzinski's sign
With the patient relaxed and supine, place your hand under the patient's head at the base of the skull and gently try to bend the head forward so that the chin touches the chest. If nuchal rigidity is present, the neck is stiff and forward flexion is reduced. If the patient flexes the hips and knees or experiences neck and back pain, Brudzinski's sign is present.

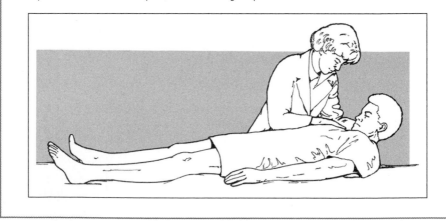

From Chipps EM, Clanin NJ, Campbell VG: *Neurologic disorders,* St Louis, 1992, Mosby.

INTERPRETING ABNORMAL FINDINGS

DETERMINING CAUSES OF HEADACHE

Headaches are common and usually harmless. Most result from stress and muscle tension. Sometimes, however, a headache can warn of a serious, even life-threatening, medical condition. The following table lists possible causes of headaches and their characteristic signs and symptoms. By assessing your patient carefully and reviewing symptoms and examination findings closely, you can help your patient obtain an accurate diagnosis and appropriate treatment.

Characteristics	Location	Possible Findings	Probable Causes
• Gradual onset • Steady ache • Progressive pain that waxes and wanes and can last for days	Usually bilateral; occipital and upper neck region; may also occur in the frontal and temporal area	• Patient may report specific triggers, such as anxiety or stress • Findings usually normal, although muscles around the face and neck may be tense or tight	• Tension • Stress • Depression • Sleep disturbance • Fatigue
• Severe, throbbing pain, typically occurring in the morning • Commonly triggered by stress, menstruation, or certain foods • Peaks in about 1 hour and may last 1 to 2 days • Commonly ends with sleep	Usually pain is unilateral and occurs in characteristic, localized regions of the head	• Photophobia • Unusual sensitivity to noise • Aura, usually visual, that precedes headache • Nausea and vomiting • Fatigue • Occasional unilateral sensory loss, hemiplegia, aphasia, or third-nerve palsy	• Migraine
• Episodes of steady, excruciating pain • Onset sudden • Lasts 30 minutes to a few hours • Occurs repeatedly (six to eight a day) for a few weeks or months, commonly followed by a headache-free period • Typically seasonal • Occurs most commonly at night, awakening the patient from sleep	Unilateral, usually orbital or behind the eye	• Unilateral rhinorrhea • Miosis • Ptosis • Flushing of the cheek on the affected side • Conjunctival redness and tearing on the affected side	• Cluster headache

continued

INTERPRETING ABNORMAL FINDINGS—cont'd

Characteristics	Location	Possible Findings	Probable Causes
• Severe pain • Worsens with stooping or bending over • Lasts for hours or days • Sudden, severe onset • Described as "the worst headache ever experienced"	Periorbital, frontal, or maxillary None specific	• Pain or tenderness over the involved sinus • Fever • General malaise • Nuchal rigidity • Photophobia • Nausea and vomiting • Focal neurologic deficits	• Sinusitis • Cerebrovascular hemorrhage (subarachnoid)
• Pain like a thunder clap • Maximum intensity immediately • May be accompanied by loss of consciousness and progression of coma • Severe, progressive • Lasts several hours or days • May develop rapidly	Diffuse or occipital pain	• Seizures • Fever, usually high • Nuchal rigidity • Photophobia • Positive Kernig's sign • Positive Brudzinski's sign • Decreased level of consciousness (LOC)	• Meningeal irritation from meningitis or encephalitis
• Severe, ripping pain in one side of face • Pain described as searing, burning, or stabbing • Onset abrupt • Pain lasts a few seconds to a few minutes	Along a branch of the trigeminal nerve: around eyes and over forehead; upper lip, nose, and cheek; side of the tongue and lower lip	• Physical examination usually normal • Patient typically identifies a trigger zone (a small area of the face, lips, gums, or forehead affected by such stimulants as brushing teeth, chewing, talking, smiling, and exposure to cold)	• Trigeminal neuralgia
• Dull, achy pain occurring days after a concussion or mild head injury • Lasts for weeks to months	No specific area	• History of concussion or mild head injury • Difficulty concentrating • Malaise • Mood alterations • Fatigue • Loss of balance • Double vision • Physical examination usually normal	• Postconcussion syndrome

- *Migraine.* This headache is severe and commonly preceded by an aura or characteristic sensation. Nausea and vomiting may ensue, and the migraine may last for several minutes, hours, or even days. The pain occurs in clusters in several parts of the head and face. It may be triggered by stress, menstruation, or eating certain foods.
- *Cluster headache.* This headache is associated with release of histamine, which causes the carotid arteries to dilate. Cluster headaches are marked by sudden, severe pain on one side of the head and excessive tearing of the eye on the same side as the pain.
- *Temporal arteritis.* This headache results from an inflammatory process that affects the cranial vessels, especially the temporal arteries. The headache is typically intractable and usually accompanied by swelling and tenderness in the temporal region, weakness, difficulty chewing, and visual changes.
- *Sinusitis.* This headache is characterized by pain and tenderness in the sinuses and worsens when the patient bends down. It may be relieved by decongestants.
- *Hypertension.* Headaches caused by hypertension are characterized by occipital pain in the morning.
- *Infection, as in meningitis or encephalitis.* This headache is accompanied by high fever, decreased LOC, and neck pain. Your patient may also have seizures.
- *Malignancy.* Brain tumors cause headaches that are dull, localized, and worsen with changes in head position.
- *Medications.* Drugs containing nitrates and others such as cyclosporine are known for causing headaches. With nitrates, headaches become less severe as the patient's tolerance to the medication increases.

NOSEBLEEDS

If your patient complains of nosebleeds, investigate further by asking the following questions:
- Would you call the amount of bleeding scant or copious? How long does it take for the nosebleed to stop?
- What color is the blood? Is it bright red, dark red, or brown, or is it blood-tinged fluid? Do the droplets have a bloody center with a clear halo?
- Does the bleeding come from one or both nostrils?
- Do you have recurrent nosebleeds, or is this the only one you have had?
- Do you have other symptoms? Do you have congestion or headaches? Do your nasal passages burn? Do you bleed easily in other areas of your body?
- When do you get the symptoms? Does the bleeding seem worse at a particular time of day or year? Does it seem to follow a particular activity, such as nose blowing?
- Was there any recent trauma or insertion of a foreign body in your nose? Have you recently inhaled any chemicals or other strong agents? Do you blow your nose often?

- Do you use nasal oxygen therapy?
- Is the air in your home or at work very dry?
- Which medications do you take, and why do you take them?

Focusing Your Assessment

When examining a patient who has nosebleeds, focus your assessment as follows:

- Inspect the nasal cavity with a bright light and speculum to confirm the bleeding and locate the site.
- Check the patient's skull, and look for recent head trauma.
- Assess the skin, and look for areas of bruising or bleeding that could indicate a bleeding disorder.
- Check your patient's blood studies for elevated prothrombin time (PT) or decreased platelet count.

Possible Causes

- *Injury or lesion.* In the anterior-inferior septum, injury or lesion causes profuse bleeding.
- *Skull injury.* This injury, especially to the basal skull, may cause CSF to leak through the nares.
- *Hypertension.* Increased blood pressure may cause fragile nasal capillaries to break and bleed.
- *Hepatic diseases.* These diseases cause thrombocytopenia (decreased platelets) and an elevated PT, decreasing the blood's ability to clot.
- *Medications.* Medications such as warfarin, heparin, or aspirin decrease the blood's ability to clot.
- *Dry, hot environments or unhumidified oxygen therapy.* Both may dry out mucous membranes and cause capillaries to break and bleed.

NECK PAIN AND STIFFNESS

If your patient complains of neck pain or stiffness, investigate further by asking the following questions:

- Did the pain occur gradually or suddenly?
- Is the pain associated with any activity or trauma? If so, can you describe the activity or trauma in as much detail as possible? If the pain is associated with an activity, does this activity require your head to be in a fixed position for a period of time?
- Is the pain constant or intermittent?
- Have you experienced associated limb pain, numbness, or weakness?
- Is the pain in front or in back of your neck?
- Do you have a fever? What about a rash, headache, or nausea?
- What, if anything, alleviates the pain?

Focusing Your Assessment

When examining a patient who complains of neck pain or stiffness, focus your assessment as follows:

- Assess neck range of motion. Look specifically for nuchal rigidity and positive Kernig's and Brudzinski's signs—possible signs of meningeal irritation.
- Assess strength of contraction of the trapezius and sternocleidomastoid muscles.
- Inspect for laceration, swelling, or bruising of the neck. Assess for torticollis (contraction of the muscles on one side of the neck).
- Check the muscle strength of both arms for flexion and extension.
- Check the reflexes of the upper extremities for symmetry.
- Palpate the neck muscles for soreness and tenderness.
- Palpate the lymph nodes for enlargement and tenderness.

Possible Causes

- *Injury from strain or whiplash.* Pain occurs in the anterior or posterior parts of the neck but usually diminishes over time.
- *Fracture of cervical vertebrae from osteoporosis, injury, or tumor.* Spinal cord injuries result in some loss of sensation, movement, and function below the site of injury.
- *Infection, especially meningitis.* Other symptoms include fever, photophobia, decreased LOC, and headache (see 🔍 Meningitis).

DISORDER CLOSE-UP

MENINGITIS

Meningitis is an acute inflammation that can affect all three meningeal membranes that cover the brain and spinal cord: (1) the dura mater, (2) arachnoid membrane, and (3) pia mater. Meningitis can result from bacterial, viral, or fungal infection; chemical irritation; or tumors. As a result of the inflammatory process, the cerebrospinal fluid (CSF) thickens and accumulates in the subarachnoid space. Eventually this raises the intracranial pressure (ICP) and causes nerve cell compression in the brain and spinal cord. Symptoms of meningitis typically appear 1 to 7 days after the onset of the primary infection, but they can be delayed for up to 3 weeks.

Viral infection is the most common cause of meningitis. Viral meningitis, also called *aseptic meningitis,* usually develops in the late summer and early fall, primarily affecting children and adults under age 30. The most common causative viruses are enteroviruses, the coxsackie virus, mumps virus, herpesvirus, and arboviruses. These viruses enter the body through the oral, oral-fecal, or respiratory pathways. Once in the body, these viruses replicate and spread to the brain through the bloodstream.

Bacterial meningitis usually follows a bacterial infection that has occurred elsewhere in the body caused by *Neisseria meningitidis, Streptococcus pneumoniae, Staphylococcus* and *Diplococcus* spp., and *Haemophilus influenzae.* Bacterial meningitis also may occur after inadvertent introduction of bacteria during neurosurgical procedures, lumbar puncture, spinal anesthesia, or from trauma.

Characteristic findings

Expect health history and physical examination findings to vary among patients with meningitis, depending on the extent and severity of the disease. It is often difficult to distinguish between bacterial and viral meningitis on the patient's symptoms alone. Use the following information to help distinguish between expected and unexpected findings.

continued

DISORDER CLOSE-UP—cont'd

Health history
- Severe headache
- Stiff neck and back
- Malaise
- Photophobia
- Chills
- Altered level of consciousness (LOC), such as confusion and delirium
- History of recent bacterial infection, such as respiratory tract, ear, or sinus
- Nausea and vomiting (more common with viral meningitis)

Inspection
- Altered LOC
- Opisthotonos
- Petechial, purpuric, or ecchymotic rash on lower portion of body with meningococcal meningitis
- Papilledema (on ophthalmoscopic examination)

Palpation
- Nuchal rigidity
- Kernig's sign
- Brudzinski's sign
- Hyperactive, symmetrical deep tendon reflexes

Vital signs
- Sudden onset of temperature elevation as high as 104° F (40° C) with viral meningitis

Complications
- Visual impairment
- Optic neuritis
- Cranial nerve palsies
- Deafness
- Personality changes
- Paresis or paralysis
- Endocarditis
- Coma
- Cerebral infarction
- Unilateral or bilateral sensory hearing loss (in children)
- Epilepsy (in children)
- Mental retardation (in children)
- Hydrocephalus (in children)

- *Musculoskeletal disorders.* Disorders such as a herniated cervical disk, ankylosing spondylitis, osteoporosis, osteoarthritis, or rheumatoid arthritis may cause neck pain and stiffness. Pain tends to be chronic, waxing and waning in intensity.

SORE THROAT

If your patient complains of a sore throat, investigate further by asking the following questions:

- Do you drink alcohol or use tobacco?
- Do you live in a dry environment? Do you work in an environment that contains chemical irritants?
- Do you use your voice constantly (as a singer, perhaps, or a teacher)?
- Do you have a history of allergies or persistent cough?
- Have you had recent surgery or an emergency that required endotracheal intubation?

Focusing Your Assessment

When examining a patient who complains of a sore throat, focus your assessment as follows:

- Inspect the throat for redness, inflammation, swollen mucous membranes, and exudate.
- Assess the patient's ability to swallow.
- Check for mild fever, headache, and muscular discomfort.
- Listen to the quality of the patient's voice. Check for hoarseness.

Possible Causes

- *Viral or bacterial pharyngitis.* Evidence includes erythema and swelling of the throat and tonsils. Fever, exudate, and severe erythema commonly accompany bacterial infections.
- *Malignancy.* The risk is highest for a smoker or former smoker. Hoarseness commonly accompanies malignancy.
- *Allergy or chemical irritation.* Exposure to offending toxins may result in a sore throat.
- *Injury.* Endotracheal intubation, nasogastric tube insertion, or overuse of the voice from shouting or singing may injure the throat. Hoarseness or loss of voice often accompany injury.

Examining the Eyes and Ears

Although an eye or ear problem rarely causes acute illness, it can result in considerable discomfort. If it impairs vision or hearing, it can also lead to psychosocial problems, such as difficulty communicating, trouble perceiving visual or auditory stimulation, or the inability to function independently. In addition, a vision or hearing impairment may make the patient especially anxious.

A nurse's ability to evaluate a patient's eye or ear disorder quickly and accurately can go a long way toward restoring health, easing discomfort, and calming fears.

EYE EXAMINATION STEPS AND FINDINGS

Preparation for accurate assessment of the eye requires the following steps:
- Make certain you are thoroughly familiar with basic eye anatomy (see Intraocular Structures).
- Review the patient's chief complaint and check the patient's history for disorders that may affect the eyes, such as diabetes mellitus, hypertension, or acquired immunodeficiency syndrome (AIDS).
- Check the patient's age, overall condition, allergies, and current medication regimen.
- Gather equipment: penlight, ophthalmoscope, Rosenbaum pocket vision screener or Snellen chart, clean opaque card for covering one eye, pupil gauge, cotton-tipped applicator and wisp of cotton, small metric ruler, sterile fluorescein strips, and a cobalt-blue light to aid corneal examination (if available and needed).
- Keep in mind that eye problems may have a neurologic component because the eye is an integral part of the brain.
- Plan to conduct the eye assessment in a quiet, well-lit room, with the patient sitting up and facing you. Be sure to note if the patient is wearing contact lenses.

INTRAOCULAR STRUCTURES

This illustration shows many of the important structures of the eye.

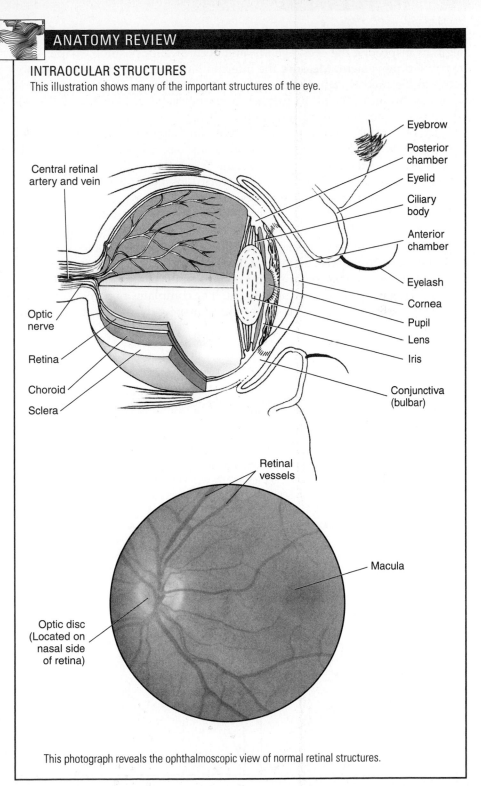

This photograph reveals the ophthalmoscopic view of normal retinal structures.

INSPECTION

Begin by inspecting the eyes, eyelids, and eyebrows for position, shape, symmetry, and movement. Measure the intercanthal space, which is the distance between the medial canthi (the angles at the medial margin of the eyelids across the bridge of the nose). Inspect for proptosis (also called *exophthalmos*), which is an abnormal protrusion of the eyeball.

Check the upper and lower lid margins for integrity, color, texture, and position. Ask the patient to close the eyes, and see whether the closed lids completely cover the eyes. Then inspect the orientation of the eyelids and eyelashes, noting if they turn outward or inward. Observe how often the patient blinks, and note any abnormal features of the blinking.

Next, inspect the conjunctiva for clarity, discharge, and inflammation. To assess the palpebral conjunctiva (the portion that lines the inside of the eyelids), gently pull down on the lower lid, and ask the patient to look up as you examine the exposed area. To inspect the bulbar conjunctiva (the portion that covers the sclera), gently pull upward on the upper lid and ask the patient to look down as you assess the exposed area. If he complains of pain or irritation beneath the upper eyelid, evert the eyelid to inspect the conjunctiva (see Performing Eyelid Eversion).

EXAMINATION TIP

PERFORMING EYELID EVERSION

You may need to evert the patient's upper eyelid when inspecting the palpebral conjunctiva. Before starting, have the patient remove contact lenses, if worn.

- Gently grasp the patient's eyelashes, and instruct the patient to look down.
- With your free hand, use a cotton-tipped applicator stick to press gently above the upper eyelid fold while pulling the lid margin up by the lashes.
- As you maintain pressure on the everted lid, shine the penlight across the conjunctival surface.
- When you have finished inspecting the conjunctiva of the everted lid, release the lid margin. The eyelid should return to its normal position when the patient looks up. If it does not, gently pull the eyelashes forward.

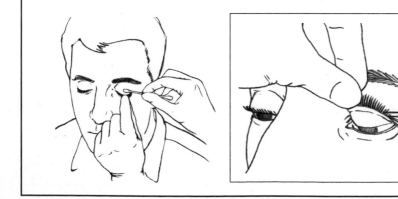

Now move on to the lacrimal apparatus, checking for adequate tear production and eye lubrication. Then inspect the sclera, noting its color and looking for scleral thinning, indicated by a bluish-gray tinge or bulging (which represents the choroid showing through the sclera).

Inspect the cornea by shining your penlight at an oblique angle onto it from the temporal side of the eye. Look for clouding, opacity, and injury.

If your patient is unconscious or has a problem with cranial nerve (CN) V (the trigeminal nerve), you will need to check the corneal reflex—a function of CN V. To do this, lightly touch the cornea with a wisp of cotton and check for appropriate blinking. In other patients, this test is rarely performed because it can cause discomfort.

To detect strabismus (deviation of one eye), perform the corneal light reflection test. Shine a penlight on the bridge of the patient's nose, and note where the spots of light fall and whether the light falls on the same location on each eye.

Next, inspect the iris, noting its shape and pigmentation (see 📋 Essentials of the Eye Examination).

EXPERT EXAMINATION CHECKLIST

ESSENTIALS OF THE EYE EXAMINATION

Use this checklist to be sure you cover the most important steps when conducting an eye exam.

❑ Inspect position, shape, and movement of eyes and associated structures.
❑ Check extraocular movements, including the six cardinal positions of gaze.
❑ Inspect eyelids for color, texture, integrity, closure, lesions, inversion, eversion, and drooping.
❑ Inspect eyelash distribution, orientation, and granulation.
❑ Check eyeball surface for lubrication, tearing, redness, and swelling.
❑ Inspect cornea for clarity, surface integrity, reflex (if needed), and light reflection.

❑ Check pupil size, shape, light response, accommodation, and red reflex.
❑ Palpate for firmness, mobility, texture, and smoothness of eyelids and orbital rim.
❑ Palpate punctum for tenderness and discharge.
❑ Test visual acuity.
❑ Perform the confrontation test.

Ophthalmoscopic examination

❑ Check lens clarity.
❑ Inspect vitreous humor for opacities, floaters, precipitates, and blood.
❑ Inspect optic disc color, shape, borders, and physiologic cup.
❑ Check retinal vessels, macula, and fovea.

---

evolve Find PDF and PDA-downloadable versions of this Expert Exam Checklist online at http://evolve.elsevier.com/Mosby/expertexam/.

Pupil Examination

With normal room light, measure your patient's pupils using a pupil gauge. Document the result in millimeters and compare the measurements of both eyes. Then assess pupil shape.

Next, check pupil accommodation by having the patient look at an object across the room. As he does this, you should check for pupil dilation. Then ask the patient to stare at your finger as you hold it about 10 cm in front of him. Check for pupil constriction and equal convergence of both eyes on your finger.

Assess the pupils' reaction to light. To evaluate direct pupillary response, stimulate one eye by briefly shining your penlight toward the pupil. Observe the reaction of the stimulated pupil as light is applied. To evaluate consensual pupillary response, stimulate the eye a second time, this time watching the response of the other (nonstimulated) pupil. Repeat the test with the other eye.

Extraocular Muscle Assessment

To evaluate the function of extraocular muscles and the cranial nerves that control them, ask the patient to follow your finger with his eyes as you move it through each of the six cardinal positions of gaze (see Six Cardinal Positions of Gaze Test).

SIX CARDINAL POSITIONS OF GAZE TEST

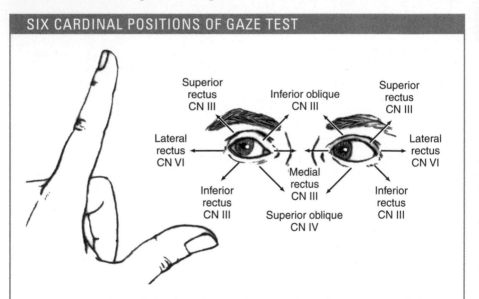

To assess extraocular muscle function, ask your patient to watch your finger as you move it through the six cardinal positions of gaze. Begin by holding your index finger about 12 to 18 inches directly in front of the patient. Then move your finger through each of these maneuvers:
- From the midline to the patient's right side
- Upward, staying to the right of the midline
- Downward, staying to the right of the midline
- Left, across the midline
- Upward, staying to the left of the midline
- Downward, staying to the left of the midline

Make sure the patient moves only the eyes, not the head, when following the movement of your finger. Observe for conjugate (parallel) eye movement and note any abnormalities, such as deviation of one eye or nystagmus. Ask the patient to report any diplopia or blurred vision during this test.

LIFESPAN CONSIDERATIONS

To check the six cardinal positions of gaze in a young child, use an appealing object, such as a doll or stuffed toy, instead of your finger.

Visual Acuity Testing

If your patient has a specific eye complaint, especially vision loss, test visual acuity by using a vision-screening card, such as the Rosenbaum pocket vision screener, and a vision chart, such as the Snellen chart. If the patient normally wears corrective lenses, make sure they are worn during this test.

To test far vision, place the chart on a wall that is 20 feet from the patient. Note the line on the chart at which the patient can accurately read the letters with each eye. Record the numeric fraction that is to the left of that line (e.g., 20/20). To test near vision, hold a pocket card at a distance of 14 inches from the patient. Record the distance equivalents to the right of the line at which the patient can accurately read.

If the patient cannot read the largest letters on the card, hold up several fingers and ask how many he sees. If the patient cannot see your fingers or answers incorrectly, wave your hand in front of his face to determine if he can detect the hand movement. If he cannot, then shine a penlight into the patient's eyes to see if he can perceive light. Document the best response.

Visual Field Testing

Evaluate your patient's visual fields and peripheral vision by conducting the confrontation test.

Standing 2 to 3 feet directly in front of the patient, with your eyes level with his eyes, ask the patient to stare straight ahead and meet your gaze. Then ask him to cover the left eye while you cover your right eye. Slowly bring your fingers from beyond the limits of the visual fields in all four quadrants, and instruct the patient to tell you when he can first see them. Repeat the test for the patient's left eye by asking him to hold his hand over the right eye and gaze into your right eye as you close your left eye. Again, test his visual fields. If you see your fingers in your peripheral vision before he does, your patient may have restricted visual fields.

Document your findings by making a circle on a piece of paper. Think of the circle as the edge of a normal visual field. Then, at each of your testing locations, record the perimeter of the patient's vision. Also record the locations of any areas of vision loss inside the visual field.

NORMAL FINDINGS

• Eyes, eyelids, and eyebrows symmetrical in shape and position and freely mobile (The eyes should align with the top of the pinnae. The skin of the eyelids should be loose, thin, and elastic. In an older patient, loose, hanging skin may cover a portion of the lid [dermatochalasis].)

- Eyelids free from inflammation and scales
- Edges of upper and lower eyelids frame upper and lower margins of irises when patient's eyes are open (The opening between the lids is wide enough to allow light through to the pupil.)
- Eyelashes curve outward from eyelid margins, which lie snugly against the eyeball (The lashes on the upper lid turn upward; on the lower lid, they turn downward. Lashes are usually longer and more abundant on the upper lid than on the lower lid.)
- Eyelashes free of mucus and scales
- Conjunctiva transparent and free of discharge or hyperemia (reddened, dilated vessels) (The eyeball surface appears moist and well lubricated.)
- Sclera white and translucent

LIFESPAN CONSIDERATIONS

In the older adult, sclera may appear bluish because of thinning.

CULTURAL CONSIDERATIONS

In dark-skinned patients, sclera may be yellowish or slightly pigmented with brown spots.

- Corneal reflex brisk, indicating intact function of CN V
- Corneal surface smooth, transparent, and free of precipitates or irregularities (In an older patient, you may note corneal arcus [arcus senilis], a grayish-white corneal ring visible around the iris.)
- Corneal light reflection at same place on each cornea in light reflection test, indicating equal eye positioning
- Irises flat and circular, with similar pigmentation in both eyes
- Pupils round, from 3 to 5mm in size (A slight difference in size [<1mm] between pupils is common.)
- Pupils respond equally and briskly to light on direct and consensual tests
- Pupils dilate appropriately when focusing on far objects and constrict and converge equally when focusing on close objects
- Eyes congruent (parallel) in all positions while testing the six cardinal positions of gaze
- Corrected visual acuity 20/20 (If not possible, then correct visual acuity to 20/30 to 20/40.)
- Full visual fields, without restriction or defects (See ▲ What to Expect When Examining the Eyes.)

NORMAL FINDINGS

WHAT TO EXPECT WHEN EXAMINING THE EYES

Use this brief review to confirm normal findings when examining the eyes.

- Orbits symmetrical in placement, shape, and position; eyeballs freely mobile
- Eyelids smooth, nontender, and free of discharge (ectropion or entropion may be seen in older adults)
- Tear ducts nontender and free of discharge
- Eyelashes free of granulation, scales
- Surface lubrication and moisture adequate
- Conjunctivae clear and moist
- Sclerae white and opaque
- Corneas smooth and transparent
- Irises flat and circular, with even bilateral pigmentation
- Pupils equal in size, round, and reactive to light, with proper accommodation (PERRLA).
- Lenses clear
- Vitreous transparent
- Optic disc flat and slightly oval or round; nasal aspect slightly darker pink
- Optic nerve border distinct; temporal border may have grayish crescent
- Physiologic cup paler than optic disc
- Retina of uniform red-orange color; macula darker than retina

ABNORMAL FINDINGS

- Proptosis or exophthalmos, possibly associated with Graves' disease. (If unilateral, it may indicate an underlying tumor.)
- Incomplete eyelid closure (lagophthalmos), from exophthalmos or weakness of CN VII (the facial nerve), as well as periorbital swelling
- Eyelids everted at the margins (This condition, called *ectropion,* may result from the loss of skin elasticity with age.)
- Eyelids inverted (This condition, called *entropion,* commonly results from aging or from palpebral conjunctival scarring.)
- Drooping eyelid (ptosis), associated with Horner's syndrome (a neurologic condition caused by a spinal cord lesion), myasthenia gravis, or weakness of CN III (the oculomotor nerve)
- Involuntary spasm of the orbicularis oculi muscle in the eyelid (Called *blepharospasm,* this condition may result from phenothiazine medications [e.g., chlorpromazine], a foreign body in the eye, or infection.)
- Eyelid swelling, possibly related to a wide range of medical conditions, including inflammation, allergic reaction, infection, heart failure, renal disease, hypothyroidism, and Graves' disease
- Red eyelid margins, with dried mucus clinging to the lashes, suggesting blepharitis, a chronic bilateral inflammation of the eyelid margins usually accompanied by itching, burning, and irritation (Causes of blepharitis include staphylococcal infection, seborrheic dermatitis, allergy, and psoriasis. Chronic blepharitis may be associated with gout, diabetes mellitus, and ectropion.)
- Acute pustular infection involving an eyelash follicle, meibomian cyst, or sebaceous gland of the eyelid (Called a *stye* or a *hordeolum,* this infection typically results from a staphylococcal organism.)

- Chalazion, an obstruction of the meibomian glands, appearing as a localized, beadlike swelling on the eyelid (Recurrent chalazions may warrant surgery for removal and biopsy to rule out malignancy.)
- Soft, yellowish, raised, waxy lesion on or beneath the eyelid (This finding, called *xanthoma* [or *xanthelasma*] *palpebrarum*, often occurs in groups. Although sometimes benign, these lesions are commonly associated with hyperlipidemia.)
- Inflammation and dilation of the conjunctival blood vessels, typically resulting from conjunctivitis, an inflammation of the conjunctiva caused by bacteria, viruses, allergies, certain drugs, or environmental factors
- Sudden onset of bright-red blood in a discrete area outside the conjunctival vessels, from subconjunctival hemorrhage (Typical causes of this condition include heavy sneezing or coughing, trauma, hypertension, and clotting disorders such as hemophilia.)
- Inadequate tear production (dry eye syndrome), possibly resulting from a systemic condition, such as Sjögren's syndrome, Stevens-Johnson syndrome, pemphigoid syndromes, or systemic lupus erythematosus
- Corneal haziness or cloudiness from edema, possibly resulting from an acute increase in intraocular pressure (IOP) or keratitis
- Red eye, accompanied by increased tearing, a foreign body sensation, moderate-to-severe eye pain, decreased visual acuity, and photophobia (This condition results from corneal abrasion, best identified by fluorescein staining [see Checking for Corneal Abrasions].)

CHECKING FOR CORNEAL ABRASIONS

If you routinely care for patients with ophthalmic conditions, you will probably perform corneal staining to check for possible corneal abrasions. This procedure involves the use of fluorescein, a fluorescent dye available in sterile filter paper strips.

To use a fluorescein strip, wet it with a drop of sterile water or saline solution; then touch it to the patient's palpebral conjunctiva. Have the patient blink a few times to distribute the fluorescein solution over the cornea.

Next, shine a light over the cornea, preferably a bright penlight with a cobalt-blue filter. Any defects in the corneal epithelium will appear bright green.

- Irregularly shaped or "keyhole" pupil, possibly resulting from surgical removal of a portion of the iris (Another cause of pupil irregularity is an adhesion resulting from iritis [inflammation of the iris]. A square pupil, an unusual finding, may result from use of an iris clip lens, a type of intraocular lens.)
- Unequal pupil diameter (anisocoria) (Usually this condition is congenital, although it is sometimes associated with CN palsy.)
- Pinpoint pupils, possibly resulting from topical miotic ophthalmic drugs (e.g., pilocarpine), systemic drugs (e.g., opiate agents), Horner's syndrome, damage to the pons, migraines, or cluster headaches
- Dilated pupils, possibly resulting from topical mydriatic ophthalmic drugs (e.g., atropine), some systemic drugs (dexfenfluramine and scopolamine), or CN III palsies

- Pupil moderately dilated and nonreactive to light, possibly signaling acute angle-closure glaucoma (A medical emergency, it may be accompanied by eye redness and pain, decreased visual acuity, blurred vision, pressure felt over the eye, corneal clouding, seeing halos around lights, and nausea and vomiting.)
- Pupil dilated and fixed or slow to respond to light (Called *tonic pupil* [or *Adie's pupil*], this condition is caused by a disturbance of autonomic innervation to one eye and often impairs accommodation, resulting in blurred vision. Decreased deep-tendon reflexes may accompany it.)
- Lack of parallel eye movement or deviation of one eye, indicating an abnormality of the extraocular muscles
- Involuntary oscillating eye movements called *nystagmus*, possibly resulting from a disorder of the labyrinth (inner ear) or the vestibular portion of CN VII (It also may result from a metabolic disorder, drug toxicity, or cerebellar disease.)
- Vision of 20/40 or less with corrective lenses, possibly caused by opacities in the cornea, lens, or vitreous humor, as well as by dysfunction of the visual pathway (retina or brain) (Cataracts or systemic disorders such as hyperglycemia may cause this.)
- Loss of central vision caused by macular degeneration
- Blind spots noted during confrontational testing, possibly resulting from vision field loss caused by glaucoma
- Loss of vision on one side of both visual fields (Called *homonymous hemianopia*, this condition results from occlusion of the cerebral arteries.)

PALPATION

To palpate the eye, have the patient sit comfortably or lie in a semi-Fowler's position. Using your thumb and index finger (or your index and middle fingers), gently palpate the eyelid and orbital rim, evaluating for firmness, mobility, texture, and smoothness. Then apply gentle pressure on the punctum, the tiny opening in the margin of each eyelid that opens into the lacrimal duct.

NORMAL FINDINGS

- Eyeball firm, smooth, and yielding slightly to pressure (somewhat like a soft rubber ball)
- Eyelid and puncta nontender and free of discharge

ABNORMAL FINDINGS

- Eyelid edema, cysts, and crepitus, suggesting mucocele, an infection resulting from sinusitis or obstructed sinus drainage
- Tenderness of the lids, possibly resulting from such disorders as seborrheic dermatitis
- Purulent discharge expressed from the punctum (This finding indicates dacryocystitis or infection of the nasolacrimal duct.)
- A palpable mass in the punctum, possibly indicating adenoma or adenocarcinoma

OPHTHALMOSCOPIC EXAMINATION

Assessment of the retina and optic disc requires an ophthalmoscope. For most patients, this examination is done only as part of the initial screening, unless the patient has a known or suspected problem involving the retina, macula, or optic disc.

Although the ophthalmoscopic examination is much easier to conduct when the patient's pupils are dilated, with practice you may be able to view the optic nerve and macula through an undilated pupil (especially in a lightly pigmented eye) in a dimly lit room. You or your patient may wear contact lenses during this examination. Your patient should not wear eyeglasses; you should wear them only if you are markedly astigmatic or myopic.

Begin by dimming the room lights. To check for a red reflex, which means the lens is free of clouding and opacities, ask the patient to stare straight ahead at a fixed point at eye level on the wall across the room.

Caution the patient to keep the eyes still; then approach him at an angle, starting about 15 inches away, moving toward him until the ophthalmoscope almost touches the patient's eyelashes. Set the lens dial of the ophthalmoscope at 0, and focus the light on the pupil of one eye. You should be able to see the red reflex as a distinct orange-red glow. Repeat the steps with the patient's other eye.

 EXAMINATION TIP

If you lose track of the red reflex, the light source has probably moved from the pupil to the iris or sclera. When this happens, redirect the ophthalmoscope and aim it at the pupil.

To view the retina and its structures, adjust the lens dial to the minus range (if the patient is myopic) or to the plus range (if the patient is hyperopic or aphakic). Turn the dial until the retina comes into clear view, and observe the color of the retina, checking for opacities, floaters, precipitates, and blood. Note any hemorrhages, exudates, or aneurysms in the background. Also inspect retinal veins and arteries for pallor, hemorrhage, distention, tortuousness, narrowing, and obliteration.

To view the optic disc, which is located on the nasal half of the retina, ask the patient to look straight ahead and focus on an object with the unexamined eye. If the disc does not come into view at first, follow the retinal arteries and veins to the point where they converge. Inspect the disc for a yellowish-orange to pink color, a slightly oval or round shape, and distinct borders (although these may be blurred on the nasal side). The temporal border may exhibit a grayish crescent, particularly in a myopic eye.

Observe the size of the physiologic cup, the yellow or white depression in the center of the optic disc. Compare the horizontal diameter of the physiologic cup to that of the optic disc. Locate the macula by looking temporal to the optic nerve to an area free of blood vessels. Highly light sensitive, the macula may appear darker and slightly more yellow than the retina. The patient may be unable to tolerate light focused on the macula for more than a few seconds.

Finally, view the fovea, a slight depression in the center of the macula used for sharpest vision. You may see a foveal reflex, a pinpoint white light reflected back to the ophthalmoscope.

Next, assess the lens, vitreous humor, and retinal structures. Begin by setting the lens dial of the ophthalmoscope in the plus range; then inspect the lens of the patient's eye for clarity and opacities. To assess the vitreous humor, observe for opacities, floaters, precipitates, and blood.

NORMAL FINDINGS

- Red reflex bright and regular
- Crystalline lens clear, translucent, and free of opacities
- Retina uniform red-orange tinge (It may appear darker and pigmented in dark-eyed and dark-skinned patients.)
- Macula free of blood vessels
- Physiologic cup half the horizontal diameter of the optic disc
- Vitreous humor clear, transparent, and free of precipitates and opacities

ABNORMAL FINDINGS

- Loss of the red reflex, possibly resulting from vitreous opacities, such as a hemorrhage
- Lens opacity, usually indicating cataracts (Typically, a cataract forms in the center of the lens [nuclear cataract] or at the periphery [cortical cataract].)
- Retinal abnormalities, such as granular areas, perivascular exudates, and hemorrhages at the optic fundus (These may result from infection, as with cytomegalovirus [CMV].)
- Retinal detachment, pallor, breaks, or folds, possibly resulting from diabetic retinopathy, vascular occlusion, or retinal or macular degeneration
- Retinal hemorrhages and narrowing, obliteration, dilation, or tortuousness of the retinal vessels, possibly resulting from retinal vascular occlusion or diabetic retinopathy (See 🔍 Diabetes Mellitus.)

🔍 DISORDER CLOSE-UP

DIABETES MELLITUS

A chronic disease complex of insulin deficiency or resistance characterized by a disturbance in the metabolism of carbohydrates, proteins, and fats, diabetes mellitus occurs in two forms: type 1, previously termed *insulin-dependent diabetes mellitus* or *juvenile-onset diabetes mellitus,* and type 2, previously termed *non–insulin-dependent diabetes mellitus* or *maturity-onset diabetes mellitus.* The exact cause of diabetes mellitus is unknown. Genetic factors and a faulty autoimmune response are thought to play a major role in type 1 diabetes mellitus, whereas genetics and obesity are considered risk factors for type 2 diabetes mellitus.

Pathophysiology

Insulin deficiency or resistance diminishes the use of glucose by the cells, leading to an increased blood glucose level, protein loss from body tissues, and increased mobilization of fats from storage areas. This results in abnormal fat metabolism and lipid deposits in vascular walls, causing atherosclerosis.

As blood glucose level rises, glucose enters the kidney tubules and spills into the urine (usually

continued

DISORDER CLOSE-UP—cont'd

when the blood glucose level reaches 180 mg/dl). Because glucose cannot diffuse through the cell wall without insulin, the osmotic pressure of extracellular fluid rises, causing water to leave the cells and subsequent tissue dehydration. Water is lost in the urine because the osmotic effect of glucose in the kidney tubules prevents tubular reabsorption of fluids. Thus the patient with diabetes mellitus experiences dehydration associated with hypovolemia.

The body attempts to supply glucose to the cells by shifting from metabolizing carbohydrates to metabolizing fats for energy. This leads to increased ketone production, which results in ketosis. Ketones are excreted in the urine. Sodium is also excreted, causing the blood sodium concentration to decrease. Hydrogen ions then replace sodium, triggering metabolic acidosis.

Type 1 diabetes mellitus
In type 1 diabetes mellitus, a marked decrease or absence of functioning beta cells (the insulin-secreting cells of the pancreas) leads to a lack of insulin and a rise in the blood glucose level. Type 1 diabetes mellitus typically comes on suddenly and causes severe symptoms.

Type 2 diabetes mellitus
In type 2 diabetes mellitus, the pancreas may produce normal, decreased, or even increased amounts of insulin, but the patient has a decreased response to it (insulin resistance). Typically, symptoms are vague and develop gradually.

Characteristic findings
Expect health history and physical examination findings to vary among patients with diabetes mellitus, depending on the extent and severity of the disease. Use the following information to help distinguish between expected and unexpected findings:

Health history
Type 1 diabetes mellitus
- Early onset (age 40 or younger)
- Frequent urination (polyuria)
- Extreme thirst (polydipsia)
- Exaggerated hunger (polyphagia)
- Weight loss despite increased food intake
- Extreme fatigue
- Weakness

Type 2 diabetes mellitus
- Late onset (typically older than age 40, although an increased prevalence of the disease is seen among children and adolescents between 10 and 19 years old who are obese and have a strong family history)
- Family history of diabetes mellitus
- Obesity
- History of gestational diabetes or delivery of newborn over 9 lb
- History of other diseases, such as severe viral infection, autoimmune dysfunction,

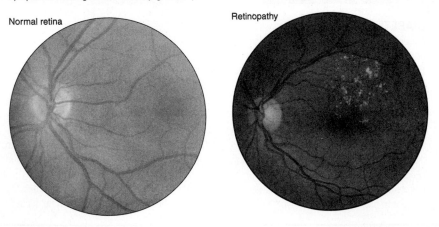

Normal retina

Retinopathy

continued

DISORDER CLOSE-UP—cont'd

other endocrine disorders, recent stress or trauma, or use of drugs that increase blood glucose levels

- History of frequent infections and slow healing
- Vaginal itching
- Pruritus
- Polyuria, polydipsia, and possibly polyphagia
- Sexual problems
- Vaginal discomfort
- Vision changes
- Tingling, pain, or numbness in extremities

Inspection
- Retinopathy
- Cataract formation
- Skin changes on legs and feet
- Muscle wasting, loss of subcutaneous fat, fruity breath odor (with ketoacidosis) in type 1 diabetes mellitus

Palpation
- Poor skin turgor
- Dry mucous membranes

- Decreased peripheral pulses
- Cool skin
- Decreased reflexes

Vital signs
- Orthostatic hypotension

Complications
- Diabetic ketoacidosis in type 1 diabetes mellitus
- Hyperosmolar nonketotic coma syndrome in type 2 diabetes mellitus
- Cardiovascular disease
- Peripheral vascular disease
- Cerebrovascular disease
- Retinopathy
- Nephropathy
- Diabetic dermopathy
- Peripheral neuropathy (numbness or pain in extremities)
- Autonomic neuropathy (gastroparesis, nocturnal diarrhea, impotence, hypotension)
- Skin, urinary tract, and vaginal infections

- Retinal exudates, typically resulting from diabetic retinopathy, vascular occlusion, or retinal or macular degeneration
- Round, white or yellow retinal deposits called *drusen,* possibly indicating macular degeneration
- Swollen optic disc with engorged retinal vessels, whitish cotton-wool spots, and a macular "star" caused by exudates, typically resulting from hypertensive retinopathy
- Bulging optic disc (papilledema), resulting from increased intracranial pressure (ICP) secondary to a brain tumor, meningitis, or pseudotumor

EXPLORING EYE COMPLAINTS

Common eye complaints include discharge, pain, vision changes, and vision loss. The following section presents pertinent health history questions to ask a patient who reports one of these symptoms, explains how to focus your assessment when examining patients with these complaints, and provides their possible causes.

EYE DISCHARGE

If your patient complains of eye discharge, investigate further by asking the following questions:

- What color and consistency is the discharge? Is it clear or purulent? Thick or thin?
- Is the discharge coming from one or both eyes?
- Does anything reduce or increase the amount of discharge?
- Is the discharge associated with a particular time of day or activity?
- Does anyone else in your household have eye discharge or other eye symptoms?
- Do your eyes itch or burn?
- Are your eyes sensitive to light?
- Do you wear contact lenses? If so, what method do you use to clean them?
- Do you have a fever, cough, or runny nose?
- Do you have allergies?

Focusing Your Assessment

When examining a patient who complains of eye discharge, focus your assessment as follows:

- Examine the eye discharge for color, consistency, and amount.
- Inspect the conjunctiva for redness and inflammation.
- Palpate the lacrimal sac for tenderness, and try to express additional discharge.
- Test your patient's visual acuity to see if it has been affected by the condition that is causing the discharge.
- If the patient wears contact lenses, examine their condition. If the patient's lens cleaning solution is available, inspect the solution for cloudiness or discoloration.

Possible Causes

- *Acute bacterial conjunctivitis.* Sometimes called *pinkeye*, this infection causes a thick, sticky, purulent or mucopurulent discharge. The conjunctiva appears inflamed, with red, dilated vessels.
- *Viral conjunctivitis.* This infection typically causes a clear or yellow discharge.
- *Allergic conjunctivitis.* This condition typically causes a scant, stringy, white discharge.
- *Corneal injury or infection.* These problems typically cause a watery or purulent discharge. Vessels surrounding the iris may appear inflamed and dilated, and visual acuity may be affected. Corneal injury or infection may result from such conditions as eye trauma, prolonged wearing of contact lenses, or improper contact lens cleaning.
- *Allergy.* Some allergies cause a clear, watery discharge and red, itchy eyes. Symptoms typically arise shortly after exposure to the allergen.

EYE PAIN

If your patient complains of eye pain, investigate further by asking the following questions:

- How would you rate the eye pain on a scale of 0 to 10, with 0 representing *no pain* and 10 representing *the worst pain you have ever felt*?
- Are your eyes unusually sensitive to light?
- Have you had a severe headache, nausea, or vomiting since the eye pain began?
- Have you experienced any vision changes? For instance, have you had double vision or reduced visual clarity?
- Do you see flashes of light?
- Have your eyes been tearing excessively?
- Have you noticed any discharge coming from your eyes?

Focusing Your Assessment
When examining a patient who complains of eye pain, focus your assessment as follows:

- Inspect the conjunctiva, check for discharge, and assess the pupils and their reaction to light.
- Using an ophthalmoscope, check for the red reflex and examine the optic disc.

Possible Causes
- *Acute angle-closure glaucoma.* This disorder causes severe eye pain accompanied by blurred vision or sudden vision loss, severe headache, and nausea and vomiting. The patient may report seeing colored halos around lights. Circumcorneal redness is also common. Expect to find the affected pupil dilated and nonreactive to light. The ophthalmoscopic examination may reveal an enlarged physiologic cup (see ⟲ Responding to Acute Angle-Closure Glaucoma).

ACTION STAT

RESPONDING TO ACUTE ANGLE-CLOSURE GLAUCOMA
Sudden onset of severe, throbbing eye pain and unilateral vision loss are classic symptoms of acute angle-closure glaucoma. If a patient complains of these symptoms, you must act fast to prevent optic nerve damage and permanent blindness.

What to look for
Typical clinical findings may include the following:

- Sudden onset of severe, throbbing eye pain (usually unilateral)
- Sudden loss of vision, usually accompanied by nausea and vomiting
- Pain radiating to the face and head along CN V (the trigeminal nerve)
- Dilated conjunctival and episcleral vessels around the corneoscleral limbus
- Steamy or hazy cornea
- Fixed and moderately dilated pupil (4 to 5 mm)
- Shallow anterior chamber
- Extremely high intraocular pressure (IOP) as determined by tonometry (60 mm Hg or higher)
- Premonitory symptoms, such as blurred vision, decreased visual acuity, seeing colored halos around lights, and pain in the head

continued

ACTION STAT—cont'd

What to do immediately

If you think your patient may have acute angle-closure glaucoma, notify the physician immediately; then take the following steps to help reduce IOP and manage other symptoms:

- Give an osmotic beverage, such as 50% glycerin in water and lime or lemon juice. Usually the physician prescribes 4 to 6 oz given over cracked ice, to be sipped slowly through a straw. In many cases, giving an osmotic beverage terminates the attack.
- Be prepared to administer an intravenous (IV) carbonic anhydrase inhibitor (e.g., acetazolamide) as prescribed.
- If the carbonic anhydrase inhibitor is ineffective, expect to give an IV osmotic (1 to 2 g/kg of mannitol 20% solution in water).
- Administer ophthalmic beta-blockers (e.g., timolol maleate) as prescribed. These drugs lower IOP by reducing aqueous humor formation and improving aqueous outflow.
- As IOP decreases, administer a miotic agent (e.g., pilocarpine) as prescribed to improve aqueous outflow.
- Administer analgesic agents as prescribed to manage eye pain.
- Give antiemetic agents as prescribed to control nausea and vomiting.
- Administer an ophthalmic topical steroid drug (e.g., prednisolone) as prescribed to reduce inflammation.
- Frequently assess the patient's pain, vision, and associated symptoms, such as nausea.

What to do next

Once your patient has been stabilized, you will need to do the following:

- Frequently monitor cardiovascular, pulmonary, gastrointestinal, and mental status.
- Administer pilocarpine as prescribed to maintain a low IOP.
- Give 250 mg of acetazolamide (Diamox) orally two or four times daily as prescribed to control IOP.
- Keep the patient's head elevated at least 45 degrees to control IOP.
- Assess the patient for fear and anxiety, and allow the patient to express any fears and anxieties regarding potential vision loss.
- Provide support, information, and comfort measures as needed.
- Keep the patient informed of planned procedures, and provide the name and purpose of any prescribed medication.
- Prepare the patient for surgery (e.g., laser surgery, surgical iridectomy) as needed.

- *Acute keratitis.* This condition typically causes mild-to-severe eye pain accompanied by blurred vision, increased tearing and blinking, and unusual sensitivity to light. The patient also may report a foreign body sensation, such as sand, in the eye.
- *Infectious conjunctivitis.* This condition may cause mild-to-moderate eye pain, typically accompanied by discharge, sticky, encrusted eyelids, and reddened conjunctiva.
- *Uveitis.* This disorder typically causes eye pain and conjunctival inflammation, misshapen pupils, and slightly blurred vision. Ophthalmoscopy may reveal corneal inflammation and opaque deposits.
- *Injury by a foreign body.* This injury typically causes sudden, severe eye pain and a foreign body sensation. The conjunctiva usually appears inflamed, and the eye tears excessively. Usually, removing the foreign body relieves the pain. An irregularly shaped pupil may indicate a penetrating ocular injury. The pupil may also become miotic.

VISION CHANGES

If your patient reports a change in vision, investigate further by asking the following questions:

- Do objects appear blurry?
- Do you see flashes of light, halos around lights, or floating spots in front of your eye?
- Have you been seeing double? If so, are the images side by side or on top of one another? Do double images occur in one eye or both eyes?
- Have you noticed recent drooping of the eyelids?
- Have you been tiring easily or feeling weak?

Focusing Your Assessment

When examining a patient who complains of vision changes, focus your assessment as follows:

- Inspect the eyelids for symmetry and appearance.
- Perform the six cardinal positions of gaze test to evaluate the extraocular muscles.
- Conduct an ophthalmoscopic examination to check for the red reflex and assess the retina.
- Test visual acuity.

Possible Causes

- *Refractive error.* Most vision changes occur gradually and indicate the need for a refractive correction. Patients with a refractive error simply need a prescription for corrective lenses.
- *Detached retina.* Signs and symptoms include seeing flashes of light or floating spots in front of one eye. (The "floaters" occur as the retina pulls away from the choroid and vitreous humor leaks between the two layers, causing blood and tissue particles to "float" in the visual field.) The ophthalmoscopic examination typically reveals absence of a red reflex, an orange or red crescent-shaped retinal tear, and black retinal vessels. As symptoms progress, the patient may describe the sensation of a shade being pulled down over the affected eye. Unless treated, vision in that eye will be lost. Retinal detachment may result from head injury, eye inflammation, severe myopia, diabetic retinopathy, or age-related changes in the vitreous chamber.
- *Cranial nerve impairment.* Horizontal diplopia—seeing side-by-side double images—indicates impairment of CN III (oculomotor) or CN VI (abducens). Vertical diplopia—seeing one image above the other—signals impairment of CN III or CN IV (the trochlear nerve). Diplopia is caused by the inability of the extraocular muscles to control eye movements. The problem may be intermittent or constant, may affect near or far vision, and may occur in one or both eyes.
- *Head injury.* If your patient with double vision has suffered a recent head injury, investigate for early signs of increasing ICP, such as appetite loss, nausea, and vomiting.

- *Neuromuscular disorder.* If diplopia has had a gradual onset, find out if the patient has other possible signs or symptoms of a neuromuscular disorder, such as myasthenia gravis or multiple sclerosis (e.g., ptosis, eyelid drooping, generalized muscle weakness).
- *Lens impairment.* Double vision in only one eye suggests a problem with the lens and generally points to a cataract.
- *Diabetes mellitus.* Signs and symptoms include blurred vision, caused by the effects of fluctuating blood glucose levels on the lens. Diplopia can result from alterations in the oculomotor nerves caused by hyperglycemia. High blood glucose levels can also cause vascular congestion in the eyes, resulting in the appearance of halos, flashing lights, and dark spots.

VISION LOSS

If your patient complains of vision loss, investigate by asking the following questions:

- Do you have no vision at all, or can you see lights or shadows?
- When did you first notice the vision loss?
- Did it start suddenly or gradually?
- Is your vision impaired all of the time or mostly at night?
- Have you lost vision only in a part of your visual field? For instance, can you see objects directly in front of you but not those to the left and right without moving your head?
- Do you have a chronic medical condition, such as diabetes mellitus, hypertension, or AIDS, or a chronic eye condition, such as glaucoma or cataracts? If so, what medication do you take?

Focusing Your Assessment

When examining a patient who complains of vision loss, focus your assessment as follows:

- Inspect the cornea for clarity, opacities, and irregular red reflex.
- Evaluate the conjunctiva for redness and excessive tearing.
- Using an ophthalmoscope, inspect the retina for hemorrhages, tears, and exudate, and the optic disc for swelling (a sign of papilledema).
- Perform the confrontation test to check for visual field defects.
- Test your patient's visual acuity. If the patient cannot read the largest letters on the eye chart, ask if he can see your hand movement. If he cannot, shine a penlight into the patient's eyes and ask if he can detect the light.

Possible Causes

- *Diabetic retinopathy.* A common complication of diabetes mellitus, diabetic retinopathy causes gradual vision loss from damage to or occlusion of retinal blood vessels (see ▨ Determining Causes of Acute Vision Loss).
- *Cataracts.* Progressive opacification of the crystalline lens, usually with age, can cause a gradual loss of vision.

INTERPRETING ABNORMAL FINDINGS

DETERMINING CAUSES OF ACUTE VISION LOSS

Acute vision loss may be temporary or permanent and may range from slightly impaired vision to total blindness. Use the following table to help determine the cause of your patient's vision loss.

Characteristics	Possible Findings	Probable Causes
• Sudden vision loss • Floating spots or flashes of light preceding vision loss • Sensation of shade being pulled over eye	• No red reflex • Detached retina that bulges inward and appears translucent and rippled	• Retinal detachment
• Sudden vision loss • Sensation of shade being pulled over eye • History of hypertension, diabetes mellitus, or heart disease	• Loss of normal transparency of retina • Diffuse retinal hemorrhages • Dilation of retinal capillaries • Macular edema	• Retinal vein occlusion
• Central vision loss • Progressive blurring of vision	• Cloudy lens • White pupil	• Nuclear cataract
• Central vision loss • Report that vertical lines appear wavy and middle of visual field is fuzzy, smudged, or empty • Possible loss of color vision	• Proliferation of a ccessory blood vessels on retina • Drusen (hyaline excrescences) • Intraretinal or subretinal hemorrhages	• Macular degeneration
• Peripheral vision loss • Severe eye pain • Nausea and vomiting • Halos seen around lights	• Reddened eye • Middilated, nonreactive pupil • Hazy cornea • Enlargement of physiologic cup	• Acute angle-closure glaucoma
• Spotty vision loss, especially at night • Scotomas (blind spots in visual field)	• Reduction in the visual field	• Lesion in retina or visual pathway
• Poor night vision • Dry skin and hair; ear, sinus, respiratory, urinary, and digestive infections; inability to gain weight; nervous disorders; skin sores	• Corneal dryness and ulceration (xerophthalmia)	• Vitamin A deficiency

continued

INTERPRETING ABNORMAL FINDINGS—cont'd

Characteristics	Possible Findings	Probable Causes
• Night blindness followed by slow loss of peripheral vision, leading to tunnel vision • Possible hearing loss	• Shrinkage of optic disc (optic atrophy), narrowing of retinal arterioles, and spotty pigmentation of retina	• Retinitis pigmentosa
• Sudden, transient vision loss • Sensation of shade being pulled over eye	• Small, glistening, yellowish red crystals at the bifurcation of the retinal arteries	• Amaurosis fugax, a disorder associated with carotid stenosis, temporal arteritis, migraines, or papilledema

- *Age-related macular degeneration.* The loss of pigmentation in epithelial photoreceptor cells in the macula causes progressive loss of central vision. On examination of the retina, you may note round, yellow or white deposits.
- *Acute angle-closure glaucoma.* This condition typically causes severe eye pain and acute vision loss.
- *Advanced open-angle glaucoma.* This condition causes gradual, painless vision loss in which the patient develops tunnel vision.
- *Retinal vein or artery occlusion.* When a thrombus blocks blood flow in a retinal vein or artery, it causes sudden, painless vision loss.
- *Vitreous hemorrhage.* When blood fills the vitreous cavity, it may cause acute vision loss. This is typically associated with diabetic retinopathy.
- *Retinal tearing or hemorrhaging.* This problem usually causes acute vision loss. The patient may describe a dark curtain being drawn over the vision in one eye. This can be caused by aphakia, myopia, diabetes mellitus, or trauma.
- *Neurologic conditions.* Those that affect the optic nerve can cause acute vision loss. Conditions include occipital lobe lesions, transient ischemic attacks, and vascular occlusions.
- *Renal disease.* This problem can cause acute vision loss as a result of papilledema or hemorrhages seen with pyelonephritis, glomerulonephritis, and diabetic nephropathy.
- *Cardiovascular problems.* Carotid stenosis and other cardiovascular problems can cause acute vision loss as a result of atherosclerotic changes that interrupt the blood supply to the eyes or hypertensive retinal disease.
- *Vitamin A deficiency.* This condition typically causes poor nighttime vision.

EAR EXAMINATION STEPS AND FINDINGS

Ear disorders range from treatable conditions, such as acute otitis externa (inflammation of the external ear canal), to more severe disorders, such as Ménière's disease (a chronic disease of the inner ear). Besides causing pain, an ear disorder can affect hearing and interfere with the patient's ability to perform daily activities. Therefore make certain you are familiar with basic ear anatomy (see Structures of the Ear).

ANATOMY REVIEW

STRUCTURES OF THE EAR

This illustration shows the structures of the external, middle, and inner ear.

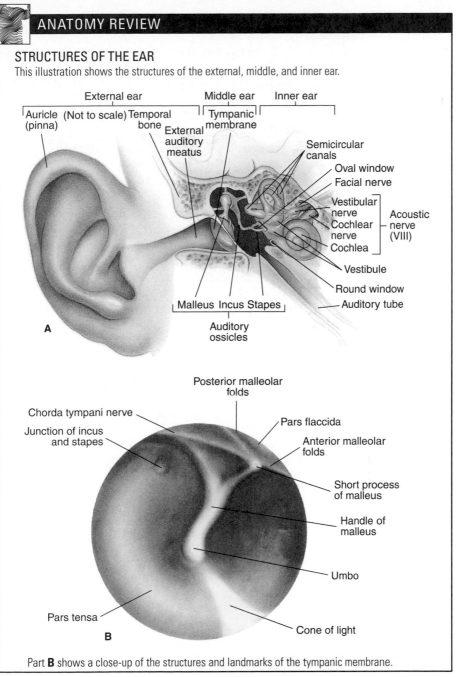

A

B

Part **B** shows a close-up of the structures and landmarks of the tympanic membrane.

A from Thibodeau G, Patton K: *Anatomy and physiology,* ed 5, St Louis, 2003, Mosby; **B** from Seidel HM, Ball JW, Dains JE, Benedict GW: *Mosby's guide to physical examination,* ed 5, St Louis, 2003, Mosby.

Preparation for accurate assessment of the eye requires the following steps:

- Seat the patient comfortably.
- Ensure adequate room lighting.
- Select a quiet area free of distractions if you are going to test the patient's hearing.
- Gather your equipment: penlight for inspection and an otoscope if you plan to examine the middle ear.

INSPECTION AND PALPATION

For optimal speed and efficiency, inspect and palpate the external ear at the same time. With your patient facing you, observe ear size and placement and assess the color and integrity of the skin on the ears. Then examine external ear structures, the auricle (pinna) and its parts (lobule, tragus, antitragus, helix, and antihelix). Observe the position of the ears on the head by imagining a line between the eye's outer canthus and the ear's pinna.

Next, palpate the auricle, checking for freedom of movement, tenderness, and lesions. Palpate behind the external ear for lesions and tenderness, and feel the preauricular and postauricular lymph nodes for tenderness and enlargement.

Using a penlight, inspect the external auditory canal. Check for nodules, cysts, abrasions, discharge, lesions, inflammation, and obstruction (see Essentials of the Ear Examination).

EXPERT EXAMINATION CHECKLIST

ESSENTIALS OF THE EAR EXAMINATION

Use this checklist to make sure you cover the most important steps when examining the ears.

❑ Check ear size, placement, skin color, texture, and integrity.

❑ Inspect auricles for mobility, color, discharge, cysts, nodules, lesions, and tenderness.

❑ Check auditory canal for nodules, cysts, abrasions, discharge, lesions, inflammation, obstruction, cerumen impaction, and tenderness.

❑ Inspect preauricular and postauricular lymph nodes for size, consistency, and tenderness.

❑ Check auditory canal for patency, integrity, cerumen impaction, swelling, bony overgrowths, redness, drainage, and pain.

❑ Inspect tympanic membrane for color, integrity, cone of light, bony landmarks, bulging, erythema, perforation, drainage, fluid, air, and lesions.

---

evolve Find PDF and PDA-downloadable versions of this Expert Exam Checklist online at http://evolve.elsevier.com/Mosby/expertexam/.

NORMAL FINDINGS

- Auricles similar in size and placement (They should move freely and painlessly. Older patients may have more prominent auricles.)
- Auricles free of scales, redness, and inflammation
- Skin over the ears dry, clean, and the same color as the skin on rest of the body
- Earlobes (lobules) soft and flexible (In an older patient, they may be pendulous.)

- Pinna aligned with outer canthus of the eye, deviating no more than 10 degrees vertically
- Preauricular and postauricular lymph nodes either nonpalpable or small, soft, and nontender
- External auditory canal free of nodules, cysts, and drainage
- Buildup in cerumen not impacted in the canal, although it may be present (Cerumen may be flaky, and its color may vary from creamy pink to black or brown. In an older patient, cerumen may appear dry from a lack of active sebaceous glands [see 🧩 What to Expect When Examining the Ears].)

NORMAL FINDINGS

WHAT TO EXPECT WHEN EXAMINING THE EARS
Use this brief review to confirm normal findings when examining the ears.
- Auricles equal in size and placement, symmetrically positioned, and freely mobile
- Skin over ears clean, dry, and same color as other skin; free of scales, redness, and inflammation
- Preauricular and postauricular lymph nodes nonpalpable or small, soft, and nontender
- External auditory canal patent and free of nodules, cysts, drainage, inflammation or obstruction; cerumen present but not excessive or impacted
- Tympanic membrane intact, shiny, translucent, and pearly gray; cone of light present; bony landmarks visible

ABNORMAL FINDINGS

- Dry, scaly skin on the external ear or in the auditory canal, indicating psoriasis or seborrhea
- Skin breakdown, abrasions, or erosions, possibly resulting from pressure caused by a person lying on the side for prolonged periods
- Eroded areas behind the external ears, sometimes developing from the pressure of oxygen tubing in patients who need chronic nasal oxygen therapy
- Painful, crusted lesions on the helix, possibly representing squamous cell carcinomas caused by frequent sun exposure (If the lesions have metastasized, nearby lymph nodes may be enlarged.)
- Hard nodules, or calculi, on the auricle rim or outside the opening of the external auditory canal, possibly representing gouty tophi (When you apply pressure to them, they may express uric acid, a white, crystalline substance.)
- Low-set ears, usually seen with Down syndrome or congenital renal disorders
- Tenderness of the external ear on palpation and movement, possibly resulting from otitis externa and accompanied by enlargement and tenderness of the postauricular lymph nodes
- Foreign body obstructing the auditory canal (A pea, a bead, or even an insect may completely or partially obstruct the canal. More common in children than adults, foreign bodies may become trapped in the canal and remain lodged there until removed. Sometimes, a foreign body leads to tympanic perforation.)

OTOSCOPIC EXAMINATION

An otoscope is used to examine internal ear structures. (For details on using the otoscope, see Chapter 1.) When examining a child, enlist the help of a parent or guardian (see 🔲 Performing an Otoscopic Examination in a Child).

LIFESPAN CONSIDERATIONS

PERFORMING AN OTOSCOPIC EXAMINATION IN A CHILD

Examining children's ears can challenge your assessment skills. If the child has symptoms of ear pain, he will likely already be uncomfortable and frightened. Therefore as you proceed with the examination, speak in soothing tones and prepare to enlist the help of a parent or guardian. Use the following guidelines to help keep the assessment on track:

- Save the otoscopic examination for last. Perform less invasive parts of a physical examination first to help establish rapport with the child and avoid upsetting him early in the process.
- If the child is small enough, have him sit facing inward on the parent or guardian's lap. Then ask the parent or guardian to restrain the child by wrapping his or her arm around the child's body, with the other arm holding the child's head.
- If the patient is too big for a lap, have him lie either supine or prone on an examination table. Ask the parent or guardian (and possibly a third person) to help restrain the child's head and legs, if needed. Under these conditions, expect to lie across the child's torso to immobilize it as you insert the otoscope.
- If the child is younger than 3 years, straighten the ear canal by grasping the lower part of the pinna and pulling down and back. This is because the ear canal is shorter and straighter at this age. As the child ages, the ear canal becomes more S shaped. Therefore, for a child older than 3 years, expect to pull the upper part of the pinna up and back as you would for an adult.
- As you insert the speculum of the otoscope in the ear canal, try to brace the lateral aspect of your hand (the one holding the pinna) against the child's head to prevent injury if the child suddenly moves.
- If the child is crying or screaming, the increased blood flow to the tympanic membrane may give it a red appearance. If you are skilled with the use of a pneumatic otoscope, use it to detect a lack of tympanic membrane movement—a sign of otitis media.
- When you have completed the otoscopic examination, comfort the child, or return the child to the parent or guardian for reassurance.

Before you begin the otoscopic examination, inspect the auditory canal for signs of inflammation and obstruction. If you note either condition, do not insert the otoscope because doing so could cause further irritation or force a foreign object farther into the canal.

If you have determined that you can safely insert the otoscope, pull the outer portion of the auricle up, back, and slightly outward (when examining an adult). Then examine the external canal, which normally contains hair and cerumen. If necessary, remove excess cerumen to improve your view of the tympanic membrane. Next, gently insert the speculum of the otoscope into the inner portion of the canal.

EXAMINATION TIP

Holding the otoscope with the handle up can provide greater stability during the examination. When you insert the speculum into the ear canal in this manner, you can brace your hand against the patient's head to prevent injury.

As you inspect the tympanic membrane, look for a cone of light—a triangular reflection visible in the left lower quadrant of the left ear and the right lower quadrant of the right ear. Then locate bony landmarks, such as the incus, umbo, and the handle and short process of the malleus.

If you have trouble seeing the tympanic membrane or its structures, gently reposition the speculum to get a better view. (Inner ear structures, such as the vestibule, semicircular canal, and cochlea, are not visible for examination.)

NORMAL FINDINGS
- Tympanic membrane intact and pearly gray
- Visible bony landmarks, such as the incus, umbo, and handle and short process of the malleus (In an older patient, these landmarks may be more pronounced because of sclerosis or atrophy.)

ABNORMAL FINDINGS
- Lesions in the canal, possibly representing boils or herpes vesicles
- Cerumen impaction, possibly blocking your view of the tympanic membrane (The impacted cerumen may vary in color and appear either shiny and wet or dry and hard.)

CULTURAL CONSIDERATIONS

Whites and blacks tend to have cerumen that is wet and dark, whereas Asians and Native Americans often have cerumen that is gray, dry, and flaky.

- Reddened tympanic membrane with purulent, foul-smelling ear drainage, suggesting acute otitis externa
- Bulging, reddened, or perforated tympanic membrane, possibly resulting from acute otitis media (This condition may be accompanied by dilated tympanic blood vessels and loss of bony landmarks. Another sign of otitis media is absence of the cone of light because of bulging or retraction of the tympanic membrane.)
- Perforated eardrum, appearing as a hole in the center of the tympanic membrane or extending to its margins (Drainage may seep through the perforation. If the perforation stems from an infection, such as otitis media, you may see a reddened ring around it.)
- Serous, amber fluid and air behind the tympanic membrane, resulting from serous effusion (This condition is caused by viral infection or barotrauma experienced during diving or air flight.)
- Vesicles on the tympanic membrane, typically reflecting bullous myringitis, a viral infection that often accompanies acute otitis media and may cause bloody ear discharge

EXPLORING EAR COMPLAINTS

Common ear complaints include ear pain, ear discharge, hearing loss, and vertigo. The following section presents pertinent health history questions to ask a patient who reports one of these symptoms, explains how to focus your physical examination appropriately, and lists possible causes for each complaint.

EAR PAIN

If your patient complains of ear pain, investigate further by asking the following questions:
- When did you first notice the pain?
- Is the pain constant or intermittent?
- How would you rate it on a scale of 0 to 10, with 0 representing *no pain* and 10 representing *the worst pain you have ever felt*?
- Does anything seem to make the pain better or worse?
- Have you recently been exposed to very loud noise, suffered an ear or a head injury, or had a foreign object inserted in your ear?
- Have you experienced fever, chills, or upper respiratory symptoms lately?
- Have you noticed any hearing loss, ringing in the ears, or dizziness?
- Do you have a sensation of fullness in your ears?
- Have you noticed any ear discharge? If so, what color was it? Was it clear or cloudy? Did it appear bloody?

Focusing Your Assessment

When examining a patient who complains of ear pain, focus your assessment as follows:
- Take the patient's temperature to check for fever (possibly indicating an ear infection).
- Palpate the external ear and mastoid process for tenderness.
- Assess the preauricular and postauricular lymph nodes for enlargement and tenderness.
- Using an otoscope, check the auditory canal for redness, drainage, trauma, and lesions (e.g., vesicles or papules).
- Gently insert the speculum and examine the canal from the meatus to the tympanic membrane. Assess the tympanic membrane for redness, bulging, perforation, and loss of bony landmarks. Also check for vesicles, fluid, or air bubbles.

Possible Causes

- *Acute otitis externa.* This condition can cause severe ear pain that typically worsens on palpation and is accompanied by a mild hearing loss; tinnitus; dizziness; purulent, foul-smelling ear discharge; and enlarged, possibly tender, postauricular lymph nodes. Otoscopic findings include inflammation of the auditory canal, possibly with abrasions or lesions, and a reddened tympanic membrane.
- *Bullous myringitis.* This disorder may cause sudden, severe ear pain with bloody ear discharge. Vesicles may appear on the tympanic membrane.
- *Acute otitis media.* This condition causes ear pain, fever, and chills. If the tympanic membrane ruptures, the patient may describe a popping sensation in the ear, followed by some relief from the pain. Otoscopic examination may reveal bulging, redness, and possibly perforation of the tympanic membrane,

with loss of bony landmarks and dilation of tympanic vessels. After membrane rupture, the ear canal appears normal and is nontender on palpation.
- *Serous effusion.* This condition causes ear pain, accompanied by serous amber fluid and air behind the tympanic membrane, mild hearing loss, a popping sensation, and a feeling of fullness in the ear.

EAR DISCHARGE
If your patient complains of ear discharge, investigate further by asking the following questions:
- What color and consistency is the discharge? Is it clear, purulent, or bloody? Is it thick or thin?
- Is the discharge coming from one ear or both ears?
- When did you first notice the discharge?
- Does anything seem to make it better or worse?
- Does the discharge tend to appear during a specific time of day or during or after a particular activity, such as swimming?
- Do you have any ear pain?
- Have you recently had a head injury, been exposed to loud noise, or inserted a foreign object into your ear?

Focusing Your Assessment
When examining a patient who complains of ear discharge, focus your assessment as follows:
- Observe any ear discharge for color, clarity, consistency, and odor.
- If your patient has experienced a recent head injury, fluid draining from the ear could be cerebrospinal fluid (CSF). Use a test strip to check the drainage for high glucose levels.
- Examine the external ear and middle ear for tympanic perforation, inflammation, and lesions.

Possible Causes
- *Otitis externa.* This condition causes a purulent, foul-smelling ear discharge.
- *Bullous myringitis.* This condition may cause bloody ear discharge.
- *Head injury.* A head injury may allow CSF to leak from the ear. The discharge will be clear, thin, watery, and odorless. It will contain high glucose concentrations.

HEARING LOSS
If your patient complains of hearing loss, investigate further by asking the following questions:
- Can you hear some sounds, or is your hearing completely lost?
- Have you lost hearing in both ears?
- Did the hearing loss occur suddenly or gradually?
- Does anything seem to make the condition better or worse?
- Do you have ear pain or discharge?
- Do you have a sensation of pressure or fullness in your ears?
- Do you get frequent ear infections?

- Have you recently been exposed to loud noises or inserted a foreign object in your ear?
- Are you taking any medications?

(Note: If the patient's hearing loss is severe, you may have to ask any questions in writing or by using another form of nonverbal communication.)

Focusing Your Assessment

When examining a patient who complains of hearing loss, focus your assessment as follows:

- Inspect the external auditory canal for discharge and cerumen impaction.
- Using an otoscope, examine the tympanic membrane for perforation, redness, bulging, scarring, or an air-fluid level (which indicates air bubbles).
- Use the whisper test or ticking-watch test to assess the extent of the patient's hearing loss.
- Perform Weber's test and the Rinne test to check for sensorineural and conductive loss.

Possible Causes

- *Injury.* Many injuries can cause hearing loss, including exposure to loud noise, tympanic perforation, repeated infections of the middle ear, cerumen impaction, or serous effusion (indicated by air bubbles behind the tympanic membrane).
- *Age-related changes* (See Determining Causes of Hearing Loss.)

LIFESPAN CONSIDERATIONS

In older adults, hearing loss commonly is sensorineural and results in difficulty hearing high-pitched sounds or the sound combinations *oso* and *ofo.* Whatever its cause, hearing loss requires further evaluation.

INTERPRETING ABNORMAL FINDINGS

DETERMINING CAUSES OF HEARING LOSS

Hearing loss may have a sudden or gradual onset and may involve one or both ears. Use the following table to help pinpoint the cause of your patient's hearing loss.

Characteristics	Possible Findings	Probable Causes
• Progressive hearing loss (usually unilateral) • Sudden, recurrent attacks of vertigo accompanied by nausea and vomiting • Tinnitus (may be constant or intermittent) • Pressure or fullness in affected ear	• Loss or impairment of thermally induced nystagmus (as shown by caloric testing) • Decreased air and bone conduction (as shown by audiometry) • Nystagmus • Unilateral or bilateral sensorineural hearing loss	• Meniere's disease

continued

INTERPRETING ABNORMAL FINDINGS—cont'd

Characteristics	Possible Findings	Probable Causes
• Hearing loss of gradual onset • Possible nausea and vomiting	• Bilateral hearing loss affecting both auditory and vestibular portions of inner ear	• Ototoxicity from such drugs as salicylate agents, aminoglycoside medications, diuretic drugs, or antineoplastic agents
• Hearing loss most pronounced when source of sound is near auditory canal • Tinnitus • Dizziness • Possible facial numbness and asymmetry	• Sensorineural hearing loss • Tumor within ear (as shown by magnetic resonance imaging or computed tomography)	• Acoustic neuroma (tumor of CN VIII)
• Unilateral hearing loss • Pain, tinnitus, and fullness or pressure in affected ear	• Cerumen buildup in auditory canal • Inability to visualize tympanic membrane	• Excessive or impacted cerumen
• Unilateral hearing loss • Acute onset of severe vertigo • Nystagmus • Tinnitus • Nausea and vomiting	• Sensorineural hearing loss • Serous or purulent ear drainage	• Labyrinthitis

VERTIGO

If your patient complains of vertigo, an abnormal sensation of movement or spinning, investigate further by asking the following questions:
- How many episodes of vertigo have you had?
- When did the first episode occur?
- How often do the episodes happen? How long do they last?
- Can you describe the sensation in detail? For instance, do you feel as if you are spinning around the room or as if the room is spinning around you?
- Does anything decrease the sensation or make it stop, such as sitting or lying down? Does anything make it worse, such as a particular movement?
- Have you ever lost consciousness or fallen during an episode of vertigo?
- Have you noticed a recent hearing loss, ringing in your ears, or involuntary eye movements?
- Have you experienced recent nausea or vomiting?

Focusing Your Assessment

When examining a patient who complains of vertigo, focus your assessment as follows:

- Rule out other disorders that cause light-headedness or fainting, such as cardiac arrhythmias.
- Check blood pressure with the patient lying down, sitting, and standing. A drop of 20 mm Hg or more in systolic pressure when the patient rises from a lying or sitting position suggests orthostatic hypotension, a cause of dizziness often related to hydration status and use of such medications as antihypertensive agents.
- Auscultate heart sounds to help rule out cardiac arrhythmias and other heart problems. Check for rhythm irregularities and extra heart sounds (S_3 or S_4) or murmurs.
- If possible, obtain an electrocardiogram (ECG).
- Evaluate the patient's respiratory rate and pattern. Hyperventilation, resulting in hypocapnia (carbon dioxide deficiency in the blood) or hypoxia (reduced oxygen supply to tissues), can cause light-headedness or dizziness.
- Check for nystagmus, which may reflect a vestibular (inner ear) disturbance. To do this, have the patient tilt the head backward and forward or move it from side to side while sitting. Watch for involuntary, rhythmic eye movements, which may be horizontal, vertical, or rotating. Then have the patient lie flat and turn onto one side and then the other. Ask whether these movements produce vertigo or nausea. Be prepared in case these movements cause vomiting.

Possible Causes
- *Acute labyrinthitis.* An inflammation of the labyrinth of the inner ear, this condition begins suddenly and lasts hours or days. It can cause nystagmus, which you may observe as the patient moves the head forward and backward or left to right. Occasionally, acute labyrinthitis causes nausea and vomiting.
- *Ménière's disease.* This disorder produces chronic, recurrent episodes of vertigo accompanied by tinnitus, pressure or fullness in the ears, and nausea or vomiting. Although it may wax and wane in severity, it ultimately progresses, leading to unilateral or bilateral sensorineural hearing loss.
- *Benign positional vertigo.* A patient with this condition experiences sudden, transient vertigo when rolling over to the side or lifting the head. Symptoms come on suddenly and last only seconds to minutes. Nausea and vomiting occasionally may occur, but hearing is not affected. Sometimes, benign positional vertigo indicates vertebrobasilar insufficiency or cervical spine dysfunction.
- *Acoustic neuroma.* A benign tumor, acoustic neuroma causes repeated episodes of vertigo, imbalance, unsteady gait, tinnitus, and sensorineural hearing loss. The tumor develops from CN VIII (the acoustic nerve) and grows in the auditory canal. Symptoms may progress to include paresthesias and gait disturbances.

CHAPTER 6

Examining the Chest and Back

A ccurate assessment of the chest and back requires a sound knowledge of the cardiac, respiratory, and musculoskeletal systems, as well as the digestive, neurologic, and renal systems (see 🔲 Structures of the Thorax).

ANATOMY REVIEW

STRUCTURES OF THE THORAX

The following illustrations present an overview of anterior and posterior thoracic landmarks and structures, the lungs, and the heart. Be sure you are familiar with all the structures of the thorax before undertaking a thorough assessment of your patient.

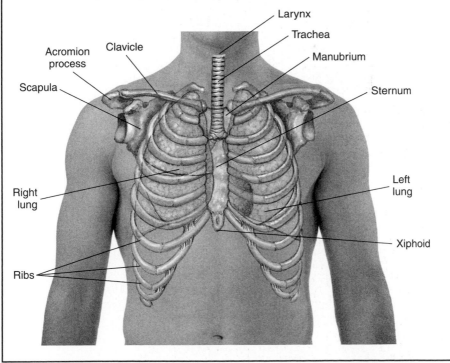

continued

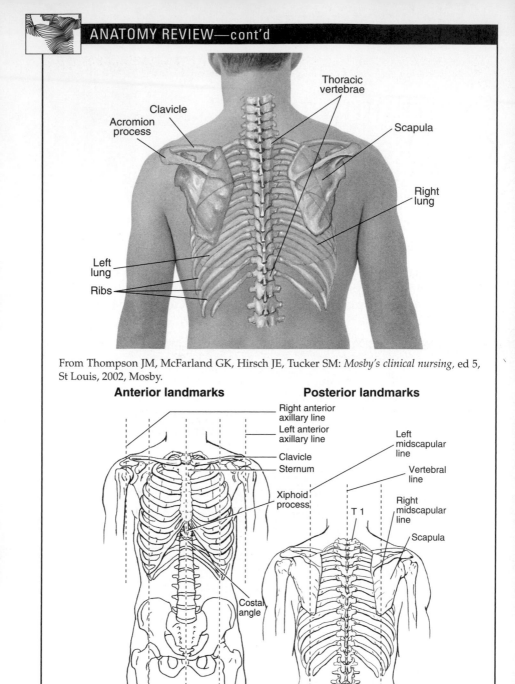

From Thompson JM, McFarland GK, Hirsch JE, Tucker SM: *Mosby's clinical nursing,* ed 5, St Louis, 2002, Mosby.

continued

Anatomy of the heart

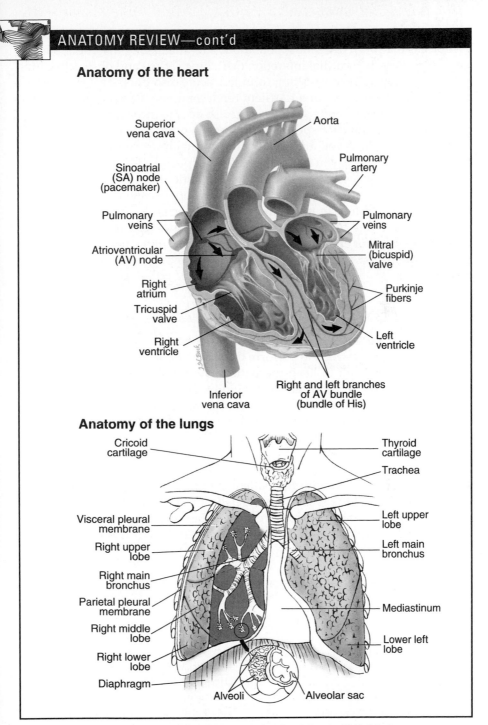

Anatomy of the lungs

From Thibodeau G, Patton K: *Anatomy and physiology*, ed 5, St Louis, 2003, Mosby.

In addition, you must be able to differentiate quickly between signs and symptoms that warn of serious, potentially life-threatening disorders, such as angina pectoris, myocardial infarction (MI), lung cancer, and obstructive lung disease, as well as those resulting from less acute disorders, such as a chronic musculoskeletal problem or a transient renal condition. Because the chest and back involve so many body systems, you also need to incorporate your examination findings with corresponding findings in other regions of the patient's body. For example, if you auscultate an abnormal heart sound that is consistent with heart failure, you need to look for peripheral edema (another sign of heart failure) when you assess the lower extremities later.

Throughout the assessment, be sure to keep pertinent points of your patient's health history in mind and focus on specific complaints the patient has identified while giving her history. You may want to combine some assessment steps for efficiency and accuracy; for example, performing inspection and palpation simultaneously before you move on to percussion and auscultation.

EXAMINATION STEPS AND FINDINGS

In preparation for assessment of the chest and back, make sure you have an appropriate room in which to perform the examination. It should be quiet and private, warm enough to keep the patient comfortable, and well lit. Bright, tangential lighting is important to highlight chest movement. Many nurses find that a revolving stool on casters offers a comfortable, mobile seat during the procedure. Also assemble needed equipment. Make sure you have examination gloves, a stethoscope, a centimeter ruler, and a washable marking pen.

INSPECTION

Begin your examination with the patient sitting upright, unsupported if possible, and undressed to the waist. If the patient is too ill to sit upright, support assistance may be necessary. Work from the upper chest downward, comparing one side to the other (see ⬛ Key Examination Steps for the Chest and Back).

EXPERT EXAMINATION CHECKLIST

KEY EXAMINATION STEPS FOR THE CHEST AND BACK

Use this checklist to make sure you cover the most important steps when examining the chest and back.

- ❑ Inspect skin integrity and color.
- ❑ Inspect the shape and symmetry of the chest.
- ❑ Inspect the spine and scapula. Look for spinal deformities and unequal scapular height.
- ❑ Watch accessory muscle use.
- ❑ Inspect the precordium for pulsations.
- ❑ Assess anterior-posterior (AP) and lateral dimensions of the thorax.
- ❑ Palpate the chest and back for masses or deformity.
- ❑ Assess the range of motion of the back and spinal column.
- ❑ Perform a full breast examination.

continued

EXPERT EXAMINATION CHECKLIST—cont'd

❑ Assess the location of the apical impulse.
❑ Palpate the anterior chest for thrills, masses, and deformities.
❑ Check for tactile fremitus.
❑ Palpate or use blunt percussion at the costovertebral angle.
❑ Measure and evaluate respiratory excursion.
❑ Percuss the lateral back and chest to assess underlying structures of the thorax.

❑ Auscultate the anterior chest for heart sounds.
❑ Auscultate to assess lung sounds.
❑ Measure diaphragmatic excursion.
❑ Auscultate the chest and back for presence and quality of breath sounds.
❑ Evaluate voice resonance.

evolve Find PDF and PDA-downloadable versions of this Expert Exam Checklist online at http://evolve.elsevier.com/Mosby/expertexam/.

Chest

Inspect your patient's chest from the front, from the side, from behind, and standing over the shoulder, looking down over the patient's anterior chest. Inspect the skin of the chest wall for cyanosis or pallor, scars, wounds, bruises, lesions, nodules, or superficial venous patterns. Observe for red or reddish-blue coloration, excoriation, or exudate.

Note the shape and symmetry of the thorax from the front and back. Estimate the anterior-posterior (AP) diameter compared with the transverse diameter.

LIFESPAN CONSIDERATIONS

Older adults can develop convexity of the thoracic spine, called *kyphosis*. This posterior curvature of the spine increases the thoracic anterior-posterior (AP) diameter and shortens the thorax.

Look at the angle of the costal margins at the xiphoid. Observe your patient's muscular development and nutritional status by noting the presence of underlying fat and the prominence of the ribs.

Assess your patient's respiratory rate, depth, and rhythm or pattern of breathing (see Assessing Your Patient's Respirations).

ASSESSING YOUR PATIENT'S RESPIRATIONS

Use the following illustrated patterns to assess and identify your patient's respirations.

Eupnea		Normal
Tachypnea		Rapid rate

continued

ASSESSING YOUR PATIENT'S RESPIRATIONS—cont'd

Bradypnea		Reduced rate
Apnea		Absence of breathing
Hyperventilation		Deep respirations, near normal rate
Kussmaul's respiration		Fast and deep, with no pauses
Cheyne-Stokes respiration		Cyclic pattern of apnea and varied breathing
Biot's respiration		Fast and deep, with periods of apnea
Apneustic respiration		Long, gasping inspirations, with ineffective expirations

Do this without your patient's knowledge so that you will be sure she is breathing in the usual manner. Compare the length of the inspiratory and expiratory phases. Note any symptoms of distress. As the patient breathes, watch for symmetry of chest wall movement, costal versus abdominal breathing, the use of accessory muscles, bulging or retraction of the inter-costal spaces (ICSs), and pulsations or heaving. Observe for the cardiac impulse in the apical area, medial to the midclavicular line in the fourth and fifth ICSs.

Inspect the patient's breasts (both male and female patients) with the arms hanging loosely at the sides. Then compare the patient's breasts, noting their size, color, symmetry, contour, texture, striae, venous patterns, dimpling, and the presence of edema or areas of redness.

LIFESPAN CONSIDERATIONS

Female patients usually have fully developed breasts by age 14; however, by age 40, breast tissue begins to atrophy as glandular tissue shrinks. At this age, supporting ligaments begin to relax, and the breasts appear to "drop" or hang more loosely.

Examine the areolae for shape, color, and texture. Observe the nipples for color, size, inversion or eversion, retraction, deviation, or evidence of bleeding, cracking, or discharge. Ask your female patient to raise the arms over her head, press the hands against her hips, and lean forward from the waist. Assess the patient's breasts again, briefly, in each position. Finally, lift the breasts to assess their lower and lateral aspects.

CULTURAL CONSIDERATIONS

The age of breast development and the appearance of the breasts vary among ethnic groups. For example, girls of African ancestry tend to develop breasts at an earlier age than other ethnic groups and also have a higher prevalence of supernumerary nipples. Asian female subjects tend to have smaller breasts than other ethnic groups. The color of the nipples and areolae may also vary among ethnic groups (usually darker in dark-skinned individuals); however, in general, the nipples are the same color as the areolae.

During your breast examination, observe the patient's axillary and supraclavicular regions for bulging, retraction, discoloration, or edema. Also inspect the axillae for signs of rash or infection.

Back

Start by having the patient expose the entire back. Ask the patient to fold the arms across her chest; then move behind her. Inspect the skin of her back for texture, lesions, scars, or sinus tract openings (tubelike, inflammatory structures that suggest infection). Observe the skin over the iliac crests and sacrum for redness and other signs of breakdown. Note any redness or nodules near the coccyx. In bedridden patients, look for edema in the sacral region.

Note the shape of the thorax and any deformities. Observe the bony framework, including the *scapulae,* as well as the angle at which the ribs slope from the vertebrae.

Now ask your patient to extend the arms in front and lower them slowly to her sides. Watch to see whether the scapulae protrude outward from her back more than normal. This condition is called *winged scapulae.* While the patient breathes, inspect the movement of her posterior chest wall for symmetry, bulging, or retraction of the ICSs.

Next ask your patient to stand. Look at the overall body posture. Assess the spinal column for alignment. Make sure the thoracic and lumbar areas curve appropriately. Observe for any abnormal curvature, such as lateral displacement. Compare the contour of the patient's shoulders and symmetry of heights of her shoulders and iliac crests.

NORMAL FINDINGS

- Skin smooth and generally uniform in color, depending on exposure to the sun; no cyanosis
- No lesions, nodules, or superficial venous patterns

- Thorax basically symmetrical, with an AP diameter less than the transverse diameter (The shape varies somewhat with the patient's body build.)
- Costal angle 90 degrees, widening on inspiration
- Respiratory rate 12 to 20 breaths per minute
- Respirations regular and quiet, neither too shallow nor too deep
- Inspiratory phase half as long as the expiratory phase
- Chest expansion symmetrical in onset and depth during respiration, without the use of accessory muscles (Male patients tend to breathe abdominally, using the diaphragm, whereas female patients tend to use the costal cage.)
- ICSs neither retracted nor bulging
- Cardiac impulse visible in about half of adults (It may be displaced upward in pregnancy or to the right in dextrocardia [a rare anomaly in which the heart is located in the right side of the chest].)
- Breast shape convex in females and even with the chest wall in males (Right and left breasts may differ in size. Skin texture is smooth and contour uninterrupted. Striae may be visible from previous changes in breast size but should be bilaterally similar.)
- Breasts free from dimpling, edema, or red areas
- Areolae round or oval and comparable in size (Color can range from pink to brown, depending on skin tone and pregnancy history. Texture should be smooth, although a peppering of Montgomery's tubercles is normal.)
- Nipples the same color as the areolae (They are either everted or have a long-standing history of inversion. They are bilaterally equal, with no deviation. They display no retraction, bleeding, cracking, or discharge.)
- Axillary and supraclavicular regions free of rash, bulging, edema, or infection

ABNORMAL FINDINGS

- Jaundice, indicating liver dysfunction or biliary obstruction
- Cyanosis or pallor, possibly indicating compromised tissue oxygenation
- Scars, possibly resulting from past injury or surgical intervention
- Bruises, possibly suggesting trauma or a bleeding disorder (If the patient has a wound, note its location, shape, size in length and depth, and the condition of any dressing.)
- Lesion or nodule that has changed shape, color, size, or texture, has become ulcerated, or has started bleeding or itching (Although it may be benign, as in pigmented nevi or fatty deposits, these signs typically suggest malignancy.)
- Spinal deformities causing asymmetry of the thorax, suggesting scoliosis (lateral curvature of the spine), kyphosis (convex curvature of the spine), or another spinal disorder
- Barrel-shaped thorax, possibly resulting from underlying respiratory disease
- Structural deformities, such as pigeon chest (prominent sternal protrusion) or funnel chest (indentation of the lower sternum)
- Protruding ribs, possibly indicating malnutrition

- Tachypnea (increased respiratory rate), possibly indicating decreased blood oxygen levels, metabolic disease, anxiety, broken ribs, pleurisy, liver enlargement, or central nervous system disease
- Bradypnea (decreased respiratory rate), possibly indicating neurologic and electrolyte disturbances, infection, or oversedation
- Abnormal respiratory pattern, possibly indicating serious underlying disease (Examples include Cheyne-Stokes respiration [crescendo-decrescendo], Kussmaul's respiration [rapid, deep], and Biot's respiration [irregular, with periods of apnea].)
- Prolonged expiratory phase, possibly indicating asthma
- Use of accessory muscles, tachypnea, orthopnea, nasal flaring, pursed lips, and cyanosis, indicating respiratory distress (See Detecting Respiratory Distress Warning Signs.)

DETECTING RESPIRATORY DISTRESS WARNING SIGNS

If your patient is in respiratory distress, you will be able to observe several characteristic signs.

A person who is having trouble breathing, and who is using accessory muscles to do so, will look anxious. The nostrils will flare, and the person will look cyanotic around the mouth. You will see the sternocleidomastoid muscles visibly contracting.

You should also see retractions at the suprasternal notch, the intercostal areas, and the substernal area. Finally, you will notice that the patient's chest is expanded more fully than normal.

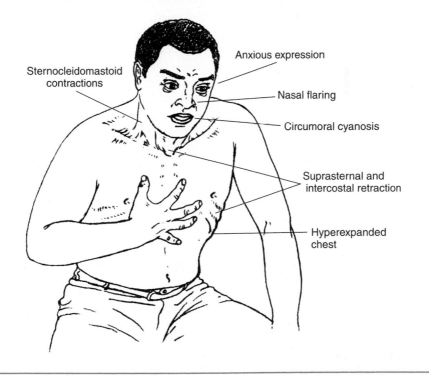

- Localized intercostal retraction during inspiration, possibly resulting from an obstruction in the large bronchi
- Generalized intercostal retraction during inspiration, indicating emphysema, asthma, or chronic bronchitis
- Intercostal bulging during expiration, suggesting emphysema, asthma, or massive pulmonary effusion
- Asymmetry, resulting from a collapsed lung or a mass
- Pulsations or heaving of the precordium, possibly indicating ventricular enlargement, valve disease, or aneurysm
- Areas of redness or tenderness on the female breast, possibly indicating mastitis
- Edema of the female breast, resulting from lymphatic blockade (from infection or carcinoma) or from radiation treatment
- Dimpling (*peau d'orange*) or unilateral discoloration or venous patterns on the female breast, possibly indicating malignancy
- Gynecomastia (enlargement of the male breast)
- Mastitis, cysts, or nodules involving the female or male breast
- Visible lymph nodes or edema in the axillary or supraclavicular regions, possibly indicating metastatic disease or infection
- Axillary rash, possibly stemming from a deodorant allergy or yeast infection

PALPATION

The chest and back are palpated with the patient in the same upright position as for inspection. In fact, inspection and palpation can be combined to decrease the time required to complete the assessment.

Chest

Begin palpation by examining your patient's breasts. Make sure your hands are warm. Palpation of male breasts can be brief but should not be omitted. Ask your female patient if she regularly performs self-examination. Give the patient instructions or reinforce her technique as you examine the breasts. Emphasize the importance of breast self-examinations in detecting cancer early in its development (see Performing a Breast Examination).

PERFORMING A BREAST EXAMINATION

To perform a breast examination, palpate each breast systematically with the pads of your fingers. Be sure to examine the entire breast, including the tail of Spence. If you feel lumps or lesions, be sure to describe fully their size, location, texture, mobility, and whether they are painful to the patient.

continued

PERFORMING A BREAST EXAMINATION—cont'd

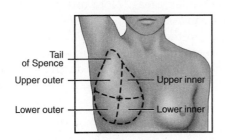

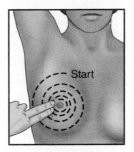

1. Before you begin, divide the breast into imaginary segments. If you find a lump or lesion, use these terms to describe its location.

2. Palpate gently but firmly in a counterclockwise pattern, starting at the outside of the breast and working slowly inward.

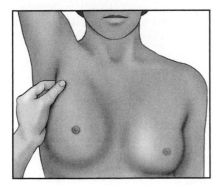

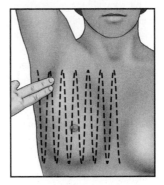

3. Now palpate the tail of Spence. Repeat the circular pattern, pushing deeper and more heavily. Do not lift your fingers off the breast as you move from point to point.

4. As an alternative, you can use a vertical-strip pattern. Start at the edge of the sternum and palpate in parallel vertical lines up one and down the next until the midaxillary line is reached. Be sure to include the tail of Spence. Finally, gently compress the nipple between your fingers to check for discharge.

Continue by palpating the lymph nodes of the axillae in both male and female patients. To examine the right axillary lymph nodes, support your patient's right forearm with your right arm and put the palm of your left hand into the axilla. Use the palmar surface of your fingers to roll the soft tissue downward against the chest wall and muscles of the axilla. Explore all sections of the axilla, and put your patient's arm through the full range of motion during your examination. Then repeat the process for the other axilla.

Next palpate the supraclavicular lymph nodes. First, bend the patient's head forward to relax the sternocleidomastoid muscle; then hook your fingers over the clavicle and palpate the entire supraclavicular area. Using both hands, palpate symmetrical areas of the thoracic muscles and skeleton. Feel the rib cage for symmetry, elasticity, and tenderness. Palpate the sternum and xiphoid process.

While palpating, pay attention to the patient's skin. Note its temperature, moistness, and turgor. Be alert for edematous areas. Note any pulsations, bulging, masses, depressions, or unusual movement.

Now palpate for conditions that relate to the patient's respiratory status. Assess for crepitus (a crackly, crinkly sensation) in the subcutaneous tissue, either localized or over the anterior thorax. Feel for vibrations during inspiration. Evaluate chest wall vibrations as the patient repeats certain sounds (see Palpating for Tactile Fremitus).

PALPATING FOR TACTILE FREMITUS

To palpate for tactile fremitus, place the palmar surfaces of both hands on the right and left sides of your patient's anterior thorax, at the second intercostal space (ICS).

Ask your patient to say "ninety-nine" repeatedly as you gradually move your hands over the patient's chest, systematically comparing the lung fields. Start at the center. Move toward the periphery, then back toward the center. Gently displace a female patient's breasts, as necessary.

Repeat this procedure on the patient's back, starting from the top of the suprascapular area to the interscapular, infrascapular, and hypochondriac areas at the level of the fifth ICS and tenth ICS, right and left of the midline.

You should feel vibrations of equal intensity on either side of the midline. Tactile fremitus is palpated most commonly in the upper chest near the bronchi. It is typically strongest around the second ICS, although the vibrations may vary in intensity with the patient's chest wall structure and voice intensity and pitch.

If you feel increased tactile fremitus in one or both lungs, your patient may have inflammation, infection, congestion, or consolidation of a lung or part of a lung. If tactile fremitus is diminished or absent in one or both lungs, this may indicate the presence of pleural effusion or pneumothorax.

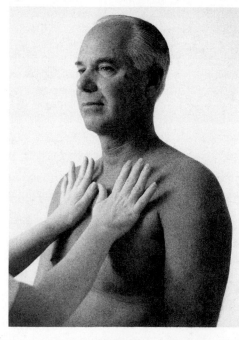

Assess respiratory excursion with the patient in the supine position. Place your thumbs along the patient's costal margins and your fingers along the lateral rib cage. Slide your thumbs medially, and raise a loose skinfold. As the patient inhales deeply, note how far your thumbs are separated by the chest expansion. Check the symmetry of respiratory movement.

If you think the patient may have a problem with lung expansion, assess respiratory excursion at two places on her anterior thorax and one on the posterior thorax. Even if you do not think a problem exists, you should be sure to assess respiratory excursion on the posterior thorax (see p. 150).

Now palpate for conditions that relate to cardiac status. With the patient in the supine position, stand at her right side and palpate the precordium using the palmar surface of your right hand. Begin at the apex, the fifth left ICS. Move to the left sternal border and then to the base (second left ICS). Feel for thrills (fine, rushing vibrations) or pulsations.

Note the location of the cardiac impulse, the point of maximal impulse (PMI). Positioning your patient on her left side may help you locate the cardiac impulse.

LIFESPAN CONSIDERATIONS

The point of maximal impulse (PMI) may be more difficult to palpate in an older adult with increased thoracic anterior-posterior (AP) diameter.

Palpate the epigastric area for pulsation. Now, with the patient in the supine position, complete your examination of the female breast. Have the patient raise one arm over her head. Place a small pillow under that shoulder and palpate the breast as described in the box on examination of the breast. Repeat for the opposite side.

Back

Continue your examination with your patient in an upright position, standing or sitting. Face the patient's back. Palpate the posterior thorax, noting any bulging, depressions, sinus tracts, nodules, masses, areas of tenderness, vibration on inspiration, or unusual movement. Palpate the scapulae, ribs, and thoracic spine for flexibility and tenderness.

Evaluate tactile fremitus in the posterior chest, comparing symmetrical areas of the lungs. Note any localized areas of increased or decreased fremitus. Move downward while noting where fremitus ends.

Assess respiratory excursion by placing your thumbs at the level of the tenth rib on either side of the vertebrae. The palms of your hands should lightly contact the posterior-lateral surface of the rib cage. Slide your thumbs medially to raise a loose skinfold between your thumbs and the spine. Watch your thumbs diverge during quiet, normal breathing; then ask your patient to inhale deeply. Feel for the range and symmetry of respiratory movement.

Palpate the costovertebral angle by placing the palm of your hand over the right costovertebral angle and striking your hand with the ulnar surface of the fist of your other hand (also known as *blunt percussion*). Repeat over the left costovertebral angle. Normally the patient should perceive this procedure as a dull thud. Make note if the patient feels any tenderness or pain (see Checking for Costovertebral Angle Tenderness).

CHECKING FOR COSTOVERTEBRAL ANGLE TENDERNESS

Check for tenderness at the costovertebral angle by percussing it during your assessment of your patient's posterior thorax.

Percussion at this site should not be painful to your patient. However, if the area does feel tender, you may need to consider other diagnostic tools to determine the source of discomfort, which may be kidney infection.

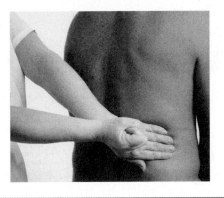

With your patient standing, check the range of spinal motion. Watch from behind while your patient bends forward (flexion). You can also place two to three fingers of the same hand adjacent to the spinal processes as the patient bends forward. Note their separation. Also inspect the spine again for normal and abnormal curvature.

Now ask your patient to bend back at the waist as far as possible (hyperflexion); then have her bend to each side as far as possible and rotate her upper trunk in a circular motion. Finally, ask the patient to lean forward and rest her weight on the examination table, with the arms straight and palms down. Palpate the paravertebral muscles and along the spinal processes. Note any tenderness, herniated disks, or muscle spasms.

NORMAL FINDINGS
- In female subjects, breast tissue dense, firm, and elastic (Generalized nodularity and tenderness is common during the menstrual cycle.)
- Axillary and supraclavicular lymph nodes not palpable

- Rib cage bilaterally symmetrical; ribs slightly elastic but sternum, xiphoid process, and thoracic spine inflexible
- Scapulae equal in height, with no "winging" on movement
- Ribs extended at about a 45-degree angle to the vertebrae
- Skin smooth, without lesions, scars, or sinus tract openings; skin over bony prominences intact; no redness or edema
- Skin warm and dry or slightly moist if the patient is anxious or has a fever; normal turgor with no edema
- No crepitus or vibration palpated on inspiration
- Fremitus prominent and symmetrical over large bronchi, except for a slight increase over the right upper lobe (Fremitus varies with the intensity and pitch of the patient's voice and chest wall structure and thickness.)
- Thorax expanded at least 5 cm and symmetrical in adults
- Costovertebral angle free of tenderness or pain
- Cardiac impulse gentle and brief, aligned with the midclavicular line in the fifth left ICS (It may be displaced upward in pregnancy or located on the right side in dextrocardia.)
- Abdominal aortic pulsation palpable in the epigastric region of a thin patient
- Diaphragm slightly higher on the right side because of the liver
- Spinal curve convex (outward) at the thorax area and concave (inward) at the lumbar area
- Spinal column with no lateral curvature
- Shoulders and iliac crests equal in height
- Back symmetrically flat, with a lumbar concavity convex on flexion (Expect forward flexion of 75 to 90 degrees. Spinous processes should separate. Hyperflexion is normally 30 degrees. Lateral bending is normally 35 degrees. The trunk should rotate 30 degrees in each direction.)
- Spinous processes with no tenderness or muscle spasms

ABNORMAL FINDINGS
- Nodules in the female or male breast, possibly indicating malignant tumor, benign cyst, or fibroadenoma (See 🔍 Breast Cancer.)

🔍 DISORDER CLOSE-UP

BREAST CANCER
Breast cancer is the leading cause of cancer deaths among female patients in the United States and Europe. Its exact cause is unknown. However, it has been linked to a number of risk factors, including a family history of breast cancer, early menarche, delayed pregnancy, and such environmental factors as exposure to radiation and use of hormone therapy.

Malignant cells usually originate in the epithelial tissue of the breast. The majority develop in the ductal system; the minority develop in the lobar system. The upper outer quadrant is the most common site of cancer. About half of all breast cancers are found here and in the tail of Spence.

continued

DISORDER CLOSE-UP—cont'd

The uncontrolled growth of cancer cells within the breast tissue begins with a single cell that divides, or doubles, in 30 to 210 days. After 16 such doublings, the mass reaches a size of 1 cm or more. At this stage, it can be clinically detected. As it continues to grow, the tumor may attach to the chest wall. It also may spread to the regional lymph nodes, primarily the axillary nodes. The cells metastasize easily, breaking away from the main tumor and traveling through the lymphatic system and bloodstream to other sites, such as the lungs, liver, and bones.

Characteristic findings

Expect health history and physical examination findings to vary among patients with breast cancer, depending on the extent and severity of the disease and its progression. Use the information that follows to help distinguish between expected and unexpected findings.

Health history

- Painless lump or mass in the breast
- Thickening of breast tissue
- Family history of breast cancer, especially among first-degree relatives, such as sisters, mother, and daughters
- Premenopausal female patient older than 45 years
- History of long menstrual cycle, early menarche, or late menopause
- First pregnancy after age of 35 years
- History of radiation exposure or estrogen hormone therapy
- History of preexisting fibrocystic breast disease

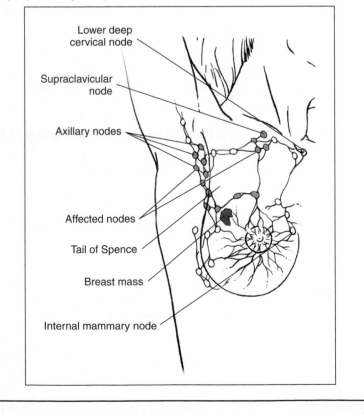

continued

DISORDER CLOSE-UP—cont'd

Inspection
- Nipple discharge (clear, milky, or bloody)
- Nipple retraction
- Scaling around nipple area
- Dimpling of breast tissue and peau d'orange appearance
- Increased vascularity
- Pain or tenderness
- Arm edema (may indicate advanced disease)

Palpation
- Hard lump, mass, or thickening of tissue
- Expression of fluid from nipple
- Enlarged supraclavicular and axillary lymph nodes, with possible palpable lumps

Complications
- Infection
- Bone metastasis, with decreased mobility and possible fractures
- Central nervous system metastasis
- Respiratory system metastasis

- Lymph node enlargement, possibly indicating infection or malignancy (Biopsy may be needed.)
- Chest asymmetry, possibly resulting from thoracic deformities or pneumothorax
- Tenderness in pectoral muscles, costal cartilages, or ribs, possibly indicating musculoskeletal inflammation, local trauma, tumor, or underlying pleural inflammation (as with pneumonia or pulmonary infarction)
- Crepitus, indicating air in the subcutaneous tissue from a rupture somewhere in the respiratory system (It may occur with emphysema or pneumothorax.)
- Intermittent bubbling sound only on inspiration and clearing with a cough, suggesting coarse crackles
- Scraping or grating sound on inspiration and possibly expiration, suggesting a pleural friction rub, caused by inflammation of the pleural surfaces
- Absent or decreased fremitus, suggesting bronchial obstruction, pneumothorax, pleural effusion, pulmonary edema, emphysema, or chest wall edema or increased thickness
- Increased fremitus, revealing areas of consolidation (as in pneumonia), heavy bronchial secretions, a tumor, or compressed lung tissue
- Respiratory excursion that reveals loss of symmetry or impairment of thoracic movement, suggesting underlying disease of the lung and pleura on one or both sides
- Forceful or widely distributed cardiac impulse, signaling increased cardiac output (as in anemia, hyperthyroidism, or fever) or left ventricular enlargement

- Thrills, possibly resulting from valve disease
- Pulsations in locations other than the cardiac impulse region, possibly indicating right ventricular enlargement, pulmonary artery dilation, or abdominal aortic aneurysm
- Skin breakdown, especially in bedridden patients and over bony prominences, possibly resulting in pressure ulcers
- Dependent edema in the sacral area of a bedridden patient
- Barrel-shaped thorax, associated with respiratory disease or possibly aging
- Chest structure abnormalities, possibly resulting from thoracic kyphoscoliosis
- Winged scapulae, indicating injury to the nerve of the anterior serratus muscle
- Horizontal slope to the ribs, possibly indicating emphysema
- Asymmetrical thoracic expansion during respiration, possibly resulting from a collapsed lung or a mass
- Intercostal bulging or retraction, possibly indicating pulmonary disease or bronchial obstruction
- Poor posture, with causes ranging from osteoporosis to poor personal habits
- Abnormal spinal curvature, possibly suggesting scoliosis, kyphosis, or lordosis (Scoliosis [lateral curvature] can be structural or functional. Kyphosis [accentuated convex thoracic curvature] may be observed in aging adults, especially female patients. Lordosis [accentuated concave lumbar curvature] occurs in pregnancy and obesity.)
- Abnormalities in shoulder contour and height, suggesting spinal column misalignment or shoulder dislocation
- Unequal heights of the iliac crests, possibly suggesting legs of different lengths or a deformity in the hips
- Persistence of lumbar concavity and failure of the spinous processes to separate on flexion, suggesting arthritis of the spine (spondylitis)
- Decreased spinal mobility, possibly resulting from degenerative joint disease or ankylosing spondylitis
- Spinal tenderness, possibly suggesting rheumatoid arthritis, osteoporosis, infection, or malignancy involving the spine
- Herniated intervertebral disks, producing tenderness of the spinous processes, intervertebral joints, sacroiliac notch, and sciatic nerve, as well as paravertebral muscle spasm and tenderness
- Costovertebral angle tenderness, possibly indicating kidney infection

PERCUSSION

Percussion of the chest and back is used to identify the left ventricular border of the heart, the depth of diaphragmatic excursion in the upper abdomen during breathing, the border between the right lung and the liver, and the border between the left lung and the stomach. Percussion can be used to help identify disorders that impair lung ventilation, such as stomach distention, hemothorax from postthoracotomy bleeding, lobar consolidation, and pneumothorax.

Chest

Begin by having your patient lie on her back in a comfortable position. You will be percussing from the supraclavicular area to the midabdominal area and out to the sides. If a female patient has large breasts, have her lift them while you percuss the area. If she cannot do so, you will need to displace each breast with your nondominant hand as you percuss with your dominant hand. Avoid percussing over the clavicles, breast tissue, and heart. Begin with the supraclavicular areas and alternate from one side to the other down the anterior chest, percussing over each ICS. Remember to percuss over the same area on each side for comparison (see Percussing the Chest and Back).

EXAMINATION TIP

PERCUSSING THE CHEST AND BACK

When percussing your patient's chest and back, work your way back and forth across the thorax in a systematic fashion, comparing one side of the body to the other as you go. Keep in mind that you will follow the same pattern when auscultating breath sounds. The following illustrations show typical percussion patterns for assessing the chest and back.

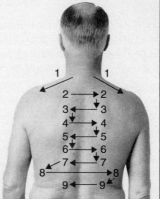

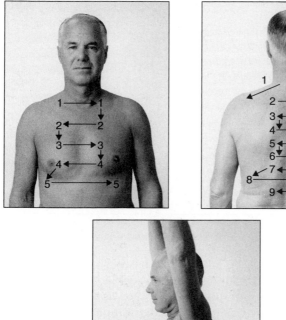

At the point on the right side where the sound changes from resonant to dull, you are percussing over the border between the lungs and the liver. As the diaphragm contracts with each inspiration, the lungs descend, and the border between the lungs and the liver moves down a few inches. This is called *diaphragmatic excursion* (see Measuring Diaphragmatic Excursion).

MEASURING DIAPHRAGMATIC EXCURSION

To assess diaphragmatic excursion, you will need a centimeter ruler and a washable marking pen. With your patient seated upright with the back exposed, ask her to take a deep breath and hold it. Then begin percussing at the base of the right scapula and move downward toward the patient's diaphragm.

When you detect a change from resonance to dullness, you will have found your first anatomic landmark. Tell your patient to breathe and place a mark at this site before continuing to the next step.

Now, ask your patient to exhale as much as possible and hold it. This time, begin percussing at your first landmark, and move upward on the posterior thorax toward the scapula. When you notice a change from dullness to resonance, you will have found the second landmark. Place a mark at this site; repeat this technique on the other side of the patient's posterior thorax so that you can compare measurements on the right and left sides.

Once you obtain your two landmarks, measure the distance from one line to the other to deter-mine diaphragmatic excursion. Normal excursion distance is 3 to 5 cm. Keep in mind that the diaphragm is usually higher on the right than on the left because of the position of the liver.

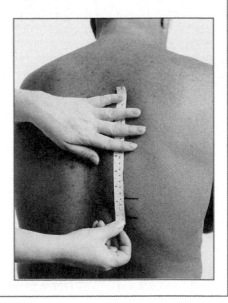

As you percuss down the left side of the chest, the sound changes from resonant to tympanic over the gastric air bubble of the stomach. Although x-rays are more accurate, percussion also can be used to identify the border of the left side of the heart to determine whether the patient's heart is enlarged or displaced. To percuss for the cardiac border, have the patient lie on her back, with the left arm over her head resting on a pillow. Locate the fourth left ICS along the axillary line; it should be just below the axilla. Starting at the axillary line, percuss medially toward the sternum, in the ICS. When the sound changes from resonant to dull, you have identified the cardiac border. Use a pen to mark this point.

Now repeat the procedure, starting at the fifth left ICS. Then use the sixth left ICS. Each time, mark the location where the sound changes. For a more detailed assessment, you can start at the second or third ICS. Because the sternum hides the right cardiac border, it cannot be percussed in most cases.

Back

To examine the back, ask the patient to sit with both arms crossed in front or resting on a bedside table. If possible, have the patient lean forward into her lap, with arms crossed and neck flexed. By separating the scapulae and ICSs, this position exposes more lung. Remember not to percuss over the scapulae or the spine.

As you percuss the back, you will again move from side to side to compare and contrast your findings. Percuss between the ICSs on each side. When you reach the lower back area, stand somewhat to the side rather than directly behind your patient. This hand position will feel more natural, and you will produce a clearer sound. Remember that, because your patient is breathing and the diaphragm is moving, you may not percuss a distinct diaphragmatic border.

With the same procedure you used for the anterior chest, measure for diaphragmatic excursion. Finally, ask your patient to rest an arm on her head, and percuss along the midaxillary line at 2-inch intervals.

NORMAL FINDINGS

- Band of resonance about 2 inches wide (also known as *Krönig's isthmus*) between the neck and shoulder on each side as you percuss the apices
- Resonant sounds over the lungs until you reach the diaphragm (This will be at about T10 on your patient's back. It may be one ICS higher on the right side because of displacement by the liver.)
- Area of dullness to the left of the sternum between the third ICS and fifth ICS that is produced by the heart
- Dullness over the diaphragm
- Diaphragmatic excursion about 1¼ to 2¼ inches and almost equal in length on both sides.

ABNORMAL FINDINGS

- Dullness over the lungs during percussion, possibly indicating a mass or consolidation (The dullness of right middle-lobe pneumonia typically occurs behind the right breast [see ◌ Pneumonia].)

DISORDER CLOSE-UP

PNEUMONIA

Pneumonia is an acute lung inflammation caused by an infection with one or more organisms, such as bacteria, viruses, and fungi. Pneumonia also may result from aspiration of food, fluids, or vomitus or inhalation of toxic or caustic chemicals, smoke, dust, or gases. The disorder may occur as a complication of immobility and chronic illnesses, and it often follows influenza. Pneumonia can involve lung

continued

DISORDER CLOSE-UP—cont'd

tissue in part or all of a lobe, or it can occur diffusely.

Pneumonia is most likely to occur when normal defense mechanisms are weakened or overcome. This is especially likely in a patient who has a decreased level of consciousness, is immunocompromised, or has a portal for microorganisms, such as an endotracheal tube.

In bacterial pneumonia, bacteria initiate a massive inflammatory reaction in the alveoli. When chemical mediators cause pulmonary capillaries and other vessels to dilate, they become more permeable to fluid, fibrin, and red and white blood cells, creating exudate. The exudate-filled airways and alveoli cause the normally air-filled lung tissue to consolidate, stiffen, and impair gas exchange. If pneumonia affects large areas of lung tissue, hypoxemia and respiratory failure can ensue.

In viral pneumonia, interstitial inflammation and desquamation occur in the bronchiolar epithelial and goblet cells and bronchial mucous glands, impairing mucociliary clearance. Eventually, the alveoli fill with exudate, which can diminish gas exchange. While viral pneumonia is usually mild and self-limiting, the patient can develop a secondary bacterial pneumonia.

Characteristic findings

Expect health history and physical examination findings to vary among patients with pneumonia, depending on the cause and severity of the disease. Use the following information to help distinguish between expected and unexpected findings.

Health history
- History of influenza
- History of exposure to noxious gases
- Immobilization
- Decreased level of consciousness
- Nasogastric tube feedings
- Endotracheal intubation and mechanical ventilation
- Complaints of fever, chills, sweats
- Headache, fatigue
- Chest pain
- Cough

Inspection
- Productive cough with sputum (color varies with type of infection)
- Dyspnea

Palpation
- Increased tactile fremitus
- Unequal chest expansion

Percussion
- Dullness over affected area
- Decreased respiratory excursion on affected side

Auscultation
- Crackles (coarse)
- Wheezes (sonorous)
- Egophony
- Bronchophony
- Whispered pectoriloquy

Vital signs
- Tachycardia
- Tachypnea
- Fever

Complications
- Septic shock
- Hypoxemia
- Respiratory failure
- Empyema, lung abscess
- Bacteremia
- Endocarditis, pericarditis
- Meningitis

- Hyperresonance over the lungs, indicating hyperinflated or emphyse-matous lungs (Hyperresonance heard on only one side may indicate a pneumothorax.)
- High diaphragmatic excursion on one side, suggesting a pleural effusion or high diaphragm, possibly resulting from diaphragmatic (phrenic nerve) paralysis, stomach distention (left side), hepatomegaly (right side), or significant atelectasis
- Bilaterally low diaphragm level at rest, indicating a depressed diaphragm, usually from a severely hyperinflated chest associated with emphysema or asthma
- Unilaterally low diaphragm level at rest, resulting from tension pneumothorax

AUSCULTATION

Ask your patient to sit up straight. If she cannot sit up, have the patient lie down and roll to one side and then the other side. Raise the head of the bed 30 to 45 degrees. In either position, ask the patient to remain still and breathe normally while you auscultate heart and breath sounds. Before listening, prepare the patient and her environment for optimal results (see ▨ Auscultating Heart and Breath Sounds: Tips for Success).

EXAMINATION TIP

AUSCULTATING HEART AND BREATH SOUNDS: TIPS FOR SUCCESS

General tips
- Make sure the patient is warm and relaxed to minimize shivering and movement, which can increase abnormal sounds.
- Avoid listening over clothing; place the stethoscope directly on the skin.
- If the patient has a hairy chest or back, moisten the hair to avoid extraneous sounds that you could mistake for abnormal heart or breath sounds.
- Try to minimize ambient sounds by closing the door to the hallway and turning off unnecessary machines. If the patient is mechanically ventilated, consider asking a colleague to manually ventilate the patient while you auscultate.
- Find anatomic landmarks, such as intercostal spaces (ICSs), to determine where you are listening at each point. Remember that many sounds, such as bronchial breath sounds, are normal only in certain locations.

Heart sounds
- With the patient in a supine position, instruct her to hold the breath momentarily as you listen for heart sounds. Signal the patient when to resume breathing.
- Listen to the entire precordium by inching from one spot to another to make sure that you have covered the major auscultatory areas.
- Take time to evaluate each area carefully before moving on. Once you have auscultated each area using the diaphragm, repeat the procedure using the bell of the stethoscope.
- When using the bell, remember to apply it to the chest wall lightly because excessive pressure will turn the bell into a diaphragm.

Breath sounds
- Have the patient sit upright, if possible, to listen to the anterior lateral and posterior thorax. Position the patient's arms over her head to listen to the lateral sites and folded across her chest for the posterior sites.

continued

EXAMINATION TIP—cont'd

- Use a zigzag motion when moving your stethoscope to each position to compare sounds on each side.
- Pay careful attention to areas where palpation and percussion revealed abnormal findings. If

the patient has dyspnea, auscultate these abnormal areas first (e.g., the lung bases) in case she experiences fatigue during the examination.

Heart Sounds

The heart makes characteristic sounds that reflect its activity. Auscultating these sounds carefully and identifying abnormal sounds accurately can detect a number of serious cardiac disorders (see Sounds of the Cardiac Cycle).

SOUNDS OF THE CARDIAC CYCLE

The sounds you hear while auscultating your patient's heart reflect the physical events happening inside your patient's chest. In a normal heart, those events produce two characteristic heart sounds: S_1 and S_2.

Just before S_1, the mitral and tricuspid valves are open, and most of the blood in the atria is filling the relaxed ventricles. The atria then contract slightly, pushing about 30% more atrial blood into the ventricles. This atrial contraction is called the *atrial kick*.

Now the ventricles contract, beginning the period called *systole*. Pressure in the ventricles increases rapidly, forcing the mitral and tricuspid valves to close. The *lubb* sound produced by the closing of the valves, S_1, is the first sound you hear in the cardiac cycle in a patient with a normal, healthy heart. Although the mitral valve closes about 0.02 to 0.03 seconds before the tricuspid valve, the time difference is so small that you hear only one sound.

As ventricular pressure continues to increase, it causes the aortic and pulmonic valves to open, and blood is pumped out of the heart into the lungs and aorta. Once the ventricle ejects most of its blood, pressure begins to fall and the aortic and pulmonic valves snap shut. The *dubb* sound produced by the closing of the valves, S_2, marks the beginning of diastole. The *dubb* of S_2 is slightly more highly pitched than the *lubb* of S_1.

S_1 and S_2 split

If enough time elapses between the closing of valves that normally close simultaneously, you may hear what is called a *split S_1* or *S_2*. The first part of the split sound is closure of the left-sided heart valves (aortic or mitral); the second part is closure of the right-sided heart valves (pulmonic or tricuspid). S_1 splitting may be normal or may indicate a conduction disorder, such as right bundle branch block. S_2 splitting that increases with inspiration and almost disappears with expiration is called *physiologic splitting* and is normal.

Before beginning auscultation, warm the diaphragm and bell of your stethoscope by rubbing them between your hands. You will use the diaphragm to hear higher-pitched heart sounds, such as S_1, S_2, murmurs of aortic and mitral regurgitation, pericardial friction rubs, and lung sounds.

You will use the bell to hear low-pitched sounds, such as S_3, S_4, and diastolic murmurs. As you auscultate, you will need to be familiar with chest landmarks to aid in positioning the stethoscope and documenting your findings (see How and Where to Listen for Heart Sounds).

HOW AND WHERE TO LISTEN FOR HEART SOUNDS

The following table provides tips on how to position your patient, what part of your stethoscope to use, and where to listen for specific heart sounds.

Heart Sound	Patient Position	Stethoscope Part	Where to Listen
S_1 (first heart sound)	Any position	Diaphragm	Heard best at apex
S_2 (second heart sound)	Sitting or supine	Diaphragm	Aortic area at second right intercostal space (ICS) to the right of the sternum Pulmonic area at second left ICS to the left of the sternum
S_3 (third heart sound)	Supine or left lateral recumbent	Bell	Apex
S_4 (fourth heart sound)	Supine or left semilateral	Bell	Apex
Murmur	High Fowler's and leaning slightly forward	Diaphragm and bell to differentiate between high-pitched and low-pitched sounds	Entire precordium Heard best over affected valve's auscultation site
Rub	Any position	Diaphragm	Entire precordium Heard best at third ICS, left sternal border

Begin auscultation by placing the diaphragm of your stethoscope over the patient's PMI, which is located at about the fifth ICS (left midclavicular line). Listen to the patient's apical pulse for 60 seconds, noting the rate, rhythm, quality of sound, and any extra or unusual sounds.

If your patient has a pacemaker, you will need to know its normal settings and whether it is a demand or fixed device to aid in assessing its function. For example, if you auscultate your patient's heart rate at 50 beats per minute (bpm), and you know her pacemaker is set to activate when the ventricular rate is less than 60 bpm, you can assume that the pacemaker is malfunctioning.

Describe the patient's rhythm as *regular, regularly irregular,* or *irregularly irregular.* In ventricular trigeminy, where every third beat is a premature ventricular contraction (PVC), you might hear *lubb-dubb, lubb-dubb-lubb* in a pattern that repeats itself. This would be considered a regularly irregular rhythm.

Atrial fibrillation, in which no pattern to the ventricular beats exists, is an example of an irregularly irregular rhythm.

If your patient has an irregular rhythm, you will hear the heart rate speed up and slow down as you listen. To get an accurate rate, you will need to listen for a full minute and carefully count the beats.

Keep in mind that some patients, such as those with a history of atrial fibrillation, normally have an irregular rhythm. To assess it accurately, you will need to know your patient's baseline rhythm and heart rate range. If you have trouble hearing the heart rate, find your patient's carotid pulse and palpate it as you listen with the stethoscope. You will hear the first heart sound, S_1, at the same time you feel the pulse.

Next, listen for heart sounds over the aortic, pulmonic, mitral, and tricuspid areas (see Identifying Key Cardiac Auscultatory Areas).

IDENTIFYING KEY CARDIAC AUSCULTATORY AREAS

When listening for normal and abnormal heart sounds, it helps to locate the aortic, pulmonic, tricuspid, and mitral valve auscultatory areas, as well as areas to where sounds can be transmitted, such as Erb's point. To identify these key areas, palpate and count the intercostal spaces (ICSs). Remember that you can easily locate the second ICS by sliding your fingers laterally from the manubriosternal junction—where the sternum meets the second rib. As you move toward the heart's apex, you may need to displace breast tissue with your nondominant hand to accurately count the ICSs.

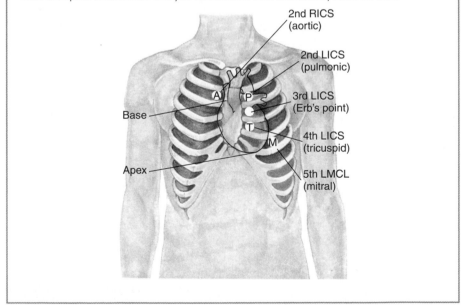

From Wilson SF, Giddens JF: *Health assessment for nursing practice,* ed 2, St Louis, 2001, Mosby. *LICS,* Left intercostal space; *LMCL,* left midclavicular line; *RICS,* right intercostal space.

Continue using the diaphragm of your stethoscope. Have your patient breathe normally, and spend 10 or 15 seconds over each area. Take longer if you hear something unusual.

Work your way down the left sternal border as you listen over each ICS between the second and fifth ribs. Remember that heart sounds may not be detected in exactly the same location with every patient. In addition, the angle of the heart can shift slightly in the chest if the patient has left or right ventricular hypertrophy, which will displace the best location to listen to the tricuspid and mitral valves.

Initially, focus on the S_1 sound. It will be loudest over the mitral and tricuspid areas. Listen to its intensity and for the presence of splitting. This is best heard at the left sternal border.

Next, focus on S_2, which is loudest over the aortic and pulmonic areas. To try to hear a split S_2, have your patient hold her breath for a few seconds while you listen; then have her exhale and listen again. You should hear the split during inspiration, and it should disappear during expiration. If the split occurs during inspiration and expiration, it is called *fixed splitting*.

Now check for S_3 and S_4, the extra heart sounds. S_3 is called a *ventricular gallop*. This faint, low-pitched sound is heard directly after S_2 and results from early, rapid filling of the ventricle with blood at the very beginning of diastole. It is heard best over the mitral valve area and sounds like *lubb-dup-ah.*

S_4 is called an *atrial gallop*. It is a low-frequency sound that occurs in conditions of increased ventricular stiffness. It is heard late in diastole, or just before S_1, and sounds like *ta-lup-dubb*. It may be hard to distinguish split heart sounds from S_3 and S_4. An occasional patient has both an S_3 and an S_4, producing a quadruple rhythm. If the heart is beating fast, you will hear one loud extra sound called a *summation gallop*.

To listen for an S_3 or S_4, have your patient roll partly onto her left side. This position helps accentuate a left-sided S_3 or S_4. Using the bell of your stethoscope, listen over the PMI. To help you determine whether you are hearing a split sound or an S_3 or S_4, have your patient sit up, lean forward, and inhale. Listen for the split S_2. Then listen while the patient exhales. If the split does not change, it may be either an S_3 or a fixed physiologic split.

S_4 is much harder to distinguish from a split S_1, but it is heard immediately before the S_1. Usually, a split heart sound is faster, and each part of the split has the same pitch. S_3 or S_4 may have a slightly lower pitch. Note the location you best hear the sounds and the timing, pitch, intensity, and effect of respirations. If the extra sounds differ from the S sounds in quality, pitch, and duration, you may be hearing a murmur. In addition, be aware that you may hear other sounds, including clicks, snaps, and rubs.

LIFESPAN CONSIDERATIONS

Heart sounds may be more faint in an older adult with increased thoracic anterior-posterior (AP) diameter.

Murmurs. Murmurs are turbulent sounds made as blood flows across a sclerotic (stiff) or incompetent valve or through an abnormal heart wall opening.

The turbulence is caused by disturbed blood flow through a small or rigid orifice. The smaller the orifice, the more resistance it creates and, often, the louder the murmur.

Most murmurs are associated with valve diseases, such as stenosis or insufficiency. Stenotic valves prevent forward blood flow. With valve insufficiency, or prolapse, the leaflets close improperly, resulting in backward blood flow.

Murmurs also can be caused by nonvalvular conditions, including ventricular septal defects (VSDs), sclerotic or aneurysmal arteries, hyperkinetic states, anemia, pregnancy, patent ductus arteriosus, narrowing of the aorta, and hypertrophic obstructive cardiomyopathy (HOCM), also known as *idiopathic hypertrophic subaortic stenosis* (IHSS).

Characterize a murmur by its timing, location, radiation, quality, pitch, shape, and duration. Start by identifying the murmur as systolic or diastolic. To do so, palpate your patient's carotid pulse as you listen. Systolic murmurs occur with S_1, or immediately after you feel the pulse, before S_2. Usually, they are harsh, high-pitched sounds in a *lubb-shh-dubb* pattern. If the patient has valve disease, the sound is produced either from forward flow through stenotic valves open during systole (the aortic and pulmonic) or from backward flow through closed but insufficient valves (the mitral and tricuspid). These are classified as *ejection* or *regurgitant murmurs*. Keep in mind that certain conditions or age-related changes can produce innocent systolic murmurs (see *Understanding Causes of Innocent Murmurs*).

LIFESPAN CONSIDERATIONS

UNDERSTANDING CAUSES OF INNOCENT MURMURS

Some murmurs have no apparent pathologic cause and are therefore known as *innocent murmurs*. These innocent murmurs occur during systole and result from normal physiologic changes related to age or pregnancy. Use this chart to help identify an innocent murmur and its cause.

Patient Characteristics	Description of Murmur	Possible Cause
Children and adolescents	Early to midsystole, grade I or II, medium pitch, blowing, short, and nonradiating; best heard in second intercostal space (ICS), left sternal border	Forceful myocardial contractions coupled with increased blood flow
Children, ages 3 to 7 years	Musical or vibrating, nonradiating murmur that becomes softer when the child is inactive and quiet, and louder with activity; best heard in third or fourth ICS, right sternal border	Increased velocity of blood flow across aortic valve; possible bands crossing the left ventricular outflow tract
Pregnant women	Systolic ejection murmur grade II to grade IV; may grow more intense with either inspiration or expiration; best heard in second ICS, right sternal border	Increased blood volume related to pregnancy
Older adults	Early systole, grade I or II; best heard in second ICS, right sternal border	Increased length, stiffening of aorta

A diastolic murmur is heard after S$_2$. It is a much softer, lower-pitched sound in a *lubb-dubb-shh* pattern. Diastolic murmurs are produced either from forward blood flow through a stenotic mitral or tricuspid valve or from backward blood flow through an insufficient aortic or pulmonic valve. The aortic and mitral valves are affected most often because of the high pressures on the left side of the heart.

Focus on the location, radiation, quality, pitch, shape, and duration of the murmur. Identify the place on the chest where you can hear the murmur best. Note whether the sound radiates to other chest areas. As you listen, remember the direction of blood flow, and try to follow the sound with your stethoscope. Include this direction in your documentation.

Note the quality of the murmur. Describe it as *swooshing, heaving, whistling, musical, rumbling, roaring,* or *blowing.* Use the most descriptive terms to document what you hear. You may need to be creative. Describe the pitch as *high, medium,* or *low.*

Next, describe the shape of the sound, a measure of the murmur's intensity over a period of time. It is described in four ways: (1) crescendo (soft to loud), (2) decrescendo (loud to soft), (3) crescendo-decrescendo (gets loud, then gets softer), and (4) plateau (same loudness throughout).

Most murmurs can be heard with the diaphragm of your stethoscope. However, if your patient has a low-pitched, soft, blowing murmur, you will hear it best if you use the bell of your stethoscope.

Keep in mind that the intensity of a murmur does not always correlate with your patient's condition. Consider a small VSD, for example. It may produce a loud murmur because the blood must travel through a small opening at high pressure. If the defect enlarges, the murmur will become softer because blood flow will meet less resistance. However, the larger defect may place your patient in greater hemodynamic compromise.

Finally, describe the murmur's duration and the place you hear it in the cycle. If you hear it only with ejection, document it as a systolic ejection murmur. You also can describe a murmur as *early, early-to-mid, mid, mid-to-late,* or *early-to-late,* followed by the word *systolic.* If you hear the murmur throughout the cycle, document it as *pansystolic* or *holosystolic.*

Clicks. A click is an extra systolic sound. Clicks are usually midsystolic or late systolic and are commonly associated with mitral valve prolapse. The best way to hear a click is to ask your patient to sit up, lean forward, and exhale while you listen with the diaphragm of the stethoscope over the apex of the heart or the left sternal border. Having your patient squat or lie in the left lateral recumbent position will also help to bring out this sound. Ask your patient to bear down (Valsalva's maneuver), and listen to see if the click intensifies.

If through your stethoscope you hear a click that sounds like cracking bone, usually at the end of inspiration and sometimes with expiration, you are probably hearing a sternal click. This is especially likely if the patient has recently had heart surgery with a thoracotomy. In fact, if the sternum has not fused yet, you may be able to palpate the sternal click.

Do not confuse this sternal click with a heart sound. If you think sternal instability could be causing your patient's click, palpate for it first. Then, as you auscultate, you will be aware of it. You can feel it by having your patient take a deep breath and cough as you place the palm of your hand over the incision area.

If your patient has a mechanical heart valve, you will hear a valve click that can sound somewhat like a ticking clock. It will have a different quality than the click of mitral valve prolapse.

Snaps. An opening snap is a very early diastolic sound caused by the opening of a thickened mitral valve. When diseased valve leaflets close, they may have a tendency to stick together. As the valve opens, the separation produces a snapping sound, something like a boat sail being suddenly filled with a gust of wind. This sound radiates toward the apex of the heart. It is softer with inspiration and louder with expiration. Its high-pitched snapping quality will help you distinguish it from an S_3 or a split S_2. It is usually accompanied by a diastolic murmur.

To hear this sound, have your patient lean onto her left side. Ask her to exhale. Starting at the left sternal border, move the diaphragm of your stethoscope toward the apex of the heart as you listen.

Rubs. A pericardial friction rub is a scratchy, scraping sound that gets louder when your patient exhales and leans forward. To hear it, listen with the diaphragm of your stethoscope over the third ICS at the left sternal border.

Commonly, the sound you hear will have two components, although occasionally it will have three. This is because the heart moves three times in the cardiac cycle: (1) during atrial systole, (2) during ventricular systole, and (3) during ventricular diastole.

Atrial systole occurs immediately before ventricular systole, so they often combine to produce a single component of the sound. Ventricular diastole then produces another component.

NORMAL FINDINGS

- S_1 and S_2 sounds producing the *lubb-dubb* associated with normal valve closing
- Ventricular rate between 60 and 100 bpm in a resting adult
- Ventricular rate less than 60 bpm (bradycardia) in some young adults, athletes, or patients taking heart-slowing medications, such as beta-blockers
- Rhythm consistent and regular, without extra beats
- Systolic murmur in a young child
- Valve click in a patient who has had a valve replacement

ABNORMAL FINDINGS

- Heart rate less than 60 bpm, possibly indicating increased intracranial pressure (late sign), cardiac arrhythmias (e.g., heart block), parasympathetic or vagal stimulation, baroreceptor (carotid artery) stimulation, digitalis toxicity, or pacemaker malfunction

- Heart rate more than 100 bpm (tachycardia), possibly indicating dehydration, sepsis, anxiety or sympathetic stimulation, cardiac arrhythmias (e.g., atrial fibrillation, ventricular tachycardia), hemorrhaging, effects of epinephrine or similar drugs, chemical stimulation (caffeine or nicotine), thyrotoxicosis, hypoxia, anemia, or heart failure
- Irregular heart rhythm, possibly resulting from atrial fibrillation, premature or delayed ventricular contractions, premature atrial contractions, or heart block (See ▦ Correlating Pulse and Heart Sounds.)

EXAMINATION TIP

CORRELATING PULSE AND HEART SOUNDS

When assessing a patient with extra heart sounds, you may get a better understanding of those sounds when you correlate them with the patient's pulse.

To perform the procedure, you will need your stethoscope and a quiet room. As you auscultate for heart sounds over the patient's apex, use your other hand to gently palpate the carotid artery at the same time. The carotid artery is best because it is closest to the heart.

As you auscultate, remember that S_1 is the sound you hear at virtually the same time you feel the patient's pulse.

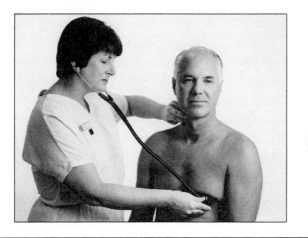

- Absent or muffled heart sounds, possibly resulting from blood or fluid collected in the pericardial sac (Even a small amount of fluid can cause a life-threatening emergency.)
- Fixed split S_2, possibly associated with right ventricular failure
- Audible S_3, possibly an early sign of heart failure in patients older than 30 (It is common in people under age 20 and is best heard in those with slow heart rates. The rapid filling of ventricles or slow filling of a ventricle that is already overfilled [as seen with heart failure] is a possible cause.)
- Audible S_4, possibly resulting from MI and ischemia and hypertension (The vibration of the forceful atrial contraction required to move blood into a stiff ventricle may cause it.)

- Murmur, typically indicating valve disease, such as stenosis, insufficiency, incompetence, or regurgitation (Nonvalvular conditions that cause murmurs include VSDs, sclerotic or aneurysmal arteries, hyperkinetic states, anemia, pregnancy, HOCM, patent ductus arteriosus, and coarctation [narrowing] of the aorta [see ▦ Determining the Cause of Murmurs].)

INTERPRETING ABNORMAL FINDINGS

DETERMINING THE CAUSE OF MURMURS

When you auscultate a murmur during your assessment of heart sounds, keep in mind that a murmur can have several causes that are usually related to an alteration in a valve or other cardiac structure. To help pinpoint the probable cause, be sure to describe the murmur's pitch, quality, shape, and whether it occurs during systole or diastole. Also look for any accompanying signs and symptoms or disorders. Use this chart to guide you.

Characteristics	Locations	Possible Findings	Probable Causes
• High-pitched, blowing, holosystolic murmur; plateau shaped	• Heard best at apex of the heart with patient lying on left side; may radiate to axilla and back	• Tachycardia, S_3 and S_4 heart sounds, split S_2; myocardial infarction (MI), papillary muscle rupture, endocarditis, heart failure	• Mitral regurgitation
• Medium-pitched, blowing, holosystolic murmur; increased intensity with inspiration; plateau shaped	• Heard best at fourth intercostal space (ICS), left sternal border, or area of xiphoid process	• Fatigue, jaundice, anorexia; MI, endocarditis, heart failure	• Tricuspid regurgitation
• High-pitched, blowing, decrescendo diastolic murmur	• Heard best at left sternal border, second right ICS or third left ICS while patient leans forward, holding the breath	• Tachycardia, S_3; fatigue, cough, dyspnea on exertion, orthopnea, paroxysmal nocturnal dyspnea (PND), pulmonary edema; endocarditis	• Aortic regurgitation
• High-pitched, blowing, decrescendo diastolic murmur	• Heard best at left sternal border, second right ICS, or third left ICS while patient leans forward, holding the breath	• Dyspnea, pulmonary hypertension, jugular venous pulsation with increased v waves; endocarditis, cardiac trauma	• Pulmonic regurgitation
• High-pitched, loud harsh, holosystolic murmur	• Heard best at third to fifth ICSs along left sternal border	• Dyspnea, chest pain, syncope, acute heart failure, shock; palpable precordial thrill, hypotension	• Ventricular septal defect

continued

INTERPRETING ABNORMAL FINDINGS—cont'd

Characteristics	Locations	Possible Findings	Probable Causes
• Medium-pitched, harsh, midsystolic murmur; crescendo-decrescendo or diamond shaped	• Heard best at second left ICS; may radiate to left shoulder and upward	• Delayed capillary refill, cyanosis, possible palpable thrill, second ICS, left sternal border; congenital heart disease	• Pulmonic stenosis
• Medium-pitched, harsh, midsystolic murmur; musical when heard at apex; crescendo-decrescendo or diamond shaped	• Heard best at second right ICS; radiates to neck and down left sternal border or apex	• Syncope, angina, exertional dyspnea, possible palpable thrill, second ICS, right sternal border; left ventricular hypertrophy, rheumatic heart disease, atherosclerosis, congenital heart disease	• Aortic stenosis
• Low-pitched sound with rumbling quality, middiastolic and late-diastolic murmur; decrescendo-crescendo shaped; intensifies with expiration	• Heard best over fifth ICS along midclavicular line; radiates very little; best heard with bell of stethoscope	• Fatigue, exertional dyspnea, atrial fibrillation, right parasternal lift, decreased pulse amplitude; may also have mitral regurgitation; rheumatic heart disease	• Mitral stenosis
• Low-pitched sound with rumbling quality; middiastolic or late-diastolic murmur; decrescendo-crescendo shaped; intensifies with stethoscope	• Heard best over fourth ICS along left sternal border; radiates very little; best heard with bell of stethoscope	• Fatigue, hepatomegaly, decreased pulse amplitude, increased jugular venous pulsation; rheumatic heart disease, right atrial myxoma	• Tricuspid stenosis

- Click, or a sharp, high-pitched sound with a "clicking" quality, usually suggesting mitral valve prolapse
- Opening snap, usually resulting from rheumatic heart disease

Breath Sounds

Breath sounds result from the flow of air in and out of the different structures of the respiratory system. The duration, pitch, and quality of normal breath sounds differ according to the location where they are auscultated because of the differences in the underlying airways. The three types of normal breath sounds are (1) bronchial (also called *tracheal* or *tracheobronchial*), (2) broncho-vesicular, and (3) vesicular (see Identifying Characteristic Breath Sounds in the Chest and Back).

IDENTIFYING CHARACTERISTIC BREATH SOUNDS IN THE CHEST AND BACK

As air enters the lungs through the upper airways, it produces different sounds at different locations based on the diameter of the airway, airway pressure, and vibrations. Depending on where you place your stethoscope on the thorax, normal breath sounds have varied pitch, intensity, and duration. To find the expected location of bronchial, bronchovesicular, and vesicular breath sounds, refer to these illustrations.

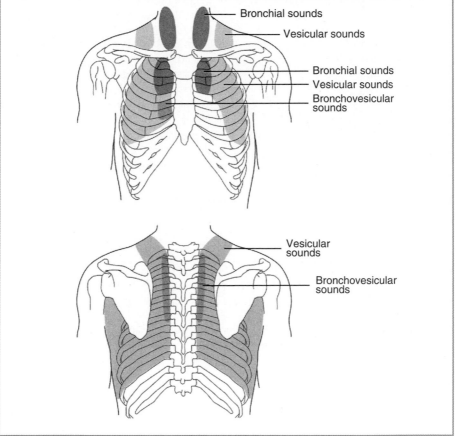

From Barkauskas VH, Baumann LC, Darling-Fisher CS: *Health and physical assessment,* ed 3, St Louis, 2002, Mosby.

When you listen for breath sounds, follow an organized, systematic pattern, as you did for percussion.

If possible, encourage your patient to sit upright, look straight ahead with her chin up, and take deep breaths through her mouth. This will ensure maximum lung inflation with each breath. If the patient is in bed, raise the head of the bed to a 45- to 90-degree angle. Adjust the angle of the bed to the most comfortable position. If your patient has emphysema or chronic obstructive pulmonary disease (COPD), she may be more comfortable leaning over the bedside table, with the lips pursed and arms resting on a pillow. As an alternative, you could ask the patient to sit on the edge of the bed and dangle the feet. If your patient is short of breath, encourage her to take slow, deep breaths. Show the patient how to perform pursed-lipped breathing, if necessary.

Begin your auscultation of breath sounds with the anterior chest. Ask your patient to take a breath each time you place your stethoscope on her chest. Listen for at least one full breath in each location. Be aware of your patient's comfort level. If she becomes light-headed, let the patient rest before you continue. Move the stethoscope from side to side, in the same position on each side, working your way down the chest. Repeat the pattern on the back. This method is used to compare and contrast what you are hearing from one side to the other.

Start by listening for bronchial breath sounds over the trachea. These are loud, high-pitched, harsh, and hollow. To hear them, listen with the diaphragm of your stethoscope just medial to the cricoid cartilage and above the supraclavicular notch as your patient takes a deep breath. Typically, the inspiratory phase is about half the duration of the expiratory phase.

As you listen over your patient's bronchial area, you should also hear bronchial breath sounds. Listen over the right bronchus and then the left. Place the diaphragm of the stethoscope just above the clavicles on each side of the sternum, between the scapulae and over the manubrium. Because the right bronchus is more parallel to the sternum than the left, bronchial sounds may be more prominent on the right side. You will hear high-pitched, blowing, muffled sounds. If you are listening to an intubated patient, expect to hear breath sounds over each bronchus. If you do not, the endotracheal tube may have slipped into one of the bronchi and only one lung is being aerated. Notify the physician immediately if this occurs.

Bronchovesicular sounds are heard at the apex of the right lung anteriorly, and posteriorly to both sides of the spine, between the scapulae. They are similar in quality to bronchial sounds but begin to take on a vesicular quality along the sides of the chest. Inspiration and expiration length are equal.

Bronchial and bronchovesicular breath sounds provide information about the middle and upper airways of the patient's lungs. Although many common pulmonary problems occur in the lobes of the lungs, the patency of the upper airways is vital. If the patient is intubated, has recently been extubated, is asthmatic, has a tracheostomy, has had upper-airway trauma or surgery, has had a pneumonectomy or a collapsed lung, or has had any condition involving tracheal or bronchial irritation, you may need to pay special attention to these breath sounds as heard over the precordial area.

Vesicular sounds are heard over most of the peripheral lung fields, in the areas away from the larger airways. They are soft, relatively low-pitched sounds that last throughout inspiration and fade quickly as expiration begins. Inspiration is three times the length of expiration, and the quality is breezy or swishing.

In addition, be sure to listen for adventitious (added) breath sounds. (The terminology has been changing over the years and is still evolving.) Adventitious breath sounds are divided into two categories: (1) crackles (noncontinuous sounds) and (2) wheezes (continuous sounds). Wheezes are divided into two categories: (1) sibilant wheezes (formerly called *wheezes*) and (2) sonorous wheezes (formerly called *rhonchi*). Listen for both normal and adventitious sounds, and document the type, duration, and location in the respiratory cycle.

Crackles and Wheezes. Crackles are distinct, noncontinuous sounds of two types: (1) fine and (2) coarse. Fine crackles are thought to be caused by two mechanisms. One type of crackling sound occurs when alveoli in the lung bases "pop" open during inspiration, as with atelectasis or pulmonary fibrosis. The other type of crackle occurs in patients with pulmonary edema, probably from air bubbling through fluid. When you listen, you will hear crinkling, popping, or even sounds like a slurping straw, usually at the beginning or end of inspiration. *Rales* and *crepitus* are older terms for fine crackles.

Typically, crackles that result from fluid are dependent. Fluid settles at the lowest portion of the lungs and the level ascends as the condition worsens. If your patient has been sitting upright, expect to hear them in the lung bases. Alternatively, if your patient has been lying on one side for several hours, the fine crackles will be more prominent in the lung on that side. In the final stages of heart failure, auscultation typically reveals continuous crackles, along with sibilant and sonorous wheezes (the so-called *washing-machine chest*).

If your patient has diffuse interstitial fibrosis, you may hear dry crackles that resemble the sound of crumpling cellophane or Velcro.

Coarse crackles and *sonorous wheezes* are current terms for what used to be called *rhonchi*. Although secretions in the tracheobronchial passages can cause both, they are dissimilar.

Coarse crackles are not continuous sounds, and they do not have a musical tone. Sonorous wheezes are low-pitched, continuous noises. They can also be heard in the presence of constriction, obstruction, or spasm of the large airways.

When you listen for coarse crackles, you will hear loud bubbling or gurgling sounds during both inspiration and expiration but more commonly on expiration. These sounds are heard primarily in the trachea and bronchi, but they are also heard in the lower lobes of the lungs.

Expect to hear these sounds if your patient has pneumonia or bronchitis. If your patient cannot easily cough up secretions or has a loose, productive cough, you will hear coarse crackles with or without a stethoscope. Often they can be remedied by suctioning, having your patient cough, respiratory treatments, or bronchodilators.

If you are not sure whether you are hearing fine or coarse crackles, listen to your patient's lungs, have her cough a few times, and then listen again. Usually, coarse crackles will clear or diminish after coughing. Fine crackles caused by fluid or secretions will remain unchanged.

Sibilant wheezes are prolonged, high-pitched, musical or whistle sounds resulting from rapid airflow through narrowed airways and intraluminal smooth muscle contractions. They may be polyphonic (consisting of several pitches) or monophonic (a single pitch).

Sibilant wheezes are heard most often during or at the very end of expiration. Sometimes, however, they can be heard throughout the respiratory cycle. If you hear them bilaterally, they may indicate bronchospasm. They may or may not be associated with crackles and are not affected by coughing.

Other Breath Sounds. Stridor, a loud musical sound produced by upper airway obstruction, is heard commonly during childhood croup and does not require a stethoscope. It is typically inspiratory, but it becomes inspiratory and expiratory as the airway becomes more obstructed. To differentiate stridor from wheezes, listen over the trachea below the cricoid cartilage on one side of the neck. Stridor sounds loudest in this location, whereas wheezing is loudest in the chest.

Less commonly, you may encounter such sounds as friction rubs, referred breath sounds, and a mediastinal crunch. A pleural friction rub occurs during or at the end of inspiration and has a high-pitched, scratchy sound. Different from a pericardial rub, a pleural rub is heard with inspiration and disappears after expiration.

To determine whether a rub is pleural or pericardial, listen over the patient's heart while she holds her breath. If you hear a rub with each heartbeat, the rub is pericardial, not pleural. Occasionally a combination of both kinds of rubs, called *pleuropericardial rub*, occurs.

Referred breath sounds are noises heard over an area where you would not normally expect to hear anything, such as on the side where your patient had a pneumonectomy or a lobectomy, or above a tracheostomy. Because sound travels through fluid and tissue, you may hear a faint inspiratory or vesicular sound over that area.

A mediastinal crunch (Hamman's sign) is a precordial crackling or crunching sound heard with each heartbeat, not with respirations. Nevertheless, it is still considered an abnormal breath sound. It has also been described as a *high-pitched clicking* or *whooping*. It is best heard with your patient in the left lateral position and usually disappears if your patient moves from the left to the right side.

Voice Resonance. Another way to use auscultation to evaluate your patient's lungs is through vocalization, or voice resonance. This technique involves having your patient speak or whisper sounds while you listen to areas of the lungs through the chest and back. Vocal sounds generate vibrations that travel through the lungs and out to the chest wall. As these sounds travel through anatomic structures, their clarity is lost. If they travel through solids or fluids, on the other hand, their clarity remains or increases.

To assess voice resonance, place the diaphragm of the stethoscope over the same areas where you listened for lung sounds. Listen from top to bottom and side to side to compare and contrast sounds. First, ask your patient to say "ninety-nine." See if the sound stays clear or softens. Next, have your patient say the letter "e." Note if "e" sounds like "e," or more like "a." Finally, have your patient whisper the words "one," "two," "three" while you listen. Note whether you can hear the sounds clearly or whether they become muffled.

NORMAL FINDINGS

- Bronchial breath sounds heard over the trachea and bronchi
- Bronchovesicular breath sounds heard at the lung's right apex anteriorly and between the scapulae to about the middle of the back (Inspiration is equal to expiration.)
- Vesicular breath sounds heard over the peripheral lung fields on the lower third of the back, out to the sides, and above the scapulae (Inspiration is three times the length of expiration.)
- Loud and muffled "ninety-nine" heard over the upper lung fields, becoming softer as you move down the back over patient's lower lobes
- Muffled "e" heard as auscultation progresses down chest
- Muffled noises heard as patient whispers "one, two, three" (See 🧩 What to Expect When Examining the Chest and Back.)

NORMAL FINDINGS

WHAT TO EXPECT WHEN EXAMINING THE CHEST AND BACK

Use this review to confirm normal findings when examining the chest and back.

Inspection
- Anterior-posterior (AP) thorax dimension less than the transverse dimension by nearly half
- Breasts free of nipple retractions, dimpling, discharge, erythema, or swelling
- Respirations even, without involving accessory muscles
- Spinal column straight
- Bony prominences, with no evidence of skin breakdown

Palpation
- Warm, dry skin free of lesions, masses, or areas of tenderness
- Breasts free of lumps
- Axillary and subclavian nodes nonpalpable
- Voice vibration (fremitus) equal on either side of the sternum and spine; fremitus may feel more intense over second intercostal space (ICS) and upper airways, less intense or absent over precordium and lung bases

- Equal respiratory excursion
- Point of maximal impulse (PMI) at fifth ICS and midclavicular line; occupies a radius of no more than 1 cm
- No tenderness at costovertebral angle

Percussion
- Resonance over the lung fields
- Dullness over the heart
- Diaphragmatic excursion 3 to 5 cm

Auscultation
- Bronchial sounds over the trachea
- Bronchovesicular sounds over mainstem bronchus and posteriorly between scapulae
- Vesicular breath sounds throughout remaining lung fields
- Voice resonance audible but muffled and best heard medially toward the spine
- S_1 loudest at apex of the heart; S_2 loudest at base; splitting of S_2 on inspiration is a normal finding
- Heart rate between 60 and 100 beats per minute (bpm) while patient is at rest
- Heart rhythm regular

ABNORMAL FINDINGS

- Pericardial friction rub, developing when irritated or inflamed pericardial and epicardial surfaces rub against each other, as from swelling of the pericardium from infection (pericarditis), trauma, cardiac tamponade, uremia, MI, and rubbing of mediastinal chest tubes (used for drainage after thoracic surgery)
- Soft, faint, wheezy, or absent breath sounds over the trachea
- Coarse crackles, wheezing, or absent breath sounds over the precordial area
- Coarse crackles or sonorous wheezes over the bronchial area, possibly indicating bronchitis when combined with a loose cough
- Fine crackles, possibly associated with heart failure, pneumonia, or pulmonary fibrosis (If the crackles are caused by heart failure, you will be able to hear them in the dependent portions of the patient's lungs [see 🔍 Heart Failure].)

DISORDER CLOSE-UP

HEART FAILURE

Heart failure occurs when the heart cannot pump enough blood to meet the body's metabolic requirements. Normally, the right and left ventricle work in synchrony to contract and eject blood in a forward fashion. To maintain a normal stroke volume (the amount of blood that the ventricle ejects with each beat) the ventricles must fill and maintain sufficient preload (tension against the ventricular walls). Then cardiac muscle cells (myocytes) must contract with enough force to overcome afterload (the pressure or resistance the heart pumps against).

In systolic heart failure, myocardial function is depressed when one or both ventricles cannot contract and eject blood sufficiently, despite elevated filling pressures. In diastolic heart failure, stiffened ventricular walls increase tension and end-diastolic pressure, and the ventricles cannot relax and expand to accept enough blood to maintain adequate stroke volume.

Heart failure can be acute or chronic and stem from many causes. Most commonly, the cause is ischemic heart disease, including MI. Other causes include viral cardiomyopa-

thy, valvular heart disease, and arrhythmias. Usually, heart failure stems from dysfunction of the left ventricle (the heart's main pumping chamber), but it can also result from right ventricular or biventricular failure. Whatever the cause, heart failure is often further complicated by the activation of compensatory mechanisms, including the sympathetic nervous system and the renin-angiotensin-aldosterone system.

When assessing a patient with heart failure, keep in mind that the patient's signs and symptoms are related to either increased blood volume and organ congestion or to low organ perfusion (or both). Signs and symptoms of organ congestion include weight gain (often sudden), hepatomegaly, increased jugular vein distention (JVD), peripheral edema, orthopnea and paroxysmal nocturnal dyspnea (PND), and pulmonary crackles. Manifestations of low organ perfusion caused by diminished cardiac output are fatigue; confusion; renal dysfunction; and cool, pale extremities.

Characteristic findings

Expect health history and physical examination findings to vary among patients with heart

continued

DISORDER CLOSE-UP—cont'd

failure, depending on the extent and severity of the disease. Use the following information to help distinguish between expected and unexpected findings.

Health history
- Shortness of breath
- Chest pain
- Palpitations
- Dyspnea on exertion and at rest
- Activity intolerance
- PND
- Orthopnea
- Cough, usually dry, often at night
- Fatigue and weakness
- Insomnia
- Nocturia
- Confusion or inability to concentrate
- Anxiety
- Unexplained weight gain
- Complaints of shoes or rings being tight
- Ankle swelling
- Anorexia and nausea

Inspection
- Mental confusion
- Diaphoresis
- Breathlessness
- Orthopnea
- Cough
- Anxiety
- Cyanosis of nail beds and lips
- Neck vein pulsations
- JVD
- Peripheral dependent edema

Palpation
- Enlarged or displaced apical impulse
- Cool, clammy skin
- Hepatomegaly
- Hepatojugular reflex
- Abdominal pain or tenderness
- Splenomegaly
- Abdominal distention

Percussion
- Dullness over lung bases (pleural effusions)
- Increased liver size
- Shifting dullness

Auscultation
- Crackles
- Gallop heart sounds S_3, S_4
- Sonorous wheezing
- Expiratory wheezing
- Diminished sounds (especially at bases)

Vital signs
- Narrowed pulse pressure
- Tachypnea
- Pulsus alternans
- Tachycardia

Complications
- Pulmonary edema
- Decreased perfusion to major body organs and ischemia
- Myocardial infarction (MI)
- Arrhythmias
- Sudden death

- Sibilant wheezes, usually resulting from edema, secretions, asthma, inhaled or mechanical irritants, or an allergic reaction
- Bronchial or vesicular breath sounds in atypical areas
- Absent breath sounds, possibly indicating a collapsed lobe or consolidation
- Stridor, suggesting upper airway obstruction as in childhood croup (It also suggests foreign body airway obstruction, laryngeal tumor, or tracheal stenosis.)
- Mediastinal crunch, resulting from air trapped in the mediastinal space, usually from surgery, trauma, or a punctured lung

- A clear and audible "ninety-nine" (bronchophony), suggesting that the sound is traveling through fluid or a mass
- Audible "a" as your patient repeats "e" (egophony), indicating a pleural effusion or lung consolidation.
- A clear and audible "one, two, three" as patient whispers it (whispered pectoriloquy), possibly indicating a consolidation

EXPLORING CHIEF COMPLAINTS

Chief complaints involving the chest and back may represent serious cardiac or respiratory disorders, including pneumonia, MI, bronchitis, or heart failure. You should focus your assessment and evaluate your patient completely. Keep your patient's health history in mind as you assess her chief complaint.

CHEST PAIN
If your patient complains of chest pain, investigate further by asking the following questions:
- When did the pain start?
- What were you doing when it started?
- How would you rate the pain on a scale of 1 to 10, with 10 representing *the worst pain you have ever felt?* Is it worse or better now?
- Where in your chest is the pain located?
- Does the pain radiate anywhere?
- What type of pain is it? Sharp, heavy, radiating, crushing?
- Are you short of breath, sweaty, or nauseated? Do you cough? Do you have a fever?
- Does anything make the pain feel better, such as resting or taking nitroglycerin?
- Does anything make it worse, such as taking deep breaths or coughing?
- Would you describe this pain as being like anything you have experienced before?
- Is this a chronic problem? Does the pain occur more frequently or less frequently with exertion? Have you had to cut back on your activities because of it?

Focusing Your Assessment
When a patient complains of chest pain, focus your assessment as follows:
- Observe general appearance. Is the patient short of breath or diaphoretic? A diaphoretic patient with cool extremities may be in cardiogenic shock.
- Check vital signs. Hypotension and tachycardia may be signs of cardiogenic shock.
- Auscultate heart sounds. Listen for irregularity, gallop, or murmur. A patient with recent infarcts may have a new murmur, indicating a life-threatening ruptured papillary muscle or VSD.

- Examine the neck veins for jugular venous distention, which could indicate heart failure.
- Auscultate breath sounds. Coarse or fine crackles may indicate heart failure.
- Palpate the chest wall. Point tenderness over the rib cartilage may indicate costochondritis.

Possible Causes

- *Myocardial infarction.* The classic symptom of MI is persistent crushing chest pain that may radiate to the left arm, jaw, neck, or shoulder blades. Pain associated with exertion or a heavy meal may also indicate ischemia. Rest or nitroglycerin may relieve the pain. An older or diabetic patient may have no pain at all (see ⛊ Myocardial Infarction).

DISORDER CLOSE-UP

MYOCARDIAL INFARCTION

A myocardial infarction (MI) occurs when a coronary artery becomes critically occluded, blocking blood flow to part of the cardiac muscle. The occlusion usually stems from a thrombus at the site of a ruptured atherosclerotic plaque or from prolonged vasospasm. If cells are deprived of oxygen and nutrients long enough, irreversible hypoxemic damage causes cell death and tissue necrosis.

Infarcted tissue has a central necrotic area surrounded by an injured zone. An ischemic zone surrounds the injured zone. Necrotic cells no longer function metabolically, and they do not produce or conduct electrical energy or participate in mechanical contraction. Tissue in the ischemic and injured areas, however, remains viable. Quick return of blood flow can minimize the amount of tissue lost. The patient's electrocardiogram (ECG) can help determine the size and location of the three zones.

Characteristic findings

Expect health history and physical examination findings to vary among patients with MI, depending on the extent and severity of the disease. Use the information that follows to help distinguish between expected and unexpected findings.

Health history

- History of atherosclerosis, coronary artery disease (CAD), or hyperlipoproteinemia
- Family history of heart disease
- Smoking
- History of hypertension
- Sedentary lifestyle, obesity
- Complaints of crushing, substernal chest pain radiating to left arm, jaw, neck, or shoulder blades
- Complaints of indigestion or heartburn
- Increasing frequency of angina
- Feeling of impending doom
- Fatigue
- Nausea and vomiting
- Shortness of breath

Inspection

- Anxiety and restlessness
- Dyspnea
- Diaphoresis
- Jugular vein distention (JVD)

Palpation

- Cool, mottled skin
- Diminished peripheral pulses

Auscultation

- S_4 or S_3 heart sounds
- Paradoxical splitting of S_2
- Systolic murmur
- Pericardial friction rub (transmural MI)

Vital signs

- Tachycardia and hypertension (anterior MI)
- Bradycardia and hypotension (inferior MI)

continued

DISORDER CLOSE-UP—cont'd

Complications
- Arrhythmias
- Cardiogenic shock
- Heart failure
- Rupture of atrial or ventricular septum

- Ventricular aneurysms
- Cerebral or pulmonary embolism
- Reinfarction
- Post-MI pericarditis

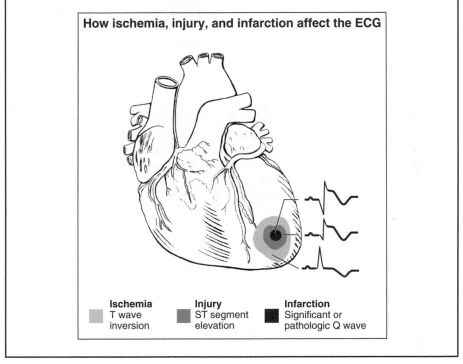

How ischemia, injury, and infarction affect the ECG

Ischemia	**Injury**	**Infarction**
T wave inversion	ST segment elevation	Significant or pathologic Q wave

- *Costochondritis (Tietze's syndrome).* One of the most common causes of chest pain, costochondritis may be associated with trauma or exercise and commonly follows viral illness. With costochondritis, pain usually occurs over the second, third, and fourth costochondral cartilages. Palpation directly over the cartilage generally produces point tenderness (see ▦ Determining Causes of Chest Pain).

INTERPRETING ABNORMAL FINDINGS

DETERMINING CAUSES OF CHEST PAIN

Although commonly associated with heart disease, chest pain can also result from pulmonary, gastrointestinal, musculoskeletal, and psychologic disorders. If your patient complains of chest pain, you will need to quickly focus your examination and intervene appropriately. Use this table to help determine its cause.

continued

INTERPRETING ABNORMAL FINDINGS—cont'd

Characteristics	Locations	Possible Findings	Probable Causes
• Squeezing or aching sensation • Feeling of heaviness or burning • Provoked by exertion, emotional stress, eating • Usually lasts 1 to 3 minutes • Relieved by rest or nitroglycerin	• Substernal or retrosternal areas • May radiate to shoulders, arms, neck, lower jaw, or upper abdomen	• Increased heart rate • Increased blood pressure • Distant heart sounds • Atrial and ventricular gallops (S_3, S_4)	• Angina pectoris
• Pressing, squeezing or stabbing sensation • Feeling of tightness, heaviness, or burning • Sudden onset • May last from 30 minutes to several hours • Not relieved by rest, position change, or nitroglycerin • May be associated with nausea and vomiting	• Substernal or retrosternal areas • May radiate to shoulders, arms, neck, lower jaw, or upper abdomen	• Anxiety, restlessness • Diaphoresis • Rapid, weak pulse • Fever • Variable blood pressure; initially elevated, unless cardiogenic shock is developing • Irregular heart rhythm • Distant heart sounds • Atrial and ventricular gallops (S_3, S_4) • Systolic murmur	• Myocardial infarction (MI)
• Stabbing pain worsened by deep inspiration, movement, or lying down • Sudden onset • May be relieved by sitting up or leaning forward	• Precordial or retrosternal areas • May radiate to shoulders, neck, arms, elbows, back	• Dyspnea • Fever accompanied by diaphoresis, chills • Irregular heart rhythm • Pericardial friction rub	• Pericarditis
• Stabbing pleuritic pain • Sudden onset • May be relieved by high-Fowler's position, other position changes, or chest splinting	• Over affected lung	• Sudden onset of dyspnea • Cough with hemoptysis • Cyanosis • Diaphoresis	• Pulmonary embolism

continued

INTERPRETING ABNORMAL FINDINGS—cont'd

Characteristics	Locations	Possible Findings	Probable Causes
		• Anxiety, restlessness • Low-grade fever • Hypotension • Tachypnea, tachycardia • Wheezing • Accentuated pulmonic heart sound • Pleural friction rub	
• Severe, tearing pain • Sudden onset • May be associated with nausea and vomiting	• Anterior chest • May radiate to the neck, back, or abdomen	• Hypotension • Diaphoresis • Decreased, unequal, or absent peripheral pulses or weakness • Aortic regurgitation murmur	• Dissecting aortic aneurysm
• Stabbing pleuritic pain • Sudden onset • May be aggravated by movement, breathing, or coughing	• Lateral thorax • May radiate across the chest, over the abdomen, or to the shoulder on the affected side	• Sudden onset of dyspnea • Asymmetrical chest wall movement • Tachypnea • Cyanosis • Tracheal deviation • Tympany on percussion • Hyperresonance on affected side • Diminished to absent breath sounds over affected area	• Pneumothorax
• Gripping, sharp colicky pain • Usually precipitated by eating fatty foods or lying down • May lessen in 2 to 3 days and usually resolves within 1 week • May be associated with nausea and vomiting	• Right epigastric area or over abdomen • May radiate to right shoulder	• Splinting during deep inspiration • Low-grade fever • Involuntary guarding of right-sided abdominal muscles • Palpable gallbladder	• Cholecystitis

continued

INTERPRETING ABNORMAL FINDINGS—cont'd

Characteristics	Locations	Possible Findings	Probable Causes
• Gnawing, burning pain that worsens with empty stomach • Occurs intermittently over a few weeks, subsides, then recurs • Temporarily relieved with food or antacid agents • May be associated with nausea or vomiting	• Epigastric area • May radiate to the back	• Belching • Abdominal bloating • Weight loss	• Peptic ulcer
• Sharp, severe pain precipitated by heavy meal, bending, or lying down • May be relieved by antacids, walking, or semi-Fowler's position	• Lower chest or upper abdominal areas	• No significant findings	• Hiatal hernia

- *Angina pectoris.* Characterized by pressing, squeezing chest pain or tightness, angina pectoris results from inadequate blood flow to the heart muscle. Typically, it is provoked by exertion, stress, or eating. It usually lasts from 1 to 3 minutes, but it can last longer. Nitroglycerin or rest will relieve the pain (see 🔍 Angina Pectoris).

DISORDER CLOSE-UP

ANGINA PECTORIS

Three types of angina pectoris exist. Stable angina usually occurs when atherosclerosis narrows one or more coronary arteries and prevents them from dilating to provide increased blood flow to meet increased myocardial oxygen demand (as with exertion or stress). Stable angina is usually transient, lasting less than 5 minutes, and subsides with rest or nitroglycerin. Unstable angina occurs when an atherosclerotic plaque ruptures and a thrombus forms that partially occludes the coronary arterial lumen, disrupting blood flow to the myocardium and causing ischemia. The thrombus dissolves within 20 minutes, preventing myocardial necrosis and infarction. Unstable angina occurs with greater frequency, duration (20 minutes or more), and severity and occurs at rest or is not relieved by rest or nitroglycerin. Variant (Prinzmetal's) angina, an atypical form of angina, occurs without an identified precipitating cause, usually at the same time each day, and is associated with coronary artery spasm.

In all three types, reduced coronary blood flow causes reversible myocardial ischemia and characteristic chest pain. Chest pain

continued

develops because reduced coronary blood flow and decreased oxygen supply cause cells to switch from aerobic metabolism to anaerobic metabolism.

In anaerobic metabolism, lactic acid builds up in the cells, altering cell membrane permeability and releasing such substances as histamine, kinins, and enzymes. These stimulate terminal nerve fibers in the cardiac muscle, which send pain impulses to the central nervous system. Typically, the pain begins in the chest and radiates down the arms or up the neck.

Characteristic findings

Expect health history and physical examination findings to vary among patients with angina, depending on the extent and severity of the disease. Use the following information to help distinguish between expected and unexpected findings.

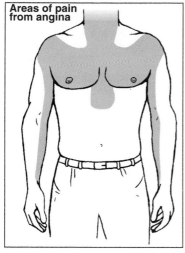

Areas of pain from angina

Health history
- History of coronary artery disease (CAD) or other risk factors for CAD, including hyperlipidemia, hypertension, hyperhomocysteinemia, cigarette smoking, diabetes mellitus, obesity, and a sedentary lifestyle
- Family history of heart disease
- Recent exposure to stress or activity
- Complaints of chest pain, described as *tight, squeezing, heavy pressure* or *constricting sensation beginning beneath the sternum and possibly radiating to the jaw, neck or arm* (lasting 1 to 5 minutes and relieved with rest or nitroglycerin [stable angina] or lasting longer than 20 minutes and unrelieved with rest or nitroglycerin [unstable angina])

Inspection
- Dyspnea
- Pallor
- Anxiety and fear
- Diaphoresis

Auscultation
- Irregular heart rhythm
- Atrial or ventricular gallop (S_3 or S_4)
- Distant heart sounds

Vital signs
- Tachycardia
- Tachypnea

Complications
- Arrhythmias
- Myocardial infarction (MI)
- Sudden cardiac death

- *Pericarditis.* Usually a stabbing pain worsened by inspiration, movement, or lying down, pericarditis results from an inflammation of the pericardial sac.
- *Thoracic aortic aneurysm.* Pain associated with an aortic aneurysm extends to the neck, shoulders, lower back, or abdomen but rarely radiates to the jaw or arms.
- *Pulmonary embolism.* Chest pain associated with a pulmonary embolism is usually accompanied by dyspnea. The pain may mimic angina, or it may

be pleuritic (worsening with a deep breath). Other signs include tachycardia, hemoptysis, and a low-grade fever. Less commonly, the patient may develop a pleural friction rub, cyanosis, or leg edema.

- *Pneumonia.* The most common signs of pneumonia are pleuritic chest pain, cough, sputum production, chills, and fever. Lung auscultation can vary from fine or coarse crackles to diminished or absent breath sounds.
- *Pneumothorax.* Sudden, sharp pleuritic pain is the classic sign of pneumothorax. The pain is usually accompanied by dyspnea and exacerbated by any movement of the chest wall, such as breathing or coughing. Chest wall movement may be asymmetrical. Breath sounds are often absent over the affected lung.
- *Cholecystitis.* The abdominal pain of gallbladder disease may radiate to the chest, back, or shoulder blades. Pain usually follows a high-fat meal or occurs at night, awakening the patient. Diaphoresis, belching, flatulence, nausea, vomiting, chills, and low-grade fever may also be present.
- *Peptic ulcer.* The pain of a peptic ulcer, usually described as *gnawing* or *burning* and worsening with an empty stomach, can radiate to the patient's chest and back, mimicking the pain a person experiences with myocardial ischemia.
- *Hiatal hernia.* Sharp, severe pain precipitated by lying down may be a sign of hiatal hernia. Antacids may relieve it.
- *Acute anxiety.* Chest pain that accompanies stress, in the absence of other physical explanations, may be a result of anxiety.

BACK PAIN

If your patient complains of back pain, investigate further by asking the following questions:
- Where is the pain located?
- When did the pain start?
- Is it getting better or worse?
- Does anything make the pain better or worse, such as changing positions?
- Does the pain radiate into either leg?
- Do you have any numbness?
- Have you had any urinary or fecal incontinence?
- Have you had any recent trauma or injury?
- Have you had a fever recently?
- What treatments have you tried to ease the pain? Have you tried heat or massage?

Focusing Your Assessment

When a patient complains of back pain, focus your assessment as follows:
- Observe the patient's posture while she is standing. Then ask the patient to bend over and touch the toes. An asymmetrical body form may indicate scoliosis.
- Auscultate the abdomen for bruits, and look for pulsating masses, which may indicate an abdominal aortic aneurysm.

- Assess the extremities and trunk for any signs of loss of sensation or motor function that may indicate such neurologic compromise as spinal cord compression.
- Have the patient perform full range of motion with the back. Limited range or pain with range-of-motion activities may indicate a problem with a vertebra or disk.
- With the patient lying flat, lift under the ankle until the leg is straight up (straight-leg test). Pain with this motion may indicate a herniated lumbar disk.
- Examine your patient for muscle weakness, decreased muscle tone, and exaggerated or diminished reflexes, which may indicate a spinal tumor.

Possible Causes
- *Abdominal aortic aneurysm.* A rapid onset of severe lower back pain, possibly radiating to the chest, suggests a rupture or dissection of an abdominal aortic aneurysm. Your patient may have a pulsating mass in the midepigastrium. Pain may radiate to the posterior thighs. With a dissecting aneurysm, repositioning does not relieve the pain. If the pain is described as *tearing* or *ripping*, and it is located in the anterior thorax and the back between the scapulae, it may indicate a dissecting thoracic aneurysm. Other signs include cold, pulseless lower extremities, and blood pressure differences between arms of greater than 10 mm Hg (see ▨ Determining Causes of Back Pain).

INTERPRETING ABNORMAL FINDINGS

DETERMINING CAUSES OF BACK PAIN
A common complaint, back pain usually stems from muscle strain or arthritis. However, it can also result from serious conditions, such as vertebral fractures and spinal cord tumors. For that reason, assess your patient's back pain carefully and thoroughly, using the following table to help determine its cause.

Characteristics	Locations	Possible Findings	Probable Causes
• Pain confined to lower back • No evidence of nerve root involvement (numbness, weakness) • Usually relieved by rest	• Lumbar and sacral area • May radiate to shoulders	• Unusual posture related to spasm • Paravertebral muscle tenderness • Restricted low-back motion	• Sprain or strain injury related to poor body mechanics • Trauma
• Sudden, severe low-back pain • Muscle spasm • Limited motion	• Lumbar or sacral areas • Thoracic spine	• Radiologic evidence of vertebral bone fractures • Paralytic ileus • Urinary retention	• Vertebral compression fractures • Heavy lifting or trauma • Metastatic tumor or myeloma • Metabolic bone disease

continued

INTERPRETING ABNORMAL FINDINGS—cont'd

Characteristics	Locations	Possible Findings	Probable Causes
• Low-back pain with limited motion • Pain improves with rest	• Lumbar and sacral areas	• Abnormal posture • Pain when straight legs are raised • Local muscle weakness, atrophy • Nerve root involvement: radicular pain, paresthesias, twitching, muscle spasms, decreased tendon reflex • L4, L5: pain to posterior thigh, calf, and foot; walking on heels may be difficult • L5, S1: pain in midluteal region, back of thigh, back of calf down to heel and bottom surface of foot and fourth and fifth toes; walking on toes may be difficult	• Prolapsed or protruded disk • Silent degeneration over several years • Flexion injury • Spinal cord tumor
• Common in lumbar or cervical spine • Pain centered in spine and increased by activity • Pain relieved by rest	• Lumbar or sacral areas • Cervical and upper shoulder	• Limited motion • Degree of radiologic changes may not correlate with symptoms	• Degenerative joint disease • Osteoarthritis
• Progressive limitation of movement • Morning stiffness	• Area affected varies with type of disorder	• Decreased mobility	• Rheumatoid arthritis: usually older female patients with pain, stiffness mainly in cervical area • Ankylosing spondylitis: usually young male patients with pain and fusion in sacroiliac region
• Dull, constant pain • Pain is unrelieved by rest and may be worse at night	• All areas of the spine and back	• Local bone tenderness	• Bone metastases from prostate, breast, lung, thyroid, or kidney cancer • Multiple myeloma

continued

INTERPRETING ABNORMAL FINDINGS—cont'd

Characteristics	Locations	Possible Findings	Probable Causes
• Severe, stabbing pain	• Lower back • Abdomen	• Dysuria, nocturia, urinary frequency, chills, and fever in male patients • Fever, lower abdominal pain, and vaginal pain in female patients • Nausea and vomiting, fever, and chills	• Gastrointestinal disease, such as peptic ulcer, pancreatitis • Genitourinary disease, such as pyelonephritis, nephrolithiasis, endometriosis, or prostatitis • Abdominal aortic aneurysm

- *Herniated or ruptured lumbar disk.* The pain associated with a herniated lumbar disk is severe and usually radiates unilaterally to the buttock, leg, and foot. Pain is intensified by Valsalva's maneuver, coughing, sneezing, or bending and is often accompanied by muscle spasm.
- *Spinal tumors.* Pain that radiates around the trunk or down the limb and cannot be relieved by bed rest may indicate a spinal tumor. The patient also may have muscle weakness or wasting, with exaggerated or diminished tendon reflexes. Urinary retention or constipation may also be present.
- *Fractured vertebra.* Pain with a fractured vertebra usually worsens with movement and may radiate to the legs. Mild paresthesia may accompany the pain.
- *Osteoarthritis.* Patients typically describe arthritic pain as *deep, aching pain.* Rest usually relieves it. Your patient may complain of morning stiffness and aching during weather changes.
- *Genitourinary problems.* In a female patient, severe back and abdominal pain associated with the menstrual period and dysmenorrhea may indicate endometriosis. In a male patient, low-back pain associated with dysuria, nocturia, urinary frequency, chills, and fever may indicate prostatitis. A pelvic infection should be considered in any female patient with a fever, lower abdominal pain, and vaginal discharge associated with low-back pain.
- *Lumbosacral strain.* Stiffness, soreness, and generalized tenderness may indicate a lumbosacral strain.
- *Kidney stone.* Severe back pain accompanied by nausea and vomiting, fever, and chills may indicate a stone obstructing a kidney or ureter.

HEMOPTYSIS
If the patient complains of coughing up blood, investigate further by asking the following questions:
- When did the hemoptysis begin?
- What color is the sputum? Does it look like fresh blood, old brown blood, or pus-filled sputum with bloody streaks?

- How often do you cough up blood?
- Does it seem to be getting better or worse?
- Have you had any associated symptoms, such as shortness of breath or chest pain?
- Have you had any recent fever or chills?
- Have you had any weight loss or night sweats?
- Have you had any recent chest surgery or trauma?

Focusing Your Assessment

When a patient complains of hemoptysis, focus your assessment as follows:

- Assess your patient for chest pain. Complaints of new-onset hemoptysis and chest pain may indicate a pulmonary embolus.
- Assess the patient's oral mucosa and nares for signs of bleeding or trauma. Hemoptysis may arise from areas other than the respiratory tract.
- Assess the skin for petechiae or bruising, which may indicate a coagulation disorder.
- Evaluate your patient's current situation. Sudden hemoptysis in a patient undergoing pulmonary artery catheter insertion could indicate pulmonary artery rupture. This is a medical emergency. In an intubated patient, it could indicate tracheal erosion.
- Assess the volume of blood.

Hemoptysis of greater than 100 ml in a 24-hour period may be life threatening.

Possible Causes

- *Bacterial infection.* Acute and chronic infections are the most common causes of hemoptysis, especially infections caused by *Staphylococcus, Klebsiella,* and *Pseudomonas* spp.
- *Tuberculosis.* Hemoptysis associated with fever or night sweats may indicate tuberculosis.
- *Coagulopathy.* The presence of petechiae or bruising of the skin along with hemoptysis may signify a coagulopathy, leukemia, or thrombocytopenia.
- *Lung cancer.* Hemoptysis in a patient with a history of smoking or occupational exposure to carcinogens may be a sign of lung cancer. Hemoptysis caused by erosion occurs in half of patients with lung cancer at some point during the disease.
- *Fungal infection.* Most pulmonary fungal infections can cause hemoptysis. Patients who are immunocompromised or have a history of tuberculosis or exposure to it are at a higher risk for fungal infections.

COUGH

If your patient complains of a cough, investigate further by asking the following questions:

- Is the cough productive or nonproductive?
- If the cough is productive, what color is the sputum?

- When did the cough start?
- Is it getting better or worse?
- Does the cough occur more frequently at a certain time of the day?
- Do you have a fever or chills?
- Are you short of breath?
- Are you taking anything for the cough?
- Do you have any other symptoms (sore throat, runny nose, hoarseness)?
- Have you noticed a recent weight loss or night sweats?
- What type of work do you do? Describe your work environment. Are you or have you been exposed to toxic chemicals, fibers, or fumes (e.g., asbestos)?

Focusing Your Assessment

When a patient complains of a cough, focus your assessment as follows:

- Auscultate breath sounds. Coarse crackles, bronchial breath sounds, or an area of consolidation may indicate pneumonia. Fine crackles may indicate heart failure. Abnormal breath sounds that clear after coughing indicate secretions rather than heart failure.
- Examine any sputum produced by the cough. Green sputum may indicate a *Pseudomonas* spp. infection. Rust-colored sputum may indicate a *Klebsiella* spp. infection. Scant sputum production may indicate a viral infection.
- Assess the results of pulmonary function testing, including the patient's 1-second forced expiratory volume (FEV1), peak flow, and vital capacity to detect obstructive pulmonary disease.

Possible Causes

- *Asthma.* Although wheezing is the characteristic symptom associated with asthma, your patient may also have an unusually tight-sounding, dry cough, with tenacious mucoid sputum. This cough may be triggered by exposure to cold or exercise.
- *Cigarette smoking.* The most common cause of a chronic cough, cigarette smoking is associated with a cough that is more severe early in the morning. Usually it produces a yellowish-brown mucus. It may disappear as quickly as 1 month after the patient stops smoking.
- *Air pollution or exposure to irritants.* Sulfur dioxide, nitrogen dioxide, and ozone are common air pollutants that cause a cough. Asbestosis is also a cause. Industrial and agricultural exposure can result in an acute or chronic cough as well. Many coughs related to air pollution begin after work or at night.
- *Bronchogenic carcinoma.* Cough is a major symptom of bronchogenic carcinoma and often is the first sign of this disease. You should consider lung carcinoma in a heavy smoker with a chronic cough.
- *Bronchitis.* Recent onset of cough and fever could indicate an acute episode of bronchitis (see ⬛ Bronchitis).

DISORDER CLOSE-UP

BRONCHITIS

Bronchitis is an acute or chronic inflammation of the mucous membranes of the bronchi. Acute bronchitis results when the larger bronchi react to an infectious agent by becoming diffusely inflamed and producing excessive amounts of mucus. The airways are otherwise normal. Acute bronchitis is common and usually causes little permanent disability.

Chronic bronchitis, by contrast, is a type of chronic obstructive pulmonary disease (COPD). Obstruction results from inflammation of major and minor airways. The submucosal glands become edematous and overgrown, secreting excess mucus into the bronchial tree.

Usually, chronic bronchitis results from prolonged exposure to bronchial irritants, such as cigarette smoke, air pollution, toxic fumes, and dust. A ventilation-perfusion imbalance develops from resistance in the small airways and because areas of inflammation and retained secretions do not occur uniformly throughout the lungs. Repeated infections with persistent obstruction can lead to scarring, necrosis, and destruction of the small bronchioles.

Characteristic findings

Expect health history and physical examination findings to vary among patients with chronic bronchitis, depending on the extent and severity of the disease. Use the information that follows to help you distinguish between expected and unexpected findings.

Health history
- Long-term smoking
- History of frequent upper respiratory infections
- History of exposure to environmental pollutants
- Cough (increasing in frequency and severity), especially at night
- Complaints of exertional dyspnea with increased time needed to recover
- Family history of COPD
- Weight gain

Inspection
- Dyspnea
- Productive cough with copious sputum (gray, white, or yellow)
- Use of accessory breathing muscles
- Cyanosis
- Finger clubbing
- Barrel chest (possible)

Palpation
- Pedal edema
- Neck vein distention

Auscultation
- Wheezing
- Prolonged expiratory time
- Decreased breath sounds
- Changes in breath sounds (variable)

Vital signs
- Tachypnea
- Elevated temperature (possible)

Complications
- Cor pulmonale
- Pulmonary hypertension
- Right ventricular hypertrophy
- Acute respiratory failure

- *Angiotensin-converting enzyme (ACE) inhibitor use.* A dry cough is a possible side effect of ACE inhibitors, which often are prescribed for heart failure and hypertension.
- *Tuberculosis.* A cough associated with fatigue, weakness, anorexia, weight loss, or night sweats may indicate tuberculosis, especially recurrent disease.

DYSPNEA

If your patient complains of dyspnea, or shortness of breath, investigate further by asking the following questions:

- Does the shortness of breath occur with rest or with activity?
- If shortness of breath occurs with activity, how much exertion causes it? Does walking 50 feet or 100 feet (or perhaps more) bring on the problem?
- Are you short of breath now?
- What helps the shortness of breath get better?
- Do you have any associated symptoms, such as dizziness or chest pain?
- Is this a new problem or a chronic problem?
- If it is a chronic problem, does it seem to be getting worse?
- Have you seen anyone for this problem? If so, what treatment are you receiving?

Focusing Your Assessment

When a patient complains of shortness of breath, focus your assessment as follows:

- Check your patient's vital signs and appearance. New-onset shortness of breath can indicate a serious underlying problem (see ▨ Determining Causes of Dyspnea).

INTERPRETING ABNORMAL FINDINGS

DETERMINING CAUSES OF DYSPNEA

A patient with dyspnea has a distressing sensation of air hunger. Because dyspnea can result from a wide variety of cardiac and pulmonary conditions, its cause can be difficult to identify quickly. Always take a detailed history when assessing a patient with dyspnea. Then use this table to help determine its cause.

Characteristics	Possible Findings	Probable Causes
• Gradual-onset dyspnea beginning as exertional • Minimal cough, usually nonproductive	• Varying degrees of respiratory distress • Tachypnea • Prolonged expiration • Expiration often begins with a grunting noise • Posture leaning forward with extended arms • Use of accessory muscles • Hyperresonance to percussion • Decreased breath sounds with faint, high-pitched wheezes at end of expiration • Weight loss • History of smoking • Carbon dioxide retention	• Emphysema

continued

INTERPRETING ABNORMAL FINDINGS—cont'd

Characteristics	Possible Findings	Probable Causes
• Gradual-onset dyspnea • Long history of cough and sputum production • Paroxysmal nocturnal dyspnea (PND) related to increased sputum production	• History of smoking, obesity, and frequent respiratory infections • Carbon dioxide retention • Coarse crackles and wheezes that change in location and intensity after cough • Late features: cyanosis, clubbing, peripheral edema, neck vein distention, right ventricular failure, cor pulmonale	• Chronic bronchitis
• Episodes of acute dyspnea • Sensation of having a lump in the throat • Hoarseness	• Stridor and retraction of supraclavicular muscles with inspiration • Respiratory distress and failure	• Aspiration of food or foreign object • Allergic reaction, resulting in angioedema • Upper airway obstruction
• Dyspnea with exertion (early), developing into dyspnea at rest • Suffocating or drowning sensation • Cough and wheezing • PND and orthopnea	• Moist inspiratory crackles • Tachypnea • Gallop rhythms and cardiac murmurs • Jugular vein distention (JVD) • Diaphoresis • Peripheral edema • Pleural effusions	• Heart failure • Myocardial infarction (MI) or ischemia • Valvular disease • Cardiomyopathies
• Dyspnea at rest • Hyperventilation	• Sharp, fleeting chest pain, variably located • Frequent sighing • Irregular breathing pattern • Normal breathing during sleep	• Anxiety • Emotional stress
• Acute-onset dyspnea • Wheezing • Cough • Commonly affects children	• Tachypnea with wheezing • Attacks can last minutes to hours • Episodic disease	• Asthma
• Dyspnea at rest • Unexplained sudden breathlessness	• Sharp or stabbing pleuritic pain • Hemoptysis • Tachycardia and tachypnea • Accentuated pulmonic heart sound • Hypotension • ST changes on electrocardiogram (ECG) • Pleural friction rub • Atelectasis after 24 hours	• Pulmonary embolus

continued

INTERPRETING ABNORMAL FINDINGS—cont'd

Characteristics	Possible Findings	Probable Causes
• Dyspnea at rest • Productive cough (mucoid, purulent, or bloody)	• Tachycardia and tachypnea • Decreased respiratory excursion on affected side • Dullness to percussion over area of infection • High-pitched, end-inspiratory crackles • Increased bronchial breath sounds • Fever • Chest pain • Increased tactile fremitus over consolidation area • Confusion or disorientation in older patients	• Pneumonia
• Exertional, gradual-onset dyspnea • Nonproductive cough	• Dry basilar crackles best heard at the end of deep inspiration • Fatigue • Malaise • Late: evidence of pulmonary hypertension, clubbing	• Interstitial fibrotic lung disease • Rheumatoid and collagen-vascular disease • Sarcoidosis
• Gradual-onset dyspnea • Productive cough	• Wheezing • Stridor • Fever • Hemoptysis • History of smoking	• Pulmonary neoplasms (primary and metastatic)

- Notify the physician immediately and consider giving oxygen if your patient is tachypneic, diaphoretic, or cyanotic.
- Check your patient's extremities to see if they are cyanotic or cold, which indicates circulatory compromise. Cold, cyanotic extremities with hypotension may indicate hypoperfusion associated with shock.
- Auscultate breath sounds. Crackles and wheezes can indicate heart failure or pulmonary edema.
- Assess your patient for chest pain, which could indicate cardiac ischemia.
- Inspect the chest for tracheal deviation, a sign of pneumothorax or pleural effusion.
- Inspect for barrel chest, a sign of emphysema.
- Check for jugular vein distention (JVD) and dependent edema (signs of pulmonary edema).
- Assess the patient's mental status. Confusion or a change in mental status may indicate hypoxia.

- Examine your patient's calves for any signs of deep vein thrombosis. A positive Homans' sign (pain when the foot is dorsiflexed) may indicate venous occlusion, which could result in a pulmonary embolus.
- Examine the color of the nail beds, gums, and conjunctivae. Pale membranes and nail beds associated with fatigue may indicate anemia, which could result in shortness of breath.

Possible Causes

- *Anemia.* Progressive weakness coupled with shortness of breath and pallor may be signs of aplastic or hypoplastic anemia.
- *Pulmonary hypertension.* Weakness, increasing shortness of breath on exertion, and fatigue may be signs of pulmonary hypertension. Signs of right-sided heart failure, such as peripheral edema, ascites, neck vein distention, and hepatomegaly, also may be present.
- *Central nervous system lesion.* Lesions in the central nervous system may press on the hypothalamus, causing an increased respiratory rate and a feeling of shortness of breath.
- *Pleural effusion.* With a large pleural effusion, the patient will complain of dyspnea and may have a visible tracheal shift. Breath sounds are diminished or absent over the effusion, and a pleural friction rub may be heard.
- *Pulmonary embolism.* Sudden dyspnea that occurs in the setting of a deep vein thrombosis could signal a pulmonary embolism. Left untreated, pulmonary infarction, severe hypoxemia, and death could ensue. Homans' sign may or may not be present.
- *Pneumonia.* Shortness of breath with a fever and cough may warn of pneumonia.
- *Pulmonary edema.* Tachypnea, tachycardia, elevated blood pressure, and shortness of breath are signs of pulmonary edema. Crackles are usually heard on auscultation of the chest. Jugular venous distention and dependent edema may also be present.
- *Lung cancer.* Occurring as squamous cell carcinoma, small cell carcinoma, or adenocarcinoma, lung cancer most commonly occurs on the wall or epithelium of the bronchial tree. Prognosis is usually poor but improves with early detection. Lung cancer should be considered in any patient who smokes and has shortness of breath.
- *Pneumothorax.* Trauma to the chest or a spontaneous leak in the lung membranes that allows air to enter the pleural space can cause the lung to collapse, resulting in a pneumothorax. Signs include absent breath sounds on one side of the chest and asymmetrical chest movements (see Telltale Signs of Tension Pneumothorax).

TELLTALE SIGNS OF TENSION PNEUMOTHORAX

Tension pneumothorax is an emergency in which the lung collapses from the force of high pressure in the pleural space. It may result from penetrating chest injury, mechanical ventilation that uses positive end-expiratory pressure, or even chest tube occlusion.

continued

TELLTALE SIGNS OF TENSION PNEUMOTHORAX—cont'd

Signs and symptoms that point to tension pneumothorax include the following:
- Sudden shortness of breath with tachypnea and tachycardia
- Anxiety
- Asymmetrical chest wall movement with mediastinal shift away from the affected side

- Absent or diminished breath sounds on the affected side
- Hyperresonance on the affected side
- Distended neck veins

The pressure causing the tension pneumothorax must be relieved rapidly so that the lung will reinflate. Prepare to assist with chest tube insertion as soon as possible.

- *Emphysema.* A leading cause of death in the United States, emphysema follows recurrent inflammation of the lung walls. Shortness of breath with a barrel chest and clubbing of the fingers are signs of emphysema (see ◳ Emphysema).

DISORDER CLOSE-UP

EMPHYSEMA

One of two major types of chronic obstructive pulmonary disease (COPD) (which also includes chronic bronchitis), emphysema is a degenerative condition characterized by destruction of alveolar walls, entrapment of air in the spaces beyond the terminal bronchioles, narrowing of small airways, and loss of alveolar elasticity.

Emphysema mainly affects expiration. Because muscles used during inspiration can pull air past most obstructions, air can enter the lungs; however, it cannot leave as easily and becomes trapped in the alveoli, severely limiting oxygen intake and ultimately leading to hypoxia.

The body uses abdominal and accessory thoracic muscles to force air past the obstruction, slowing expiration. As a result, the patient retains carbon dioxide, which leads to hypercapnia.

Besides overworking respiratory muscles, emphysema strains the heart's right side, which provides pulmonary circulation. The heart compensates for hypoxemia by pumping faster to deliver more blood to the lungs and harder to push blood through constricted capillaries. As a result, the heart's right side hypertrophies (cor pulmonale).

Characteristic findings

Expect health history and physical examination findings to vary among emphysema patients, depending on the extent and severity of the disease. Use the information that follows to help distinguish between expected and unexpected findings.

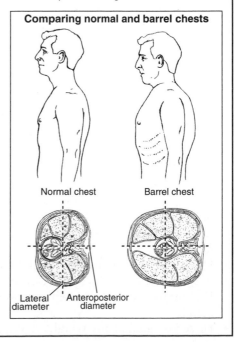

Comparing normal and barrel chests

Normal chest

Barrel chest

Lateral diameter

Anteroposterior diameter

continued

DISORDER CLOSE-UP—cont'd

Health history
- Long-term smoking
- Alpha,-antitrypsin deficiency
- Family history of COPD
- Dyspnea during daily activities
- Anorexia
- Feeling of general malaise
- Chronic nonproductive cough

Inspection
- Increased anterior-posterior (AP) and lateral chest diameters, forming the typical barrel chest
- Forward-leaning posture
- Pursed-lip breathing
- Dyspnea
- Minimal cough (may develop productive cough in late stages secondary to chronic bronchitis)
- Audible expiratory wheeze
- Cyanosis of nail beds and mucous membranes
- Finger clubbing
- Use of accessory muscles during breathing
- Emaciation
- Restlessness and anxiety

Palpation
- Decreased tactile fremitus

- Downward displacement of liver's edge
- Nonpalpable apical pulse

Percussion
- Hyperresonance
- Decreased diaphragmatic excursion

Auscultation
- Wheezing
- Decreased breath and heart sounds
- Decreased voice sounds
- Prolonged expiration

Vital signs
- Elevated temperature
- Increased pulse rate
- Decreased blood pressure
- Pulsus paradoxus
- Increased respiratory rate

Complications
- Acute respiratory failure
- Arrhythmias
- Cor pulmonale
- Peptic ulcer and gastroesophageal reflux
- Pneumonia
- Polycythemia

ORTHOPNEA OR PAROXYSMAL NOCTURNAL DYSPNEA

If your patient complains that she needs to sleep propped up on several pillows (orthopnea) or awakens at night feeling short of breath (paroxysmal nocturnal dyspnea [PND]), investigate further by asking the following questions:

- When did you first notice these symptoms?
- How many pillows do you sleep on at night? Have you increased the number recently?
- Do you sleep on extra pillows to help your breathing or for another reason?
- How often do you awaken at night with shortness of breath?
- Are these episodes increasing in frequency?
- Do you have any associated symptoms, such as chest pain, leg swelling, or cough?
- Have you gained any weight recently?

Focusing Your Assessment

When a patient complains of orthopnea or nocturnal dyspnea, focus your assessment as follows:

- Auscultate the lungs for crackles, which may indicate pulmonary edema.
- Auscultate the lungs for diminished breath sounds, which may indicate a pleural effusion.
- Auscultate the lungs for wheezes, which may indicate asthma.
- Assess the extremities for edema, a sign of fluid overload.
- Examine your patient's chest for a barrel shape, a sign of COPD.
- Assess your patient for JVD or an S_3, S_4 gallop (signs of pulmonary edema associated with heart failure and cardiac compromise).

Possible Causes

- *Pulmonary edema and heart failure.* When a patient with heart failure lies down flat, interstitial fluid from the legs and the lung bases accumulates around the lungs. Consequently, the patient typically feels more comfortable if she elevates her upper body on several pillows to sleep. If the patient falls asleep in a flat position, the respiratory compromise from fluid accumulated around the lungs often awakens her.
- *COPD.* Secretions pooling in the throat and airways can cause a patient with COPD to awaken at night with shortness of breath.
- *Cardiac disease.* Compromised cardiac pumping function causes congestion in the pulmonary vasculature system, which can awaken the patient with shortness of breath.

WHEEZING

If your patient complains of wheezing, investigate further by asking the following questions:

- When did you first notice the wheezing?
- Have you had wheezing in the past?
- Does anything seem to bring on the wheezing, such as exercise or cold?
- Do you have any associated symptoms, such as fever, chills, cough, or shortness of breath?
- Have you ever been evaluated for wheezing before? If so, did you receive any treatment?

Focusing Your Assessment

When a patient complains of wheezing, focus your assessment as follows:

- Observe the patient for signs of respiratory distress. The patient may be having an asthma attack or have an obstructed airway (see ◪ Responding to Airway Obstruction).
- Assess for signs of cyanosis in the nail beds and mucous membranes. Check the patient's pulse oximetry. If the patient is hypoxic, the physician may order oxygen.

ACTION STAT

RESPONDING TO AIRWAY OBSTRUCTION

Airway obstruction may result from a wide variety of objects, including an aspirated foreign body, a mucus plug, or, in some cases, the patient's tongue. Whatever its cause, airway obstruction must be corrected quickly. Maintaining a patent airway is the single most important nursing intervention you can perform for your patient. How you respond to acute airway obstruction depends on whether you know the cause of the obstruction and whether your patient is conscious.

What to look for

Clinical findings may include the following:
- Distressed, panicked appearance on your patient's face
- Inability to speak
- Wheezing, stridor, noisy respirations, sonorous wheezing over large airways
- Nasal flaring or use of accessory breathing muscles
- Decreased or absent breath sounds
- Excessive secretions (mucus or blood) around the mouth
- Cardiac arrhythmias
- Cyanosis
- Hypoxemia

What to do immediately

If your patient develops an airway obstruction, begin by calling for assistance first; then follow these measures:
- Rapidly try to determine the probable cause of the obstruction, possibly a foreign body or food, excessive pulmonary secretions, or mechanical obstruction, such as the patient's tongue.
- If the patient is conscious and a foreign body, such as food or an object, obstructs the airway, perform the abdominal thrust maneuver (formerly known as the Heimlich maneuver). You may have to modify your technique of performing abdominal thrusts if your patient is supine in bed or upright in a bed or chair.
- If your patient is unconscious, immediately open the airway using the head-tilt/chin-lift method. This will pull your patient's tongue away from her oropharynx and open the airway. If the patient is in bed, raise the head of the bed to semi-Fowler's position.
- If changing the patient's airway position does not relieve the obstruction, use a gloved finger to perform a tongue sweep to check for a foreign body.
- Prepare to follow the American Heart Association's basic life support recommendations, which include rescue breathing and cardiac compressions.
- If indicated, prepare to suction the anterior and posterior portion of your patient's mouth, her oropharynx, trachea, and mainstem bronchus.

What to do next

Once your patient has been stabilized and the airway is patent, you will need to do the following:
- Maintain airway patency. Use an appropriate airway device, such as an oropharyngeal or nasopharyngeal airway, as necessary.
- Obtain additional emergency respiratory equipment, such as endotracheal intubation or tracheostomy supplies and supplemental oxygen, as indicated.
- Obtain arterial blood gas levels, if ordered, to further assess the patient's oxygenation.
- Administer oxygen as prescribed.
- Maintain the patient in a comfortable position that promotes airway clearance, with the head of her bed elevated.

- Check your patient's vital signs. A tachypnic patient may need oxygen, even if the pulse oximetry reading is within a normal range.
- Auscultate the lungs. Wheezes on expiration may indicate asthma. Wheezes on inspiration may indicate bronchitis. Crackles are a sign of pulmonary edema.

- Assess for a cough with sputum production. Clear or yellow sputum may indicate asthma. Purulent sputum may indicate pneumonia.

Possible Causes
- *Asthma.* Inflammation of the bronchioles accompanied by bronchiole constriction characterizes an asthma episode. Wheezing accompanied by respiratory distress (tachypnea, use of accessory breathing muscles) may occur suddenly or gradually after exposure to an allergen. The patient also may complain of a cough with clear or yellow sputum. The peak flow and FEV1 will be decreased (see 🔍 Asthma).

DISORDER CLOSE-UP

ASTHMA

Asthma is a chronic lung disorder characterized by reversible airway obstruction, inflamed airways, and an increased responsiveness of the airways to certain stimuli. During an asthma attack, airways sensitized by allergens become reactive to bronchospastic or inflammatory triggers. Bronchospastic triggers include cold air, exercise, emotional upset, variations in temperature and humidity, and exposure to irritants, such as cigarette smoke. Most episodes of this type are preceded by a severe respiratory tract infection. Inflammatory triggers include such allergens as pollen, animal dander, house dust, mold, and food additives. Patients with allergic asthma may respond to both types of triggers.

Contact with a trigger causes bronchoconstriction. Histamine and related substances are released and initiate contraction of smooth muscle in the bronchi, edema of bronchial mucous membranes, and secretion of copious mucus in the bronchi. This activity causes epithelial injury and edema, changes in mucociliary function, reduced clearance of respiratory tract secretions, and increased airway responsiveness. Expiratory airflow decreases and gas is trapped in the airways, causing alveolar hyperinflation. The increased airway resistance initiates labored breathing.

Characteristic findings

Expect health history and physical examination findings to vary among patients with asthma, depending on the extent and severity of the disease. Use the information that follows to help distinguish between expected and unexpected findings.

Health history
- History of allergic reactions
- History of other atopic diseases, such as allergic rhinitis or eczema
- Family history of atopic diseases
- Exposure to allergen
- Sudden onset of dyspnea
- Complaints of chest tightness and feeling of suffocation
- Cough

Inspection
- Prolonged expiration
- Pursed-lip breathing
- Perspiration
- Ability to speak only a few words before stopping to catch breath
- Use of accessory muscles to breathe
- Chest muscle retractions
- Increased anterior-posterior (AP) thoracic diameter
- Cyanosis
- Confusion
- Lethargy

continued

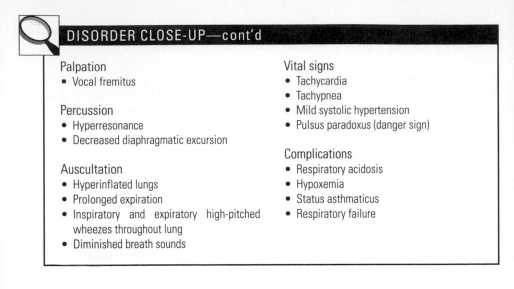

DISORDER CLOSE-UP—cont'd

Palpation
- Vocal fremitus

Percussion
- Hyperresonance
- Decreased diaphragmatic excursion

Auscultation
- Hyperinflated lungs
- Prolonged expiration
- Inspiratory and expiratory high-pitched wheezes throughout lung
- Diminished breath sounds

Vital signs
- Tachycardia
- Tachypnea
- Mild systolic hypertension
- Pulsus paradoxus (danger sign)

Complications
- Respiratory acidosis
- Hypoxemia
- Status asthmaticus
- Respiratory failure

- *Pulmonary edema.* Fluid overload may produce wheezing. Other signs include pedal edema; JVD; or S_3, S_4 gallop.
- *Pneumonia.* Secretions blocking the upper airways may result in wheezes.
- *Reaction to medications.* A common example of this would be an allergic reaction to penicillin.

Focusing Your Assessment

When a patient complains of lumps or lesions, focus your assessment as follows:
- Perform a full breast examination, including the axillae. Check both nipples for discharge. Lumps or lesions on the breasts can indicate breast cancer in both female and male subjects. Use the opportunity to educate the female patient on the technique and importance of performing a monthly breast self-examination.
- Inspect the lesion and note any drainage or scabbing.
- Note the location and size of the lesion.
- For a sacral or iliac lesion, note any sacral edema that could compromise blood supply and delay healing.
- When assessing lumps under the skin, palpate them to determine if they are hard or soft and if they are movable or attached to an underlying structure.

Possible Causes

- *Breast cancer.* Occurring most often in female subjects, breast cancer has a good prognosis when diagnosed early. Most lesions are found in the upper outer quadrant of the breast and the axillary region. A nipple discharge may indicate intraductal carcinoma.
- *Shingles.* Caused by a herpes zoster virus, shingles appears after reactivation of the dormant virus in the cerebral ganglia or the ganglia of posterior nerve roots. The patient usually complains of a 2- or 3-day history of fever

and malaise. Painful, fluid-filled vesicles develop along the dermatome. They typically dry and form scabs after about 10 days.

- *Hodgkin's disease.* Characterized by painless, progressive enlargement of the lymph nodes, spleen, and other lymphoid tissue, Hodgkin's disease results from proliferation of lymphocytes, histiocytes, eosinophils, and Reed-Sternberg cells. Common early signs include swelling in a cervical, axillary, or groin lymph node and fever, often accompanied by night sweats.
- *Malignant nevi.* Nevi (moles) begin to grow in childhood and increase in number in young adulthood. Up to 70% of malignant melanomas occur from existing nevi that undergo changes in color, size, shape, or texture. They may ulcerate, bleed, or itch. Melanomas commonly occur on the backs of persons exposed to the sun.

Examining the Upper Extremities

Examination of the upper extremities must be thorough and effective because hands, arms, and shoulders are vital to a person's ability to function. To examine the upper extremities properly, you need to perform an integrated, systematic assessment of various aspects of the musculoskeletal, neurologic, and vascular systems, as well as the skin. This requires a clear understanding of the anatomy of the upper extremities, including supporting bones and muscles, their vascular and lymphatic supply, and the relationship between these parts of the body and the neurologic system (see ▶ *Structures of the Upper Extremities*).

ANATOMY REVIEW

STRUCTURES OF THE UPPER EXTREMITIES

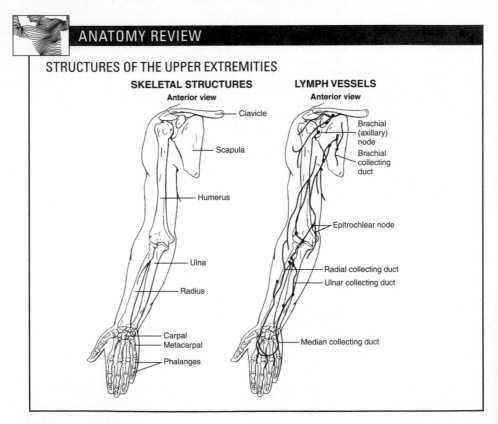

SKELETAL STRUCTURES
Anterior view

- Clavicle
- Scapula
- Humerus
- Ulna
- Radius
- Carpal
- Metacarpal
- Phalanges

LYMPH VESSELS
Anterior view

- Brachial (axillary) node
- Brachial collecting duct
- Epitrochlear node
- Radial collecting duct
- Ulnar collecting duct
- Median collecting duct

MUSCLES

Anterior view　　　**Posterior view**

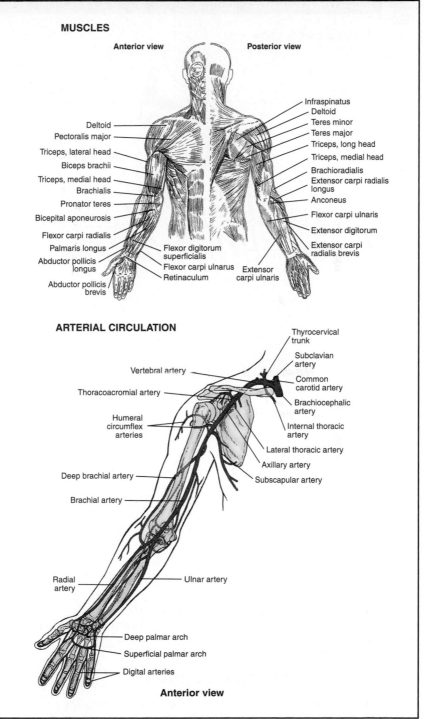

Anterior view labels:
Deltoid
Pectoralis major
Triceps, lateral head
Biceps brachii
Triceps, medial head
Brachialis
Pronator teres
Bicepital aponeurosis
Flexor carpi radialis
Palmaris longus
Abductor pollicis longus
Abductor pollicis brevis
Flexor digitorum superficialis
Flexor carpi ulnarus
Retinaculum
Extensor carpi ulnaris

Posterior view labels:
Infraspinatus
Deltoid
Teres minor
Teres major
Triceps, long head
Triceps, medial head
Brachioradialis
Extensor carpi radialis longus
Anconeus
Flexor carpi ulnaris
Extensor digitorum
Extensor carpi radialis brevis

ARTERIAL CIRCULATION

Thyrocervical trunk
Subclavian artery
Common carotid artery
Brachiocephalic artery
Internal thoracic artery
Lateral thoracic artery
Axillary artery
Subscapular artery
Vertebral artery
Thoracoacromial artery
Humeral circumflex arteries
Deep brachial artery
Brachial artery
Radial artery
Ulnar artery
Deep palmar arch
Superficial palmar arch
Digital arteries

Anterior view

From Thibodeau G, Patton K: *Anatomy and physiology,* ed 6, St Louis, 2007, Mosby.

continued

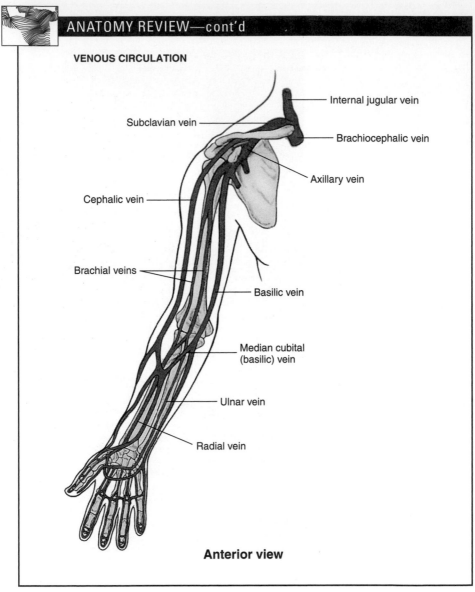

ANATOMY REVIEW—cont'd

VENOUS CIRCULATION

Internal jugular vein

Subclavian vein

Brachiocephalic vein

Axillary vein

Cephalic vein

Brachial veins

Basilic vein

Median cubital
(basilic) vein

Ulnar vein

Radial vein

Anterior view

From Thibodeau G, Patton K: *Anatomy and physiology,* ed 6, St Louis, 2007, Mosby.

In addition, you must palpate pulses, lymph nodes, and muscles; evaluate muscle strength; and test your patient's deep tendon reflexes (DTRs), sensory ability, and range of motion (ROM).

EXAMINATION STEPS AND FINDINGS

Examination of the upper extremities primarily involves the skills of inspection and palpation, which can be performed simultaneously for expediency (see ▨ *Key Examination Steps for the Upper Extremities*).

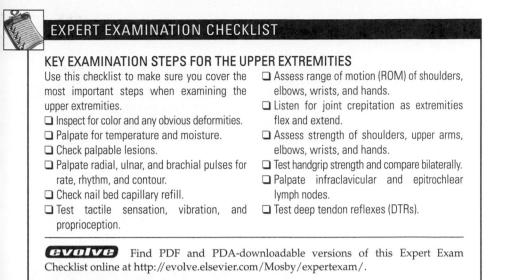

KEY EXAMINATION STEPS FOR THE UPPER EXTREMITIES

Use this checklist to make sure you cover the most important steps when examining the upper extremities.

❏ Inspect for color and any obvious deformities.
❏ Palpate for temperature and moisture.
❏ Check palpable lesions.
❏ Palpate radial, ulnar, and brachial pulses for rate, rhythm, and contour.
❏ Check nail bed capillary refill.
❏ Test tactile sensation, vibration, and proprioception.
❏ Assess range of motion (ROM) of shoulders, elbows, wrists, and hands.
❏ Listen for joint crepitation as extremities flex and extend.
❏ Assess strength of shoulders, upper arms, elbows, wrists, and hands.
❏ Test handgrip strength and compare bilaterally.
❏ Palpate infraclavicular and epitrochlear lymph nodes.
❏ Test deep tendon reflexes (DTRs).

evolve Find PDF and PDA-downloadable versions of this Expert Exam Checklist online at http://evolve.elsevier.com/Mosby/expertexam/.

Before beginning your examination, make sure the room is well lit and warm enough to keep your patient comfortable. In addition, have the following equipment readily available: a stethoscope, tape measure, reflex hammer, piece of cotton, cotton-tipped swab or paper clip (or both), and low-frequency tuning fork.

If the patient has a complaint involving one extremity, examine the unaffected one first. Doing so will give you a better idea of the normal appearance and function of the patient's extremities. It will also allow your patient to relax while you begin your examination.

INSPECTION

Inspect the skin of the upper extremities for ecchymosis, abnormal markings, changes in color, and swelling. In addition, note any unusual bruises or marks, such as needle injection sites or track marks. If your patient has an intravenous (IV) catheter in one arm, inspect the insertion site for evidence of infection and inflammation, including redness, swelling, tenderness, heat, drainage, or red streaks along the course of the vein.

Look for scratch marks and other evidence of pruritus, which may offer clues to possible liver disease, diabetes mellitus, kidney disease, or thyroid disorders.

Examine the color and shape of your patient's nails, looking for pallor, cyanosis, hemorrhages, and clubbing.

Compare the size of your patient's arms for bilateral symmetry. Note any unilateral or bilateral edema. If you suspect asymmetry or your patient has obvious edema in one arm, measure and record arm circumference. Be sure to note the measurement site in your notes so that you can compare arm circumference measurements later, using the same location.

Inspect the shoulder joints at all angles. Carefully observe their anterior, posterior, and lateral aspects. Note any swelling, deformity, or surrounding muscle atrophy. Also inspect all remaining joints, including the elbows, wrists, and interphalangeal joints.

Inspect the upper extremity muscles, looking for obvious deformity, asymmetry, gross hypertrophy or atrophy, and obvious spasms.

Evaluating Reflexes

To evaluate your patient's motor reflexes and sensory pathways, you will use a reflex hammer to elicit DTRs. When testing reflexes, position the patient's extremity so that the tendon is slightly stretched. Typically, you can accomplish this by deviating the joint (elbow or wrist) away from you.

To use the reflex hammer properly, swing it briskly downward to strike the tendon. Then quickly snap your wrist back. Be sure to hold the handle of the hammer loosely between your thumb and index finger so that you can achieve a full swinging motion.

Test the biceps, triceps, and brachioradialis (supinator) reflexes (see 🔲 *Testing Reflexes in the Upper Extremities*).

EXAMINATION TIP

TESTING REFLEXES IN THE UPPER EXTREMITIES

The following directions explain how to accurately test deep tendon reflexes (DTRs) of the upper extremities and also the grasp reflex.

Biceps reflex

With your patient's arm bent 45 degrees at the elbow, place your finger on the inside of the elbow over the tendon of the biceps muscle. Now tap your finger. The biceps should contract and the forearm should flex at the elbow. The biceps reflex, present at birth, is mediated by the spinal cord at the C5-C6 segmental level.

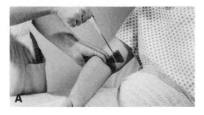

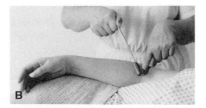

Testing biceps reflex in a sitting patient.

Testing biceps reflex in a recumbent patient.

Triceps reflex

With your patient's arm bent 90 degrees at the elbow, tap the short tendon of the triceps muscle close to its insertion near the tip of the elbow. The muscle should contract in response, and the forearm should extend. This reflex is mediated by the spinal cord at the C7-C8 segmental level. It is present 6 weeks after birth.

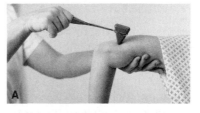

Testing triceps reflex in a sitting patient.

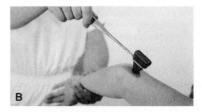

Testing triceps reflex in a recumbent patient.

If you have trouble eliciting the triceps reflex, try this alternative method. With your patient sitting up, hold his upper arm away from the

continued

body and ask the patient to let the forearm hang limp. Now test the reflex again with the arm in this position.

Brachioradialis reflex

To elicit this reflex (also called the *supinator reflex*), tap about 2 inches (5 cm) from the styloid process of the radius. In a normal response, the patient's arm flexes at the elbow and the forearm pronates. This reflex is mediated by the spinal cord at the C5-C6 segmental level.

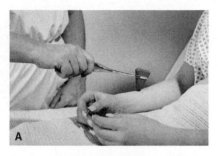

A

Testing brachioradialis reflex in a sitting patient.

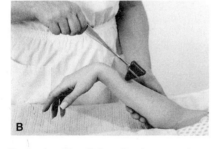

B

Testing brachioradialis reflex in a recumbent patient.

Grasp reflex

A normal reflex in infants up to about 8 months old, the grasp reflex is also an important test for patients who are unconscious or have weakened upper extremities. To test the grasp reflex, place your index and middle fingers in your patient's palm, between the thumb and index finger. Gently withdraw your fingers, pulling them across the skin of your patient's palm. If your patient's hand tightens to grasp your fingers, he has a positive grasp reflex. In an adult, this reflex indicates widespread brain damage or cortical lesions, especially in the frontal lobe area.

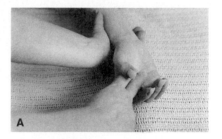

A

Testing grasp reflex by dragging index and middle fingers across the patient's palm.

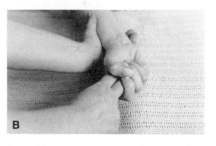

B

A positive response occurs if your patient grasps your hand.

Be sure to compare the response with the corresponding reflex on the opposite side of the body.

You can record your patient's reflex response several different ways, but many nurses use the following scale:

++++   Brisk, hyperactive, clonus of tendon associated with disease
+++   More brisk than normal, but not necessarily associated with disease
++   Normal
+   Low normal, slightly diminished response
0   No response

To increase the speed with which you record your patient's reflex responses, consider using a stick figure diagram. Write each reflex result, in plus signs, at the proper location on the stick figure. This method not only spares you from writing down all the reflex names and locations but it also gives you an easy visual comparison of reflex response at various body locations and testing times.

If you suspect hepatic disease, especially hepatic encephalopathy, ask your patient to hold the arms in front, with the wrists hyperextended as if trying to stop traffic. Ask the patient to hold this position for at least 1 minute. If abnormal movements appear, the patient may have hepatic disease.

Sensory Testing

After testing and documenting your patient's reflexes, turn to the sensory examination. This is a subjective test used to evaluate tactile sensation (superficial pain), vibration, and proprioception.

Peripheral nerve damage causes sensory deficits in consistent and predictable locations on the upper extremities. To refresh your memory, look at a dermatome chart to locate the approximate body areas innervated by the sensory portion of each spinal nerve. This way, if you detect a deficit, or your patient complains of sensory changes, you can determine which spinal nerve might be involved by comparing sensory test results in each extremity (see *Tracking the Source of Sensory Loss*).

TRACKING THE SOURCE OF SENSORY LOSS

Peripheral nerve damage causes sensory deficits in consistent and predictable locations on the upper extremities, as shown here in the shaded areas.

If your patient has an area of sensory loss, you may be able to use its location to determine which peripheral nerve is involved. Use this illustration as a key to helping track sources of sensory loss.

To track sensory loss, ask your patient to close his eyes. Then, using the stick end of a cotton-tipped swab and warm and cool objects, touch the patient in random areas and ask the patient to identify each sensation.

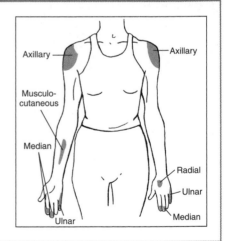

While performing the sensory portion of your examination, you will want your patient's eyes to be closed so that he responds only to what is felt. To reassure the patient, first tell him that you are going to perform some painless tests of feeling in the arms. Then ask the patient to close his eyes.

To assess tactile sensation, ask the patient to tell you when and where he feels you touching him; then touch a cotton wisp to corresponding areas of each extremity. Compare the sensitivity of both arms, and compare the sensitivity of proximal and distal parts of each arm.

Because pain and temperature sensations are transmitted together in the lateral part of the spinal cord, usually you will not have to test temperature recognition. If you decide to test it anyway, then systematically touch cool and warm objects to your patient's arms, and record the responses to temperature identification. Try using test tubes filled with cold and warm water for this part of the examination.

Assess your patient's ability to recognize superficial pain by touching various locations on the arms with the sharp and rounded ends of a paper clip or with the sharp and dull ends of a cotton-tipped swab that has been snapped in two. While your patient's eyes are closed, ask him to tell you whether you are touching him with something sharp or something dull. Be sure to apply the same amount of pressure each time and compare pain sensations between arms.

Vibration and proprioception sensations are transmitted together in the posterior segment of the spinal cord. To test vibration sensation, you can use a low-frequency tuning fork. Place the handle of the vibrating fork against the most distal bony prominence, such as the interphalangeal joint, and ask your patient to tell you when he feels vibration and when it stops vibrating. If your patient does not feel any vibrations, then move the tuning fork proximally until he does. As with all measurements of sensation, compare each extremity.

LIFESPAN CONSIDERATIONS

Older adults can sometimes have a diminished sense of superficial pain, vibration, and proprioception. Plan to use a stronger stimulus with these individuals.

To test position sense, tell your patient that you are going to move some of the fingers so they point up or down. Show the patient what you mean; then ask the patient to close his eyes. Take one of the fingers or thumbs and move it so it is pointing up or down. Ask the patient to tell you which direction the finger is pointing. Repeat this test several times on each side.

NORMAL FINDINGS
- Skin color uniform, with fingernails of equal thickness (With age, skin becomes thinner and drier, and nails take on a yellowish overtone.)
- Fine, bright-red, irregularly shaped blood vessels, called *telangiectasis,* visible through the skin (As the dermis thins, these small blood vessels dilate and sometimes burst. The resulting marks may be called *broken blood vessels, venous stars, spider bursts,* or *angioids.*)
- Flat, tan-to-brown maculae on the dorsal surface of the hands and other areas of sun-exposed skin (Common in middle-aged and older adults, these lesions are usually actinic keratoses or senile lentigo, also called *liver spots.* Most are benign, although actinic keratoses may be premalignant.)

- Bright-red, soft, dome-shaped lesions with a diameter of 1 mm or greater (They are called *cherry angiomas* and result from proliferation and dilation of superficial skin capillaries. Trauma resulting in extravasation from the capillaries or clotting in the vessels may cause the lesions to appear black. Although cherry angiomas may be observed in early adulthood, they are most numerous after age 40. They are benign.)
- Arms symmetrical in length, circumference, and alignment
- Muscle mass symmetrical, with good tone

LIFESPAN CONSIDERATIONS

Symmetrical loss of muscle strength occurs normally with aging. In addition, bilateral, symmetrical loss of muscle mass can occur and is easily observed in the bone spaces of the dorsal surface of the hands.

- Joints equal in size and shape bilaterally, without obvious deformity or lesions
- DTRs equal bilaterally; absence of finger flexor response bilaterally
- Sensory abilities allowing detection of light touch, vibration, and position (The patient can differentiate between sharp and dull sensations.)

ABNORMAL FINDINGS

- Pruritus or itching, a common symptom of dry skin (Be alert for systemic diseases associated with pruritus, such as liver disease, diabetes mellitus, kidney disease, and thyroid disorders.)
- Trauma to the skin, including abrasions, incised wounds (incisions), puncture wounds, lacerations, and burns
- Joint swelling, especially if normal bony landmarks are obscured, indicating excess fluid
- Joint deformity, possibly resulting from contracture (shortening of surrounding joint structures), subluxation (partial separation of joint surfaces), or disruption of structures surrounding the joint
- Joint weakness or disruption of joint-supporting structures, possibly resulting in a joint that is too weak to function as designed (It may require external supporting devices.)
- Thickened sheath on the palmar surface of the wrist, possibly indicating carpal tunnel syndrome (Thickening of the flexor tendon sheath of the median nerve can lead to numbness and paresthesia. Sustained palmar flexion produces symptoms of numbness and paresthesia over the palmar surface of the hand, the first three fingers, and part of the fourth finger [called *Phalen's sign*].)
- Edema, possibly resulting from an injury, cellulitis, lymphedema, venous obstruction (as might occur with thrombophlebitis, an inflammation of the walls of the veins), or heart failure
- Flattening of the anterior aspect of the shoulder, possibly indicating dislocation

- Intermittent pallor and cyanosis of the skin on the hands and fingers, possibly caused by episodic constriction of peripheral small arteries or arterioles characteristic of Raynaud's disease or Raynaud's phenomenon (After an episode of constriction, hyperemia may produce a red color [rubor].)
- Ischemic changes and gangrene of the hands and fingers, possibly accompanying Buerger's disease (thromboangiitis obliterans), an occlusive vascular condition affecting the medium-sized arteries and medium-sized, mostly superficial, veins of the extremities (Distal pulses are often diminished.)
- Streaky redness, tenderness, and warmth along the course of a vein, possibly resulting from thrombophlebitis
- Limited ROM, possibly resulting from an injury or arthritis
- Hyporeflexia (diminished reflexes) on one side, possibly indicating a lower motor neuron disorder, such as poliomyelitis (Tendon reflexes are diminished in muscular dystrophy and polymyositis in proportion to the loss of muscle strength. DTRs are diminished or absent with loss of sensation or damage to the spinal cord. Loss of sensation in an extremity, coupled with loss of reflexes, suggests lesions in the sensory arc, as seen with neurosyphilis.)
- Hyperreflexia (increased reflexes) on one side, occurring with upper motor neuron diseases, such as cerebrovascular accident (CVA) or the initial stages of amyotrophic lateral sclerosis (ALS)
- Impaired sensory testing, possibly indicating several neurologic disorders (Loss of position sense may suggest a spinal cord lesion when associated with other neurologic complaints. Vibration is the first sense to be lost in peripheral neuropathies such as that caused by diabetes mellitus. This loss also occurs with alcoholism, tertiary syphilis, and vitamin B_{12} deficiency.)
- Nonrhythmic flapping of the wrists and hands, with arms extended and wrists hyperflexed, called *asterixis* (Sometimes termed a *liver flap*, this is associated with such disorders as hepatic encephalopathy, uremia, and respiratory acidosis [see 📷 *Three Ways to Check for Asterixis*].)

EXAMINATION TIP

THREE WAYS TO CHECK FOR ASTERIXIS

An excessive involuntary flapping tremor, asterixis is most commonly seen in the wrists and fingers. This sign may be elicited when the patient is asked to sustain a fixed position or posture; then brief, irregular relaxation of the muscles used to sustain the position cause the affected body part to display a flapping tremor. Although the exact underlying mechanism of this loss of muscle tone is unknown, asterixis is believed to be the result of a build-up of metabolic toxins, such as ammonia, in the brain. These toxins may cause cerebral metabolic changes that affect the motor neurons in the brain. To confirm asterixis, use one of the following assessment techniques. Your ability to elicit asterixis will depend on your patient's level of consciousness because he will need to be alert enough to sustain a fixed position.

- If your patient is awake and alert, instruct him to stretch the arms out in front, maintaining

continued

EXAMINATION TIP—cont'd

dorsiflexion of both wrists. Look for intermittent relaxation of the wrists and flapping of the hands.

- If the patient's level of consciousness is diminished, lift one of the legs off of the bed and dorsiflex the foot at the ankle. Look

for intermittent relaxation of the ankle and flapping of the foot.

- If the patient is lethargic and weak but can follow commands, ask him to squeeze your fingers. Look for involuntary clenching and unclenching of the fist.

PALPATION

Palpate the skin of the upper extremities for temperature, moisture, and lesions or nodules. Compare between arms, noting differences and similarities, as needed. Then move on to test the patient's pulses, lymph nodes, muscles, and ROM.

Palpating Pulses

The axillary artery is the major arterial structure of the upper extremity. It is a continuation of the subclavian. As it passes into the shoulder area and begins traveling downward, it becomes the brachial artery. The brachial artery sends branches to the humerus, the muscles, and the skin of the area. About 1 cm below the bend of the elbow, the brachial splits off and becomes the radial and ulnar arteries. The radial artery continues down the lateral aspect of the forearm, but it is smaller in caliber than the ulnar. The ulnar artery is the larger of the two and courses down the medial aspect of the forearm and the wrist.

Palpate the brachial, radial, and ulnar pulses for rate, strength, contour, and amplitude (see 🖼 *Performing Allen's Test*).

EXAMINATION TIP

PERFORMING ALLEN'S TEST

Before your patient undergoes arterial blood gas sampling or insertion of an arterial catheter, you will need to check the patency of the radial and ulnar arteries by performing Allen's test.

Ask your patient to open the hand into a relaxed, slightly flexed position. Then ask the patient to make a tight fist while you use both hands to occlude the radial and ulnar arteries, as shown in the first illustration.

Now have your patient open the hand, as shown in the second illustration. Because of the temporary lack of blood supply, it will look blanched. Be sure your patient does not

spread the fingers too widely or forcefully, because this may compress the palmar arches between the fascial planes and give a false-positive result.

Now release the pressure over one artery. Most nurses release the ulnar artery first, as shown in the third illustration, but the sequence is not important. Within 3 to 5 seconds after you release the artery, your patient's palm should flush with color as it fills with blood. This result means that the patient's ulnar artery is patent.

After several minutes, repeat the test, but release the radial artery this time. The results should be the same, indicating that the patient's radial artery is patent.

---

continued

EXAMINATION TIP—cont'd

If you release an artery and your patient's hand is not infused with color within 5 to 10 seconds, the artery or one of its distal branches is occluded. Consequently, you should not puncture either artery.

If your patient is unconscious or anesthetized and cannot make a clenched fist, you can still perform Allen's test. Just use an elastic bandage to blanch the hand.

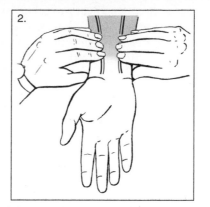

Ask your patient to open the fist. The palm should be blanched.

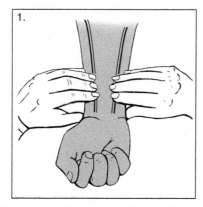

Compress both arteries while the patient makes a clenched fist.

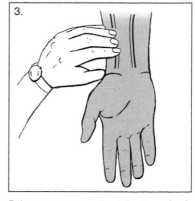

Release one artery and wait for the patient's palm to flush within a few seconds.

Document pulse amplitude using the following scale:
+4   Bounding, hyperkinetic pulse
+3   Normal pulse
+2   Diminished pulse
+1   Weak, thready, hypokinetic pulse
0   Absent pulse

Test the compliance of vein walls by compressing prominent veins with the pads of your fingers. Note resilience, texture, and the presence of valves.

If you have not done so earlier in the examination, check capillary refill time by pressing on a nail bed for several seconds. Then release the pressure, and note how long it takes for the nail to regain its normal color.

Palpating Lymph Nodes

To detect possible infection, you will want to palpate the lymph nodes (the axillary and epitrochlear nodes) for size, consistency, and tenderness. The axillary nodes are located along the chest wall, high in the axilla and midway between the anterior and posterior axillary folds. The epitrochlear nodes are located superficially on the medial side of the elbow.

Palpating Muscles

When palpating the muscles of the upper extremities, focus on their bulk (or mass), tone, and strength. Ask your patient to tell you if he feels pain or other abnormal sensations at any time while you are palpating the limbs. Be sure to document it if your patient reports any of these feelings.

Muscle bulk can be determined by bilateral examination of the upper extremities. Remember that your patient's dominant side may tend to have a larger muscle mass than the nondominant side. Examine upper extremity muscles for gross hypertrophy or atrophy. This may be difficult if your patient is markedly obese. Remember that muscle mass declines normally with age.

Upper extremity strength can be evaluated in various ways, based on your patient's age, sex, and level of muscular training. To perform a quick test of muscular strength, ask your patient to move the upper extremities through their full ROM without applying any resistance beyond what is already provided by gravity. For example, ask your patient to fully extend the elbows and place the arms palms up, in front. Ask the patient to hold this position for about 10 seconds. Watch to see whether one of the extremities drifts or falls and whether he begins to pronate the wrists, which indicates weakness.

Another way to test muscle strength is with resistance. First, ask your patient to flex the elbow and curl the arm inward as you apply resistance by trying to pull his forearm toward you. This exercise tests the biceps. Then, with your patient's elbow still flexed, ask him to extend the arm while you try to keep it in the flexed position. This exercise tests the triceps.

You can test wrist extension by having the patient make a fist and then resist your attempts to pull it down.

Evaluate finger abduction by having your patient place the palms down and spread the fingers apart. Ask the patient to resist you as you try to push his fingers back together. Test the thumb by asking your patient to touch the thumb to the tip of the little finger.

To test handgrip strength, have your patient grasp both of your hands and squeeze them as hard as possible. Note bilateral strength. Remember, however, that your patient's dominant hand may be slightly stronger than the non-dominant hand. To avoid confusion, cross your arms so that the patient's right hand grips your right hand and his left hand grips your left hand (see 🖼 *Assessing Handgrip Strength Safely*).

EXAMINATION TIP

ASSESSING HANDGRIP STRENGTH SAFELY

When testing your patient's handgrip strength, you can help prevent pain or injury to your hands and fingers by following these suggestions:

- Remove any rings or hand jewelry that could pinch or compress your fingers.
- Cross your index and middle fingers, and ask your patient to squeeze only these fingers, as shown in the photograph. This technique will prevent your fingers from being painfully squeezed together, but you will still be able to assess the patient's bilateral handgrip strength.

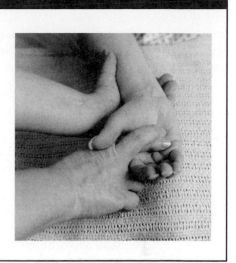

Testing for Range of Motion

Evaluate ROM in the patient's shoulder by asking him to perform three simple maneuvers. First, ask the patient to raise both arms to a vertical position at the sides of the head to check shoulder flexion. Next, ask the patient to place both hands behind the neck, with elbows out to the sides to demonstrate external rotation and abduction. Finally, ask the patient to place both hands behind the small of the back to test internal rotation.

To test elbow ROM, ask the patient to bend and straighten the elbow. Next, ask him to place the arms at the sides with elbows flexed. Then have the patient supinate and pronate the arms. Finally, ask the patient to flex and extend the arms at the elbows.

To test wrist ROM, ask the patient to flex and hyperextend the wrists. In addition, ask him to bend the wrists to the radial side, then to the ulnar side. As the patient performs these maneuvers, palpate the wrist with both of your thumbs on the wrist dorsum and your fingers underneath. Note any swelling, bogginess, or tenderness.

To test ROM in the hand joints, ask the patient to make a fist with each hand and then extend and spread the fingers. Note any decreased mobility or pain on movement.

Palpation during ROM tests gives information about joint integrity. A normal joint moves easily through its ROM. A snap or a crack may indicate that a ligament is slipping over a bony prominence.

To assess the shoulder for tenderness, palpate the sternoclavicular joint, acromioclavicular joint, subacromial area, and bicipital groove. Also palpate the tendons of the teres minor and infraspinatus muscles (sometimes called the *rotator cuff*) for swelling, nodes, tears, and pain. To do this, ask the patient to adduct the arm by bringing it over the chest. Facing the patient, place your thumb on the anterior surface of the shoulder joint and the tips of your fingers on the posterior surface. Ask the patient to move the humerus backward about 20 degrees. Now move behind the patient and, with your fingertips over the head of the humerus and your other hand between the scapulae, ask your patient to move the arm behind the body so that the dorsum of the hand rests on the small of the back (internal rotation).

To palpate the elbow, flex your patient's arm about 70 degrees and support it in that position with your nondominant hand. If the joint is swollen, you will probably be able to palpate the swelling in the medial groove. With your dominant hand, palpate the joint with your fingertips while applying pressure with your thumb on the opposite side.

Proceed to gently palpate the interphalangeal, metacarpophalangeal, and wrist joints between your thumb and fingers, noting any swelling, bogginess, or tenderness. Assess for nodule formation, which accompanies rheumatoid arthritis, gout, rheumatic fever, and osteoarthritis.

Palpate the brachial pulse, and check for an enlarged epitrochlear lymph node in the depression above and behind the medial condyle of the humerus.

Grading Muscle Strength and Range of Motion

You can grade muscle strength and ROM on a numeric scale from 0 to 5. Use the following key to grade muscle strength accurately:

0   Complete paralysis—No visible or palpable muscle contraction or movement of the extremity

1   Very severe weakness—Weak muscle contraction visible, but the extremity does not move

2   Severe weakness—Patient can roll the extremity but cannot lift it; patient can perform full ROM but not against gravity

3   Moderate weakness—Patient can perform full ROM against gravity but not against resistance

4   Slight weakness—Patient can perform full ROM against gravity and slight resistance

5   Normal muscle strength—Patient can perform full ROM against gravity and resistance

NORMAL FINDINGS

- Skin temperature cool to warm, with minimal moisture and a smooth, even texture (Stimulation of the sympathetic nervous system, as when the patient is embarrassed or anxious, causes diaphoresis and moist skin.)
- Pulses strong and equal bilaterally
- Joints free of obvious deformity, tenderness, or swelling (No crepitus is heard.)
- Muscle strength equal bilaterally, with full movement against resistance
- Veins soft and pliable
- Capillary refill brisk, less than 4 seconds
- Thrill on palpation or a bruit on auscultation over renal shunt or fistula (These findings reflect turbulent blood flow in the area and are considered normal [see ▪ *What to Expect When Examining the Upper Extremities*].)

NORMAL FINDINGS

WHAT TO EXPECT WHEN EXAMINING THE UPPER EXTREMITIES

Use this quick review to confirm normal findings when examining the upper extremities.

- Skin color of upper extremities matches skin color of rest of body, except in areas routinely exposed to sunlight
- No edema or any obvious deformities
- Skin warm and smooth, with minimal moisture
- Radial, ulnar, and brachial pulses easily palpated and bilaterally equal in strength and amplitude
- Capillary refill time less than 2 seconds
- Full range of motion (ROM) in all joints, without pain

- Symmetrical upper extremities
- Shoulder muscle strength equal bilaterally
- Handgrip strength equal bilaterally
- Brachioradialis, biceps, triceps, and deep tendon reflexes (DTRs) ++ bilaterally
- Subclavian and epitrochlear lymph nodes either nonpalpable or small, soft, mobile, and nontender
- Superficial touch and pain sensations normal bilaterally, with intact vibratory and position senses

ABNORMAL FINDINGS

- Abnormal bony growths on the distal interphalangeal joints (Heberden's nodes) or the proximal interphalangeal joints (Bouchard's nodes), indicating osteoarthritic joint changes (These growths are firm and usually nontender.)
- Subcutaneous nodules (rheumatoid nodules) over bony prominences or along the extensor surface of the ulna, indicating rheumatoid arthritis (These nodules are firm, mobile, and nontender. They may accompany other symptoms of rheumatoid arthritis, such as morning stiffness, pain on motion, or tenderness and swelling in at least one joint.)
- Firm, erythematous, painful nodules (tophi) (These form over joints during acute flare-ups of gout and, if ulcerated, leak a white, chalky substance composed of uric acid crystals.)
- Crepitus (an audible creaking sound as the joint moves through its ROM), possibly indicating pain or limitation of movement (Crepitation may be benign or associated with such joint diseases as arthritis or inflamed tendon sheaths.)
- Pulselessness, pallor, pain, or paresthesias of the distal upper extremities, indicating arterial occlusion
- Arterial compression, occurring with compartment syndrome and possibly resulting from casts, tight dressings, and infiltrated IV fluids (If arterial compression is left untreated, the patient may lose limb function and mobility.)
- Swelling of the extremity, along with pallor or cyanosis and dilation of superficial veins, warning of thrombosis of the axillary or subclavian veins (Diminished or absent pulses may occur as well, from associated arterial spasm. The patient also may have moderate-to-severe pain in the arm and shoulder, diffuse pain through the involved extremity, and fever.)

- Swelling or bogginess felt over the joint, especially the elbow, possibly accompanied by tenderness and erythema (This indicates an effusion, sometimes called *water on the elbow,* which is caused by synovitis, an inflammation of the synovial membrane resulting from trauma.)
- Decreased joint mobility and ROM, indicating arthritis, trauma, tendinitis, or bursitis (Decreased joint mobility and ROM arise as a complication of immobility or as a normal variant of aging.)
- Extreme pain on movement of the wrist, elbow, and shoulder, along with joint heat, redness, or inflammation related to tenosynovitis (an inflammation of the tendon sheath and the enclosed tendons that primarily affects the wrist, shoulder, and ankle)
- Muscle atrophy and weakness, possibly related to malnutrition or disuse, as seen with paralysis and prolonged periods of immobility (Muscles appear flattened or concave when atrophy has affected the extremity. Tremors or fasciculations also may be observed in the atrophic limb. Fasciculations indicate lower motor neuron damage as the cause of the atrophy.)
- Paralysis, possibly resulting from such conditions as Guillain-Barré syndrome, spinal cord injury, CVA, diabetic neuropathy, multiple sclerosis, or poliomyelitis
- Inflamed lymphatic vessels, possibly resulting from bacterial infection (When this occurs in superficial vessels, painful reddish streaks appear beneath the skin [lymphangitis] and are typically followed by an inflammation of the lymph nodes [lymphadenitis]. Affected nodes become enlarged and tender.)
- Veins that feel hard and cordlike, possibly indicating sclerosis (They may also feel tortuous, with prominent, beadlike valves palpable through the skin.)
- Delayed capillary refill, characterized by blanching of the nail beds for more than 4 seconds after being released from pressure (This is usually a warning of compromised circulation, as in diminished cardiac output, hypotension, or arterial occlusion.)
- Loss of a palpable thrill or an audible bruit over an arteriovenous fistula, possibly indicating thrombosis or clotting of the fistula

EXPLORING CHIEF COMPLAINTS

When examining your patient's upper extremities, your first task is to determine the chief complaint. Doing so will help you set your assessment priorities and allow you to focus your assessment appropriately.

Help your patient describe the chief complaint by asking open-ended questions and listening carefully to the answers. Allow the patient to describe the problem in his own words. Based on your patient's answers, you can focus on areas that need further assessment.

MUSCLE STIFFNESS OR SPASM

If your patient complains of muscle stiffness or spasm, investigate further by asking the following questions:
- When did your symptoms start? How long do they usually last?

- Does the stiffness or spasm tend to start after you have been performing certain activities or when you have been sitting, sleeping, or standing in certain positions?
- If the muscle stiffness or spasm occurs at night, does it ever wake you from sleep? If you wake up with it in the morning, in what position were you sleeping?
- How would you describe the stiffness or spasm? Is it sharp, dull, aching, stabbing, or throbbing?
- Did the stiffness or spasm start after an injury or after doing anything unusual?
- Does it tend to worsen with weather changes, especially when conditions become cold and damp or hot and humid?
- Does a fever, headache, or chest pain accompany the stiffness or spasm?

Focusing Your Assessment

When examining a patient who complains of muscle stiffness or spasm in the upper extremity, focus your assessment as follows:
- Look for muscle atrophy in the major muscle groups of the arms. Compare them bilaterally.
- Assess muscle tone and strength by testing each major muscle group with resistance.
- Test the patient's DTRs.

Possible Causes

- *Muscle fatigue.* Painful muscle contractions, or spasms, typically are the result of muscle fatigue. Spasms are usually relieved by rest or stretching. They can be found in neurologic disorders and electrolyte imbalances.
- *Muscle rigidity.* Rigidity is seen with such disorders as Parkinson's disease. Symptoms may progress and affect movement.
- *Muscle sprain.* Sprain follows unusual or prolonged exercise or injury. Symptoms improve with rest.
- *Hypocalcemic tetany.* This condition produces frequent spasms in many muscles and is accompanied by paresthesias in the hands and feet. If you suspect this condition, check for Trousseau's and Chvostek's signs (see 🔲 *Detecting Trousseau's and Chvostek's Signs*).

EXAMINATION TIP

DETECTING TROUSSEAU'S AND CHVOSTEK'S SIGNS
Low serum calcium (and sometimes magnesium) levels can result in tetany, a life-threatening condition characterized by muscle twitching, cramps, seizures, and sharp wrist and ankle flexion. If you suspect either disorder, evaluate your patient for the classic signs: Trousseau's and Chvostek's signs.

continued

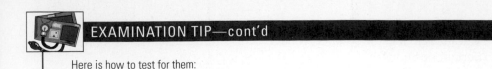

Here is how to test for them:

Trousseau's sign
- Place a blood pressure cuff on your patient's upper arm, and inflate the cuff to a point above the systolic blood pressure. Then watch the hand.
- If within 4 minutes the patient experiences a carpopedal spasm with ventral contraction of the thumb and fingers, the sign is positive.

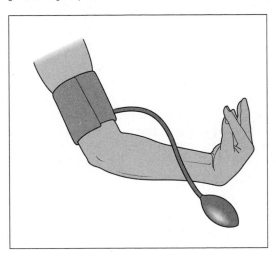

Chvostek's sign
- Tap the patient's cheek over the facial nerve, just in front of the ear.
- Watch for abnormal contraction of the facial muscles, twitching of the lips, or possible contraction of all the muscles on one side of the face. If any of these occur, the sign is positive.

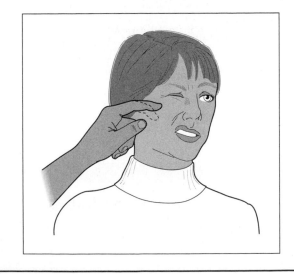

From Mosby: *Expert rapid response,* St Louis, 1999, Mosby.

- *Cervical nerve root compression.* This condition follows injury or strain to the neck. Muscular pain may be accompanied by pain that follows the distribution of the involved nerve root. The patient's DTRs may be diminished.
- *Upper motor neuron disorders.* An example of an upper motor neuron disorder is CVA, in which the patient has increased muscle tone, spasticity, and increased DTRs.
- *Lower motor neuron disorders.* An example is ALS, in which the patient has decreased muscle tone and strength, as well as decreased DTRs.

JOINT PAIN OR STIFFNESS

If your patient complains of joint stiffness or pain, investigate further by asking the following questions:

- When are your joints stiff and painful? How long do they stay that way? Does the problem tend to occur more in the morning, during the day, or at night?
- How would you describe the stiffness or pain? Is it sharp, dull, aching, stabbing, or throbbing?
- Did the stiffness or pain start after you were injured or you had done something unusual?
- Do you (the patient who is of African or Mediterranean descent) have a history of sickle cell disease?
- Do you have a family or personal history of rheumatoid or degenerative arthritis or heart disease?
- Does a fever accompany the stiffness or pain?
- Does your skin change color, or do you get a rash before, during, or after the symptoms?
- Do you remember receiving any insect bites, especially tick bites, in the past 7 months or so?
- Have you had any surgery in the affected area (particularly a joint replacement)?

Focusing Your Assessment

When examining a patient who complains of upper extremity joint stiffness or pain, focus your assessment as follows:

- Inspect the joints for swelling, ecchymosis, or deformity. Are both arms symmetrical?
- Find out if the joints are tender to the touch.
- Is there pain with ROM? Is ROM restricted because of pain?
- Take the patient's temperature to see if he has a fever.
- Assess the skin for insect bites or rashes.
- Investigate whether the pain might be referred, such as from the chest. If necessary, obtain electrocardiogram (ECG) tracings to look for patterns of cardiac ischemia or infarction.

Possible Causes

- *Rheumatoid arthritis.* Patients with rheumatoid arthritis typically have morning stiffness, joint tenderness, swelling in at least two joint groups, and subcutaneous nodules over bony prominences (see ☒ *Rheumatoid Arthritis*).

DISORDER CLOSE-UP

RHEUMATOID ARTHRITIS

A chronic, systemic, inflammatory disorder, rheumatoid arthritis is characterized by persistent synovitis of multiple joints. It is found worldwide and affects about 1% of the population. It strikes females three times more often than males.

Rheumatoid arthritis is believed to be an autoimmune process with both genetic and environmental factors playing a role in its development. Both *Helicobacter pylori* and the Epstein-Barr virus are among the possible causes of altered immune response being investigated. Rheumatoid arthritis is known by its persistent immunologic activity. T lymphocytes infiltrate the synovial membrane of the joint and proliferate, initiating an immune response. The release of cytokines further stimulates macrophage activity, and B cells produce autoantibodies to immunoglobulin G (IgG). These antibodies, called *rheumatoid factors,* are found in nearly all patients who have the disease.

An antigen-antibody reaction sparks formation of immune complexes that generate lysosomal enzymes, which can destroy joint tissue. Vasodilation from the immune response causes tissues to become warm and erythematous. Increased capillary permeability produces swelling of the affected area. The extensive network of new blood vessels (vascular granulation tissue called *pannus*) in the synovial membrane destroys the joints. Pannus erodes the cartilage and bone of affected joints and invades surrounding tissues, including ligaments and tendons.

Characteristic findings

Expect health history and physical examination findings to vary among patients with rheumatoid arthritis, depending on the extent and severity of the disease. Use the information that follows to help distinguish between expected and unexpected findings.

Health history

- Insidious onset of nonspecific symptoms
- Fatigue, malaise
- Anorexia, weight loss
- Persistent low-grade fever
- Bilateral and symmetrical stiffening of joints, beginning in the fingers and possibly extending to the wrists, elbows, knees, and ankles
- Stiffening after inactivity, especially on arising
- Tender and painful joints, initially on movement but eventually at rest
- Paresthesias of the fingers or toes
- Stiff, weak, or painful muscles
- Shortness of breath (with pulmonary nodules or fibrosis)
- Neck pain (with cervical vertebral involvement)

Inspection

- Ulnar deviation of the fingers and subluxation at the metacarpophalangeal joints
- Boutonnière deformities (flexion deformity of the proximal interphalangeal joint with extension of distal joint)
- Swan-neck deformities (hyperextension of the proximal interphalangeal joint with compensatory flexion of the distal joint)
- Limited range of movement (ROM) in affected joints
- Flexion contractures of the elbows
- Joint swelling and redness

continued

DISORDER CLOSE-UP—cont'd

Palpation
- Rheumatoid nodules (firm granulomatous lesions, either fixed or mobile) in subcutaneous tissue of areas subject to pressure
- Joints warm or hot to touch
- Muscle weakness (with spinal cord involvement)
- Positive Babinski's sign (with spinal cord involvement)

Auscultation
- Pericardial friction rub (with pericarditis)

Complications
- Fibrous or bony ankylosis
- Soft-tissue contractures
- Joint deformities
- Vasculitis
- Pleural disease
- Pericarditis
- Episcleritis or scleritis

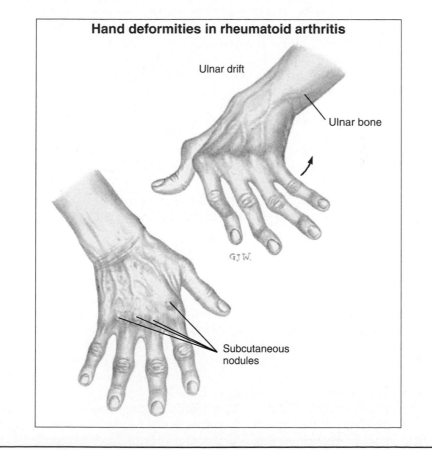

Hand deformities in rheumatoid arthritis

Ulnar drift

Ulnar bone

GJW.

Subcutaneous nodules

From Mourad L: *Orthopedic disorders*, St Louis, 1991, Mosby.

- *Osteoarthritis.* Also called *degenerative joint disease,* osteoarthritis becomes more common with age. Characterized by joint pain that worsens throughout the day, it is aggravated by exercise. Onset is gradual and usually involves only a few joints.
- *Fracture.* Your patient will most likely feel intense pain at a fracture site. Pain may radiate through the arm and will be aggravated by movement.
- *Tendinitis.* This condition produces intense localized pain, aggravated by movement and relieved by rest.
- *Septic arthritis.* An acute bacterial infection of a joint, septic arthritis usually results from contamination during surgery or from bacterial migration from an infection elsewhere in the body. It is characterized by acute pain, redness, swelling, fever, and immobility of the joint.
- *Bursitis.* Symptoms of this disorder may develop after unusually vigorous exercise or strain. The patient will complain of pain, localized tenderness, and limitation of movement.
- *Sickle cell anemia.* Chronic fatigue and painful, swollen joints mark a form of hemolytic anemia, sickle cell anemia. This disease commonly affects people of African or Mediterranean descent.
- *Lyme disease.* This is an infectious disease caused by a spirochete transmitted through tick bites. The insect bite initially produces a red mark that eventually forms a pink or red rash resembling a bull's-eye. Complications are far-reaching and range from meningitis to pericarditis. At least half the victims suffer from joint pain and swelling.
- *Angina or myocardial infarction (MI).* Both of these conditions can refer pain to the shoulder and arm. Your patient may have chest pain as well.

PARESTHESIA OR NUMBNESS
If your patient complains of paresthesia or numbness, investigate further by asking the following questions:

- When did your symptoms begin? Did they follow any type of trauma or strenuous activity?
- What is the exact location of the paresthesia or numbness? Is it the same in both arms, or do you have it only in one arm?
- Is this the first time you have experienced this problem?
- If this is a recurrence, did anything seem to provoke or start up the symptoms this time?
- How long do the symptoms last? Does anything seem to make them better or worse?
- How would you describe the paresthesia or numbness? What does it feel like? Do you have a heavy, achy, or sharp feeling? If so, does it radiate?
- Do you have any associated conditions, such as long-term alcohol or substance abuse, diabetes mellitus, chronic anemia, sickle cell disease, a recent viral syndrome, a recent immunization or injection, a recent animal bite or scratch, or a recent insect bite (especially ticks)?
- Do you have any associated symptoms, such as temperature change, altered color, swelling, slurred speech, dizziness, fever, headache, respiratory distress (particularly tachypnea), loss of motor control, or chest pain?
- Have you ever experienced anything like this before?

Focusing Your Assessment

When examining a patient who complains of paresthesia or numbness, focus your assessment as follows:

- Evaluate the sensory system, including the patient's sensitivity to pain, temperature, position, vibration, and light touch, in conjunction with evaluating the motor system (muscle tone, muscle strength, and DTRs).

Possible Causes

- *Fracture, tumor, or swelling.* This can compress a nerve, resulting in numbness or paresthesia.
- *Occlusive vascular diseases.* Raynaud's or Buerger's diseases may cause sensory changes, such as numbness or tingling.
- *Neurologic disorders.* Disorders such as multiple sclerosis and ALS cause paresthesia.
- *Neuropathy.* Degeneration of peripheral nerves can result from many systemic diseases, such as diabetes mellitus, chronic alcoholism, and lead poisoning. Paresthesia often leads to diminished or absent sensation in the most distal parts of the extremities.
- *Vitamin B$_6$ deficiency.* Pyridoxine (vitamin B$_6$) deficiency produces symptoms similar to neuropathy.
- *Hyperventilation.* This condition commonly causes a pins-and-needles sensation because of hypocapnia.
- *Carpal tunnel syndrome.* An occupation-related condition caused by repetitive wrist flexure, this disorder is characterized by paresthesia in the hand and pain in the wrist joint, palm, and sometimes the forearm. The patient may have a sensory deficit in the first three fingers and weakness in the thumb.

PARALYSIS OR WEAKNESS

If your patient complains of paralysis or weakness of the upper extremity, investigate further by asking the following questions:

- When did the problem first occur? Did it follow an event or an injury?
- Have you ever experienced anything like this before?
- Is the paralysis or weakness associated with a specific area of your arm, such as the shoulder or elbow joint, wrist, or fingers?
- Does it affect both of your arms or just one?
- If the paralysis or weakness is a transient occurrence, how long does it usually last?
- Does the paralysis or weakness tend to occur after certain activities, such as a sport? Does it tend to occur in the morning, after sleeping in a certain position?
- If the problem occurs more at night, does it ever wake you?
- What are the characteristics of the paralysis or weakness? Do you have a heavy or achy feeling associated with it? If so, does the feeling radiate?
- Does it tend to get worse with temperature changes either indoors or outdoors? (Examples include a severe decrease or increase in temperature or when the weather becomes wet or humid.)

• Do you have any other symptoms associated with the paralysis or weakness, such as swelling, slurred speech, dizziness, fever, headache, or chest pain?

Focusing Your Assessment
When examining a patient who complains of paralysis or weakness, focus your assessment as follows:
• Look for muscle atrophy in the major muscle groups of the arms. Compare them side to side.
• Assess muscle tone and strength by testing each major muscle group against resistance. This evaluates both the musculoskeletal and neurologic systems.
• Test DTRs. Absent or decreased muscle tone and strength and absent or decreased DTRs are observed in such lower motor neuron disorders as ALS and Guillain-Barré syndrome. In upper motor neuron disorders, expect increased muscle tone, spasticity, and increased DTRs.

Possible Causes
• *Systemic disorder.* Extremity weakness may be caused by many systemic disorders, such as hypokalemia, hypothyroidism, dehydration, vascular disorders, and B-complex vitamin deficiencies. Paralysis can also result from a number of conditions, including Guillain-Barré syndrome, spinal cord injury, CVA, diabetic neuropathy, multiple sclerosis, or poliomyelitis (see 🔍 *Cerebrovascular Accident*).

🔍 DISORDER CLOSE-UP

CEREBROVASCULAR ACCIDENT
During a cerebrovascular accident (CVA), commonly called a *stroke*, decreased blood flow in one or more cerebral blood vessels results in infarcted brain tissue and permanent neurologic deficit. This decreased blood flow can result when a thrombus or embolism occludes a cerebral blood vessel. It also can result from a ruptured cerebral blood vessel, in which case hemorrhage causes cellular ischemia and necrosis.

When cerebral blood flow declines or stops, oxygenation also stops. Within 4 or 5 minutes, pathophysiologic changes begin at the cellular level. Metabolism ceases when glucose, glycogen, and adenosine triphosphate are depleted, and the sodium-potassium pump fails. Cells swell as sodium draws water into them. Cerebral blood vessel walls swell, further decreasing blood flow. Even if circulation is restored, vasospasm and increased blood viscosity can continue to impede blood flow. Severe or prolonged ischemia leads to cellular death and loss of consciousness. Other neurologic deficits caused by a CVA vary with the area involved and the duration of reduced or halted blood flow. Symptoms may become slightly less severe a few days after the CVA, when brain swelling subsides. When assessing the neurologic deficits and sensory motor functions that result from a CVA, remember that they occur on the side of the body opposite the side of the brain that was damaged.

Characteristic findings
Expect health history and physical examination findings to vary among CVA patients, depending on the extent and severity of the disease. Use the information that follows to help distinguish between expected and unexpected findings.

continued

DISORDER CLOSE-UP—cont'd

Health history
- Personal or family history of CVAs
- Obesity
- Sedentary lifestyle
- History of hypertension, diabetes mellitus, atherosclerosis, hyperlipidemia, or atrial fibrillation
- Oral contraceptive use
- Complaints of motor deficits, such as gait changes, weakness, paralysis, or spasticity
- Speech problems
- Sudden onset of hemiparesis or hemiplegia
- Gradual onset of dizziness, mental disturbance, or seizures
- Complaints of numbness or tingling

Inspection
- Altered level of consciousness
- Decreased attention span
- Anxiety
- Mobility and communication difficulties
- Possible incontinence
- Agnosia
- Apraxia
- Emotional lability
- Motor deficits
- Visual field deficits

Palpation
- Diminished muscle strength
- Diminished deep tendon reflexes (DTRs) (initially)
- Sensory losses ranging from slight impairment of touch to inability to perceive position and motion of body parts

Auscultation
- Diminished breath sounds

Vital signs
- Hyperthermia
- Unstable blood pressure
- Irregular respiratory rhythm
- Irregular pulse and heart rhythm

Complications
- Fluid imbalances
- Pulmonary embolism
- Malnutrition
- Aspiration
- Sensory impairment
- Contractures
- Encephalitis
- Coma
- Brain abscess
- Pneumonia

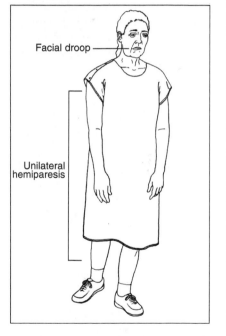

Facial droop

Unilateral hemiparesis

- *Transient ischemia.* Transient or temporary weakness in an extremity or body part may result from temporary interruption of blood supply to the brain, as seen with transient ischemic attacks (TIAs). Other symptoms include blurred vision, aphasia, and dizziness.

SWELLING

If your patient complains of upper extremity swelling, investigate further by asking the following questions:

- When did you first notice the swelling or any change in your arm?
- How did it first start? Did it occur in one location and spread, or did your arm become swollen at one time?
- Has this swelling happened before? How long ago? How long did it last? If it recurs, how often, and what provokes it?
- Does anything make the swelling better or worse?
- Do you have any associated symptoms, such as pain, fever, numbness, or tingling?
- Do you have a history of trauma, a clotting disorder, leukemia, or another neoplasm? Have you had recent exposure to an infection or had an IV or any type of puncture (including insect and animal bites)?

Focusing Your Assessment

When examining a patient who complains of swelling, focus your assessment as follows:

- Note whether the edema is unilateral or bilateral.
- Palpate the swollen area for temperature and tenderness.
- Determine whether the edema is pitting or nonpitting.
- Record the size of the swollen area by measuring the circumference of the extremity at the point of swelling.
- If a joint is involved, assess its ROM for limitation and pain on movement.

Possible Causes

- *Injury.* Fracture, sprain, or strain may cause swelling, which is typically relieved by elevation. Other associated signs and symptoms include deformity, localized ecchymosis or bleeding, pain, immobility, or paresthesia. Joint swelling indicates synovial inflammation or increased synovial fluid.
- *Infiltrated IV fluids.* This is indicated by swelling, coolness, tenderness, and redness at and above the IV catheter insertion site (see ◔ *Responding to Intravenous Fluid Extravasation*).

ACTION STAT

RESPONDING TO INTRAVENOUS FLUID EXTRAVASATION

When an intravenous (IV) catheter slips out of a vein or passes through a vein, fluids infusing through the catheter enter surrounding tissues rather than entering the intended blood vessel. Called *extravasation* or *infiltration,* this can arise even with the catheter in proper position. In this case, extravasation may occur if fluid passes through the vessel wall or backs up through the insertion site.

The consequences of IV extravasation depend on the substance that is being infused and how long the extravasation continues. Adverse reactions range from mild redness and tenderness to pain and tissue destruction that can cause infection or loss of mobility of the extremity.

continued

ACTION STAT—cont'd

Chemotherapeutic agents (e.g., doxorubicin) are among a group of IV medications known as *vesicants* because they can cause blistering, tissue destruction, or both. Other agents (e.g., dopamine) cause vasoconstriction at the site of extravasation, resulting in tissue destruction. Whatever the agent, be sure to follow your institution's policy for treatments and antidotes.

What to look for
Signs and symptoms of IV extravasation include:
- An infusion rate that slows or stops
- Swelling, redness, pain, and coolness around and proximal to the catheter insertion site
- Decreased pulse distal to the insertion site
- Failure of blood to flush back into the tubing when you lower the IV bag below the level of the needle (not always a reliable sign)
- Signs of tissue necrosis (with vesicants or vasoconstrictive drugs)

What to do immediately
If you think that IV fluid may have extravasated into the soft tissue of your patient's arm, notify the physician, and follow these measures:
- Immediately stop the infusion. Identify the IV solution and any additives or medications.
- If the infiltrated substance is a vesicant, try aspirating it back through the catheter and prepare to instill an antidote, such as sodium bicarbonate and saline, through the catheter according to your institution's policy. If you cannot aspirate the medication, remove the catheter.
- Consult the pharmacist to determine how toxic the additives are to soft tissue.
- If the IV solution contained a potent vasoconstrictor, such as norepinephrine or dopamine, add 5 to 10 mg of phentolamine to

0.9% saline to make 1 ml of solution. Inject it subcutaneously (SC) into the extravasation site, as prescribed.
- Remove constrictive clothing or devices (blood pressure cuff, dressings, or tape) distal or proximal to the catheter site within 12 hours. Otherwise, they could obstruct circulation to the area.
- Assess skin color and temperature at the site for early signs of tissue necrosis.
- Measure the circumference of the swollen area, noting the exact point of measurement so that you can compare readings later.
- Check vital signs, looking specifically for signs and symptoms of sepsis, such as fever, tachycardia, and hypotension.

What to do next
Once you have completed these steps, you will need to do the following:
- Restart the infusion at another site, if necessary (preferably not in the same extremity). If you must use the same extremity, choose a site proximal to the site of extravasation.
- Apply warm compresses to the swollen area. If the infiltrated substance is a vesicant, apply cold compresses or ice.
- Continuously assess the extremity for increased pain and redness along the vein (a sign of thrombophlebitis or infection).
- Continuously assess the extremity for evidence of compartment syndrome, including loss of distal pulses, coolness, pale and mottled skin, and paresthesias.
- Photograph the site of extravasation according to policy, especially if the patient has tissue destruction.
- Document your assessment findings and interventions promptly and carefully.

- *Insect bites or stings.* These cause localized swelling that ranges from mild to severe, depending on the patient's reaction to the venom.
- *Infection.* Swelling may be caused by infection, usually bacterial, resulting from injury, surgery, or even IV catheters. The infected tissue may be super-

ficial or deep. It may extend to the bone and result in osteomyelitis. Other symptoms include pain, redness, and decreased function or mobility. Fever also usually occurs.

- *Lymphedema.* An accumulation of lymph in the soft tissue of the extremity, lymphedema commonly results from surgical removal of lymph nodes. It also may result from obstructed lymph channels. Swelling may affect the extremity or only the most distal portion. Usually elevation of the arm improves lymph drainage and reduces swelling.
- *Tumor.* Superior vena cava syndrome may be caused by tumor compression of the superior vena cava. This results in swelling, flushing, and venous engorgement of the face, chest, and arms.
- *Thrombophlebitis.* Acute inflammation of a vein, thrombophlebitis is marked by redness and tenderness along the course of a vein, as well as by localized swelling and warmth.

Examining the Abdominal Region

The very nature of the abdominal region, its structures, and associated health complaints make assessing this area of the body a challenge. Most people are embarrassed by signs and symptoms related to what they consider "private" matters, such as bowel or bladder dysfunction and gynecologic or urologic disorders. Similarly, many people have an almost irrational fear of cancer, permanent loss of bladder or bowel control, venereal disease, or erectile dysfunction. What is worse, these fears may trigger feelings of guilt or shame.

Your goal is to create an atmosphere of openness, mutual trust, and compassion and to make your examination of the abdominal region as comfortable for the patient as possible. To do this, detailed knowledge of the structures involved, including the lower pelvis, rectum, external genitalia, liver, gallbladder, stomach, spleen, intestines, and reproductive organs is needed (see *Structures of the Abdominal Region*).

STRUCTURES OF THE ABDOMINAL REGION

The following illustrations present the abdominal structures in their normal positions.

Major Structures of the Abdominal Cavity

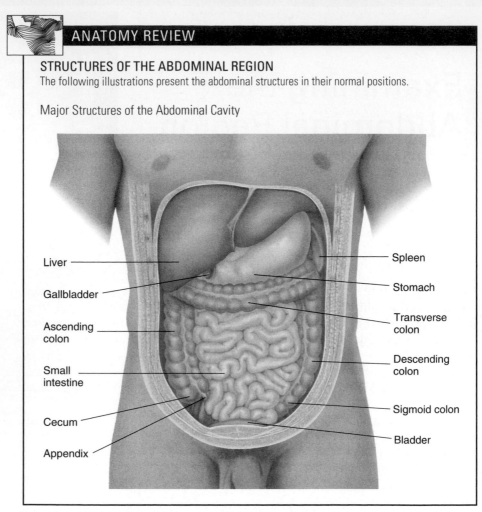

From Seidel H, Ball J, Dains JE, Benedict GW: *Mosby's guide to physical examination*, ed 6, St Louis, 2006, Mosby.

continued

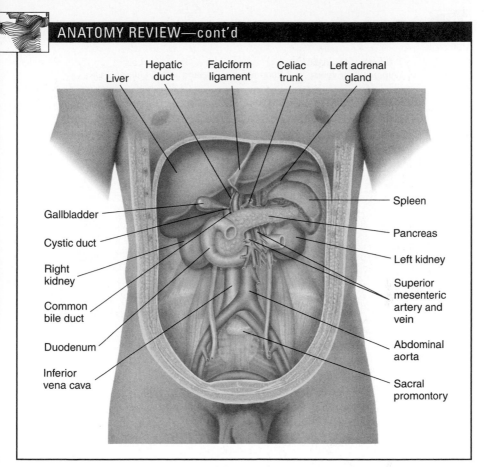

From Seidel H, Ball J, Dains JE, Benedict GW: *Mosby's guide to physical examination,* ed 6, St Louis, 2006, Mosby.

continued

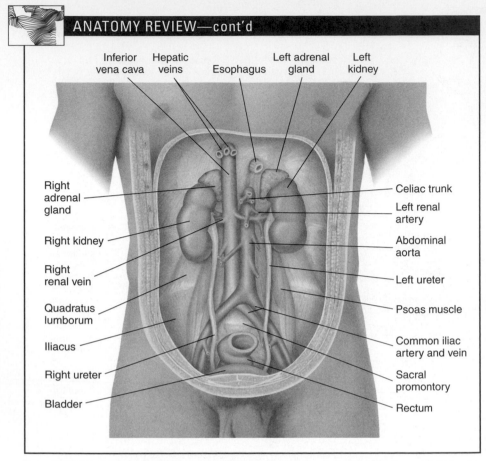

From Seidel H, Ball J, Dains JE, Benedict GW: *Mosby's guide to physical examination*, ed 6, St Louis, 2006, Mosby.

continued

Female Genitourinary System

Lateral cross-section view

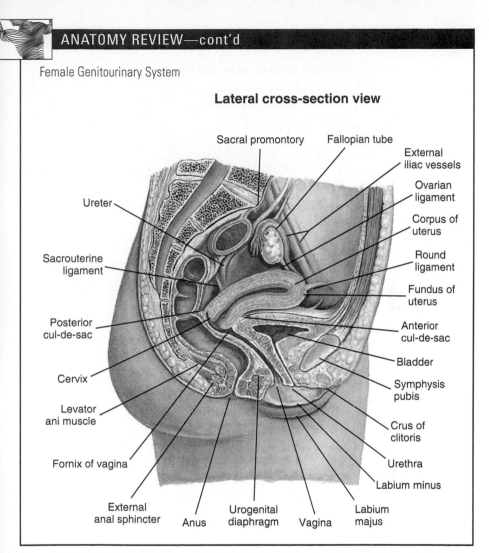

From Seidel H, Ball J, Dains JE, Benedict GW: *Mosby's guide to physical examination,* ed 6, St Louis, 2006, Mosby.

continued

ANATOMY REVIEW—cont'd

Inferior view of external genitalia

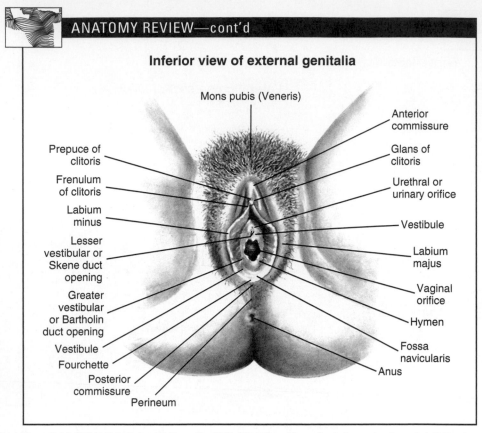

Mons pubis (Veneris)

Anterior commissure

Prepuce of clitoris

Glans of clitoris

Frenulum of clitoris

Urethral or urinary orifice

Labium minus

Vestibule

Lesser vestibular or Skene duct opening

Labium majus

Greater vestibular or Bartholin duct opening

Vaginal orifice

Vestibule

Hymen

Fourchette

Fossa navicularis

Posterior commissure

Anus

Perineum

From Seidel H, Ball J, Dains JE, Benedict GW: *Mosby's guide to physical examination,* ed 6, St Louis, 2006, Mosby.

continued

Male Genitourinary System

Lateral cross-section view

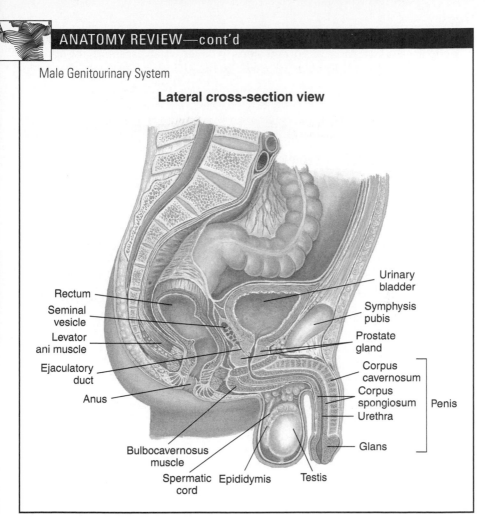

Rectum
Seminal vesicle
Levator ani muscle
Ejaculatory duct
Anus

Bulbocavernosus muscle
Spermatic cord   Epididymis   Testis

Urinary bladder
Symphysis pubis
Prostate gland
Corpus cavernosum
Corpus spongiosum
Urethra
Glans

Penis

From Seidel H, Ball J, Dains JE, Benedict GW: *Mosby's guide to physical examination,* ed 6, St Louis, 2006, Mosby.

EXAMINATION STEPS AND FINDINGS

To examine the abdominal region effectively you will need to do the following:

- Gather needed assessment equipment: stethoscope, examination drape, examination gloves, water-soluble jelly, flashlight, Hematest slide and reagent, and an examination light.
- Make sure the examination room provides absolute privacy because it will be necessary to expose male patients from the chest to the pubis and female patients from below the breasts to the pubis.
- Keep the patient fully draped, except for the areas you are examining during auscultation, palpation, and percussion.
- Arrange for adequate lighting to assess the abdominal wall.

- Ensure the room is warm and comfortable.
- Keep in mind the most important steps to cover when assessing the abdominal area (see 📋 *Key Examination Steps for the Abdominal Region*).

EXPERT EXAMINATION CHECKLIST

KEY EXAMINATION STEPS FOR THE ABDOMINAL REGION

Use this checklist to make sure you cover the most important steps when examining the abdominal region.
- ❑ Inspect for scars, striae, petechiae, and spider angiomas.
- ❑ Observe contour for symmetry, distention, shifting with position changes.
- ❑ Observe the density and pattern of pubic hair.
- ❑ Inspect genitalia for redness, swelling, lesions, and discharge.
- ❑ Inspect anus for lesions, hemorrhoids, and prolapsed rectal tissue.
- ❑ Perform digital rectal examination.
- ❑ Auscultate for bowel sounds.
- ❑ Auscultate for rubs and vascular sounds.
- ❑ Percuss the abdominal wall.

- ❑ If the patient's abdomen is distended, assess for a fluid wave.
- ❑ Palpate quadrants using a light palpation technique.
- ❑ Palpate lymph nodes and femoral arteries.
- ❑ Assess for rebound tenderness.
- ❑ Palpate quadrants using a deep palpation technique.
- ❑ If you identify a mass, determine its size, shape, consistency, surface, pulsatility, and mobility.
- ❑ Palpate external genitalia. Note any nodules or masses.
- ❑ Assess male patients for femoral and inguinal hernias.
- ❑ Milk urethra, and assess discharge.

evolve Find PDF and PDA-downloadable versions of this Expert Exam Checklist online at http://evolve.elsevier.com/Mosby/expertexam/.

INSPECTION

Begin your examination with inspection to assess abdominal contour. Place the patient in a supine position, and position yourself at the patient's side with the abdomen at eye level. Note the shape of the abdominal outline. A slender patient will have a flat or slightly concave outline. An obese patient will have a protruding abdomen. Observe for any irregularities in the outline. Assess abdominal symmetry by standing at the end of the bed.

While performing this first inspection, pay attention to the patient's apparent comfort level. If the patient seems tense or adjusts her position frequently, she may be uncomfortable. If the abdomen is distended, the patient may have trouble breathing because the abdominal contents are pressing against the diaphragm. If this is the case, you can increase comfort by having the patient turn from the supine position to a lateral one, and assess abdominal contour by looking down.

Now observe the contour of the skin and any peristaltic movement or pulsations. Normally, peristaltic movements are not visible. Some patients may have visible aortic pulsations. Note any superficial veins, petechiae, spider angiomas, striae, or scars.

Note the shape and location of the umbilicus and the hair density and pattern in the pubic region. To check for an umbilical or incisional hernia, ask your patient to raise the head and shoulders while remaining supine. A true hernia will protrude during this maneuver.

CULTURAL CONSIDERATIONS

Umbilical hernias are common in black children before the age of 7 years and in white children before the age of 2 years.

To inspect a male patient's genitals, observe the dorsal, lateral, and ventral surfaces of the penis for color, lesions, moles, size, and shape. If the patient is uncircumcised, retract the prepuce (foreskin) by grasping the penis behind the glans with your thumb and index finger and moving your fingers in the direction of the penile root. Be sure to replace the foreskin after your examination. The urethral opening (meatus) should be slitlike and have no discharge.

Spread the rugae (wrinkles) of the scrotum between your fingers to inspect the scrotal skin. Observe the scrotum for size and symmetry. Keep in mind that the left testis is normally lower than the right in the scrotal sac and that the scrotum appears more pendulous in warm temperatures because of relaxation of the dartos muscle. The scrotum also appears more pendulous in the aged because of atrophy of the dartos. To examine a female patient's genitals, spread the labia majora and inspect them and the labia minora. Note any lesions or discharge. Inspect the vestibule, especially the area around Bartholin's and Skene's glands. Look for swelling, redness, lesions, or discharge. Inspect the urethral opening and the vaginal opening.

Now ask your patient, whether male or female, to turn to the side in a lateral position. Watch the abdomen as your patient turns. Note any fluid shifting or abnormal protrusions. Help your patient draw the knees to the chest, and gently spread the buttocks to expose the anus. Observe for lesions. Note any hemorrhoids or prolapsed rectal tissue.

NORMAL FINDINGS

- Abdominal contour flat, scaphoid (concave), or round
- Abdominal veins barely visible (They may be more prominent in older adults and pregnant patients from a loss of subcutaneous tissue.)
- Involuntary undulations under the abdominal skin of a thin adult (These are normal peristaltic waves and usually move downward and to the right.)
- Arterial pulsations at the midline over the aorta in thin adults
- Respirations producing abdominal movement, mostly in male patients
- Slight abdominal shift when your patient turns from the supine to the lateral position
- Anal opening puckered and dark, with intact perianal skin
- In a male patient, a soft but not flabby penile shaft (In an older adult, the penis may be slightly flabby.)
- Glans smooth and cone shaped, without protrusions or induration
- Glans pink in white males, more pigmented in males with darker skin

- Meatus slitlike and producing no discharge
- Scrotal skin intact, with rugae (folds and creases) (The left side of the scrotum usually hangs lower than the right.)
- Pubic hair usually thick, appearing on the mons pubis and inner aspects of the upper thighs in a female patient (In an older female patient, pubic hair will appear thin and sparse. In a prepubescent female patient, hair will be absent or thin, depending on the patient's age.)
- Labia pink and moist, with no lesions
- Vestibule and urethral opening free of swelling, redness, lesions, or discharge
- Vaginal opening a thin vertical slit in a female patient with an intact hymen; a larger opening with irregular edges in a female patient with a perforated hymen
- Cervical discharge normal in quantity and character (Before ovulation, the discharge will be clear and stringy. After ovulation, it will be white and opaque.)
- Striae marks, which may be visible in patients who are now or were obese or pregnant or in those with ascites or abdominal tumor

ABNORMAL FINDINGS

- Abdominal contour indrawn (indicating high muscular tension), distended, asymmetrical, or bulging at the flanks when supine, or hollow (indicating malnutrition)
- Bulges on the abdominal wall or groin area or a grossly distended testicle, indicating an intestinal hernia
- Fluid shifting or unusual protrusions when the patient changes position from supine to lateral (Gravity causes fluid in the abdominal cavity to shift when the patient changes position, altering abdominal contour. Fluid accumulation in the gastrointestinal [GI] tract also may cause some shifting but not to the same degree. Accumulated air does not shift when the patient changes position.)
- Diastasis recti, an abnormal separation of abdominal rectus muscles (You may notice this first as abdominal distention. To confirm it, have your patient raise the head from the bed, and watch to see if the rectus muscle separates.)

CULTURAL CONSIDERATIONS

Diastasis recti is a common finding in black children, but it usually disappears by the age of 4 or 5 years.

- Visible, active peristaltic waves in normal adults, possibly indicating hyperactive bowel activity and impending bowel obstruction
- Bluish discoloration around the umbilicus (Cullen's sign) or along the lower abdomen and flanks (Grey Turner's sign), possibly indicating a retroperitoneal bleed (The color may be a shade of blue-red, blue-purple, or green-brown, depending on the stage of hemoglobin breakdown.)
- Tense, shiny abdominal skin, possibly resulting from ascites or edema
- Jaundice (yellow color) of the abdominal wall, caused by staining of tissue with bile pigments and usually seen with liver dysfunction

- Caput medusae (engorged veins around the umbilicus), indicating portal hypertension
- Scars on the abdominal wall, possibly resulting from surgery or injury
- Visible pulsations, possibly a sign of an aneurysm (These require further assessment with auscultation and light palpation.)
- Abdominal respirations in the female patient, possibly indicating respiratory distress
- Umbilical fistula, possibly draining pus, urine, or feces, depending on where the tract formed
- Umbilical calculus (a hard mass of dirt and desquamated epithelium in the umbilicus, causing inflammation and resulting from poor hygiene)
- Hemorrhoids (reddish protrusions from the anus containing distended veins)
- Prolapsed rectal mucosa (reddish velvety tissue projecting from the anus)
- Organisms attached to the pubic hair, indicating infestation by the *Pediculus pubis* louse or its nits (small, white lice eggs)
- Discharge from the penile meatus and urethra, with or without compression, indicating infection
- Penile lesions, possibly indicating a sexually transmitted disease
- Phimosis (an abnormal tightness of the prepuce preventing its retraction over the glans)
- Paraphimosis (a strangulation of the glans caused by a prepuce that will not retract over the glans)
- Epispadias (a congenital defect in which the urethral meatus opens on the dorsal surface of the penis)
- Hypospadias (a congenital defect in which the urethral meatus opens on the ventral surface of the penis)
- Absence of pubic hair in a postpubescent adult or bald spots in the pubic hair, possibly indicating a vascular or hormonal problem
- Enlarged testicle, possibly indicating hernia (if bowel loops appear on illumination) or a cyst (if fluid is present)
- Hypertrophic, indurated, soft or hard tissue of the labia majora
- Varicosities (distended superficial vessels) on the labia, possibly a sign of increased pressure in the pelvic region (This problem occurs with increased uterine size, as in pregnancy or uterine cancer.)
- Lesions, possibly indicating genital infection
- Edema of the mons pubis, labia majora, labia minora, urethral orifice, vaginal introitus, or surrounding skin, possibly indicating vaginal infection or infestation
- Purulent vaginal discharge, which may be green, gray, yellow, or white, indicating infection

AUSCULTATION

The next step in your examination, auscultation, allows you to assess the function of your patient's GI tract. Always auscultate the abdomen before percussing or palpating it because manipulating the abdominal wall may increase bowel sounds or produce sounds that usually are not present.

Before you begin, make sure the room, your hands, and your stethoscope are warm. Placing cold hands or a cold stethoscope on your patient's abdomen can make the muscles contract. If your patient has a nasogastric (NG) tube attached to low suction, turn the suction off or clamp the tube during auscultation to keep it from producing misleading sounds or interfering with your ability to hear.

Begin by mentally dividing the patient's abdomen into four quadrants, then systematically auscultate all four using the diaphragm of your stethoscope. Never drag your stethoscope across the patient's abdominal wall because doing so could increase irritation and cause muscle spasm.

Normal bowel sounds occur intermittently; they are not constant. Therefore you need to listen for about a minute over each quadrant (for a total of 3 to 5 minutes) before concluding bowel sounds are absent.

Remember that the thickness of the abdominal wall may affect what you can hear. Bowel sounds are more difficult to auscultate in obese patients. After auscultating bowel sounds, use the bell of your stethoscope to auscultate vascular sounds, bruits, or friction rubs. To assess the abdominal vascular system, auscultate over the aortic site and the iliac, femoral, and renal arteries (see 🖼️ *Identifying Vascular Sounds in the Abdomen*).

EXAMINATION TIP

IDENTIFYING VASCULAR SOUNDS IN THE ABDOMEN

You can detect abdominal vascular problems by auscultating your patient's abdomen with the bell of your stethoscope.

Listen for bruits over major abdominal blood vessels, including the aorta, renal arteries, iliac arteries, and femoral arteries.

Listen for venous hums in the umbilical and epigastric regions. Venous hums are generally softer than aortic bruits.

Finally, listen for a grating or scratching noise above and below the right and left costal borders. These sounds, known as *friction rubs,* may indicate inflammation of the kidneys or spleen.

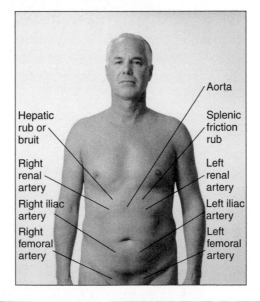

Labels: Aorta; Hepatic rub or bruit; Splenic friction rub; Right renal artery; Left renal artery; Right iliac artery; Left iliac artery; Right femoral artery; Left femoral artery

NORMAL FINDINGS

- Peristaltic sounds (high-pitched, gurgling noises) heard about every 5 to 15 seconds in an irregular pattern (They may be loud when your patient is hungry or has missed a meal.)
- Continuous sounds over the ileocecal valve if it has been more than 4 hours since the patient last ate

ABNORMAL FINDINGS

- Absent or infrequent bowel sounds, possibly indicating peritonitis, ileus, or late bowel obstruction
- Frequent, loud, rushing, high-pitched sounds, possibly indicating early mechanical obstruction or GI hypermotility (You may see peristaltic waves on the surface of the patient's abdomen.)
- Borborygmus (loud intestinal rumbling) (This is abnormal, except when the patient is hungry. Borborygmi signal passage of flatus through the large intestine.)
- Bruits, resulting from narrowing of an artery or turbulent blood flow (They are described as blowing sounds and may indicate an aneurysm or a constricted vessel. If you auscultate a midline abdominal bruit, the patient may have an aortic aneurysm. Do not perform deep palpation.)
- Friction rubs, possibly sounding like a grating noise or like two pieces of leather being rubbed together (A peritoneal friction rub may indicate peritoneal inflammation. A friction rub over the liver may indicate inflammation of the organ surface.)
- Venous hum (a continuous soft sound heard in both systole and diastole), indicating collateral circulation between the portal and systemic venous systems and usually heard over the epigastric region and umbilicus

PERCUSSION

Use percussion to determine the size and density of structures and organs in the abdominal cavity and to detect the presence of fluid or air. You may use direct or indirect percussion, but indirect percussion is more comfortable for the patient. It is also easier to perform over a large area. To perform indirect percussion, you will rest one hand on the abdominal wall and sharply tap your middle finger with the index finger of the other hand.

Percussion is contraindicated in patients with suspected abdominal aortic aneurysm or those who have received abdominal organ transplants. Use caution when percussing the abdomen of a patient who might have appendicitis.

As in auscultation, begin by mentally dividing the abdomen into four quadrants, and proceed to systematically percuss all four. As you percuss each quadrant, keep a mental image of the abdominal structures beneath your fingers. Percussion sounds vary, depending on the underlying structures. Solid structures, such as the liver, produce dull sounds. So do fluid-filled structures, such as a full urinary bladder. Air-filled structures, such as the stomach, produce tympanic sounds.

Once you have percussed all four abdominal quadrants, go back and percuss the liver and spleen, noting their size and position. To percuss the liver and determine its size, begin on the right side, at the midclavicular line, just above the patient's right nipple. Percuss downward until the sound becomes dull. This spot is the liver's upper margin. Usually, you will find it between the fifth and seventh intercostal spaces (ICSs). If you need to, mark the location to help you remember it. To find the liver's lower margin, begin percussing at a point in the abdomen where you hear tympanic sounds. Work upward along the midclavicular line until the sound becomes dull. This spot is the liver's lower margin. Usually you will find it at the costal margin. Mark this spot as well, and measure the distance between the two marks. Record the measurement in centimeters. Keep in mind that excess air in the large intestine will produce a tympanic sound that may obscure the dullness of the liver.

The spleen is more difficult to percuss. Beginning on the left side, posterior to the midaxillary line, percuss toward the umbilicus at a level between the sixth and tenth ribs. Percussion sounds should change from resonance (over the left lung) to dullness (indicating the spleen).

If your patient has a distended abdomen, check for excess fluid accumulation by percussing for a fluid wave. You will need an assistant to perform this procedure (see ▣ *Percussing for a Fluid Wave*).

EXAMINATION TIP

PERCUSSING FOR A FLUID WAVE

If you want to find out whether your patient's abdominal distention results from fluid or air, percuss the abdomen for a fluid wave. This procedure requires three hands, so you will have to ask a colleague for help.

To perform the procedure, place the patient in a supine position and ask your colleague to place the arm and hand along the midline of the patient's abdomen, as shown in the photograph. Your colleague should press the arm gently but firmly against the patient's abdomen to prevent transmission of fat waves.

Next, place your fingertips along the sides of your patient's lower abdomen, in the lumbar region. Keeping your nondominant hand in place, use the fingertips of your dominant hand to thrust quickly into the patient's side, as shown. Do you feel a wave with your nondominant hand? If so, your patient's abdominal distention probably results from excess fluid.

By contrast, if your patient's distention is caused by air, you will not feel a wave.

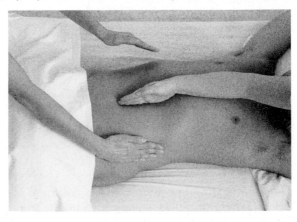

NORMAL FINDINGS

- Tympany over the stomach, epigastric area, and upper midline
- Dullness over the liver, a full bladder, a pregnant uterus, and the left lower quadrant over the sigmoid colon (shortly before a bowel movement)
- Upper and lower liver margins about 6 to 12 cm apart
- Spleen, if located, percussed in the area between the sixth and tenth ribs

ABNORMAL FINDINGS

- Flat percussion sounds over the abdominal cavity, possibly indicating a tumor
- Fluid wave, indicating accumulated fluid in the abdominal cavity
- More than 12 cm between the upper and lower margins of the liver, indicating hepatomegaly
- Large area of dullness in the left upper quadrant, indicating splenomegaly
- High-pitched tympany sound in association with abdominal distention, indicating air in the bowel
- Dull sounds in the flank area, present with ascites
- Tenderness with percussion, possibly indicating peritoneal inflammation

PALPATION

Abdominal palpation, which should include both light and deep methods, is most effective when the abdominal muscles are relaxed. Promote muscle relaxation by use of the following measures:

- Keep the areas you are not examining draped for privacy.
- Make sure your hands are warm; wash them in hot water, if necessary.
- Explain the examination before you begin, and talk to the patient soothingly and quietly throughout the process.
- Position the patient in a supine position with a pillow under the head, knees slightly bent, and arms at sides rather than over the head.
- Ask the patient to breathe through the mouth during the examination.
- Ask the patient not to talk or raise the head during the examination.

Keep in mind that sometimes a position other than supine is needed. A lateral position may help you locate abdominal masses not palpable with the patient supine. A standing position can help identify hernias. If the patient is prone to respiratory distress when supine, raise the backrest. If the patient has kyphosis, try elevating the head and shoulders for comfort.

Your positioning in relation to your patient depends on which of your hands is dominant. If you are right-handed, stand on your patient's right side for palpation. Keep your fingers close together, with the palmar surface down.

As with the other abdominal assessment techniques, divide the patient's abdomen into quadrants and palpate all four. If the patient complains of abdominal pain, begin with quadrants that are not painful, saving painful areas for last. If your patient tightens the abdominal muscles or becomes uncomfortable, proceed more slowly, or switch to another assessment and then return to palpation.

EXAMINATION TIP

ABDOMINAL PALPATION
If your patient is ticklish, have her place a hand on top of yours as you palpate. Alternatively, try distracting the patient by pressing on the lower half of the sternum with your nondominant hand.

Begin the examination with a light touch, pressing only ¼ to ½ inch (0.5 to 1 cm) into the patient's abdomen. Light palpation is used to determine characteristics of skin and subcutaneous tissue and to note temperature, tenderness, and large masses. Move your fingers in a circular motion. Proceed slowly and gently. Avoid any sudden movements. As you move over the femoral area, note the femoral pulse and palpate the inguinal lymph nodes (see *Locating the Inguinal Lymph Nodes*).

LOCATING THE INGUINAL LYMPH NODES

Located on both sides of the pubic region along the inguinal canal, the inguinal lymph nodes consist of two discrete chains: (1) the superficial superior chain and (2) the superficial inferior chain.

Palpating your patient's inguinal lymph nodes can provide clues to infectious processes in the abdominal and genital areas. Use this illustration as a guide in locating these nodes.

If you feel any nodes during palpation, make sure that you note their size and consistency and whether or not they are tender.

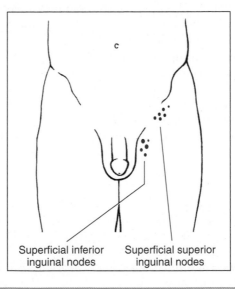

Superficial inferior inguinal nodes   Superficial superior inguinal nodes

Watch your patient's face for grimacing during light palpation. If you identify any tenderness with light palpation, remember to reassess the area when you get to the deep palpation part of your examination.

⧗ **LIFESPAN CONSIDERATIONS**

Older adults can have a diminished sense of pain and a blunted febrile response. Therefore do not assume that an older adult does not have an abdominal condition, such as appendicitis, because she does not complain of pain or have a fever.

If you find that your patient's abdominal muscles are contracted, determine whether the contraction is voluntary or involuntary. Do this by correlating the contraction with the patient's respirations. If the muscles are contracted during both inspiration and expiration, the condition probably is involuntary, indicating an underlying abdominal problem. If the muscles contract more strongly during inspiration and less strongly during expiration, the condition probably is voluntary and related to your patient's anxiety level.

Once you have lightly palpated the entire abdomen, begin deep palpation. This method is used to locate normal structures, identify masses, and assess for tenderness. Do not perform deep palpation if the patient has a suspected abdominal aortic aneurysm or appendicitis, a tender spleen, kidney transplantation, or polycystic kidneys.

During deep palpation, you are going to be pressing 1½ to 2 inches (3 to 4 cm) into the patient's abdomen. You can do so using one hand alone or with one hand on top of the other. The two-handed method is often preferred because it allows pressure to be added with the nonexamining hand while the muscles of the examining hand remain relatively passive.

As you palpate the abdomen, keep in mind you probably will not be able to feel abdominal organs in an obese but otherwise healthy individual. In a relatively thin person, you may feel the muscular structures of the abdomen, such as the rectus muscle, the bowel (which is soft, unless filled with feces), and aortic pulsations.

To palpate the liver as you feel deeply beneath the costal margin, tell the patient to take a deep breath. During inspiration the liver will descend, and you may be able to feel its edge move against your hand. Usually it is firm and rubbery. Alternatively, you can try hooking the liver by standing near your patient's head and, as she takes a deep breath, curling your fingers over the costal margin.

To palpate the kidneys, place your nondominant hand beneath the patient's right flank as you press downward with your other hand against the right outer edge of the abdomen, attempting to sandwich the kidney between your hands. Normally it feels firm and smooth. Repeat this procedure on the left flank, keeping in mind that the left kidney is usually nonpalpable because of its position beneath the bowel. In fact, usually all remaining abdominal structures, including the spleen (beneath the left costal margin) and the gallbladder (beneath the liver's margin), are nonpalpable, unless they are enlarged.

If you find a mass during abdominal palpation, document its size, shape, consistency (solid or soft), surface (smooth or irregular), tenderness, pulsatility, and mobility. If the mass is small, you can make these determinations by grasping it between your thumb and index finger. If the mass is large, you will need to perform bimanual palpation to assess it fully (see 🖳 *Performing Bimanual Abdominal Palpation*).

EXAMINATION TIP

PERFORMING BIMANUAL ABDOMINAL PALPATION

If you find a large mass in your patient's abdomen, you will want to perform bimanual palpation to accurately determine its position and size.

To perform bimanual palpation of the upper abdomen, place your patient in the supine position and stand on the side opposite the mass. Now place your nondominant hand on the outside of the patient's rib cage farthest from you, as shown in the illustration. Ask your patient to take a deep breath and, while the rib cage expands, press your dominant hand under the costal margin to probe for the mass. Angle your dominant hand in the direction of your nondominant hand, as shown. Adjust the positions of both hands as needed to fully assess the mass.

You can perform bimanual palpation on the lower abdomen as well. Simply position your nondominant hand on the patient's flank, and use your dominant hand to probe the abdomen, keeping the mass positioned between your two hands.

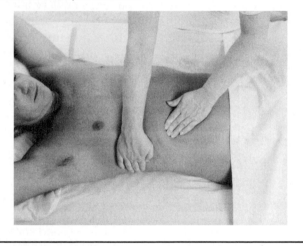

To determine if the mass is mobile, press suddenly and deeply into the region. A mobile mass will bound upward and touch the fingers of your examining hand.

To check for rebound tenderness, have your patient flex the knees to relax the abdominal muscles. Now place your hands lightly on the abdominal wall, midway between the umbilicus and the anterior-superior iliac spine (at McBurney's point). Press your fingers slowly and deeply into the abdomen; then release the pressure in a quick, smooth motion. If the patient feels pain when you release pressure, she has rebound tenderness, possibly from an inflamed appendix. The pain may radiate to the umbilicus. To minimize the risk of rupturing the appendix, do not repeat the test for rebound tenderness if you get a positive result.

Another way to check for peritoneal inflammation is to test for tenderness when the heels are jarred. Have your patient stand on the toes with the legs straight; then ask the patient to relax suddenly and allow the heels to strike the floor. If this maneuver produces abdominal pain, the patient may have peritoneal inflammation. Some patients with peritoneal inflammation complain of abdominal pain when walking.

EXAMINATION TIP

IDENTIFYING PERITONEAL INFLAMMATION

If your patient cannot stand, try to extend the patient's leg and strike the heel with the lateral aspect of your fist while she is supine. If the patient experiences abdominal pain, consider peritoneal inflammation.

Once you have palpated the patient's abdomen, move on to the genitalia. Again, be aware that your patient may be nervous and embarrassed. Use draping whenever possible, and proceed gently but firmly. Be sure to wear examination gloves.

For a male patient, palpate the bulb of the penis to note consistency and the presence or absence of induration. Use both hands to palpate the penile shaft, working from the base toward the tip to milk the urethra. Watch for urethral discharge at the meatus.

Palpate each testicle for size, shape, symmetry, mobility, and consistency. If one testicle is larger than the other, is hard, or has a fluid consistency, you will need to illuminate the scrotal sac to differentiate fluid from a mass. Darken the room and hold a flashlight close behind the affected testicle. You will be able to see the light shining through fluid. If the scrotum contains a loop of bowel, indicating intestinal herniation, the light will not shine through, and the area will appear opaque.

If you feel a mass, try to press your fingers together above it. If your fingers meet, you can conclude that the mass is confined to the scrotum. If they do not meet, the mass probably started in the abdomen and extends through the inguinal ring and into the scrotal sac.

Next, palpate each epididymis between your index finger and thumb. Locate the spermatic cord near the root of the scrotum and, with gentle pressure, roll the cord between your thumb and finger as you move downward toward the testicle. Be careful not to pinch the skin or the cord because it will cause a sharp pain.

Finally, evaluate the inguinal ring, and palpate for inguinal and femoral hernias.

For a female patient, palpate the labia majora and labia minora. Palpate the area of Bartholin's gland. Moisten your gloved index finger with water. Separate the labia with your other gloved hand, and gently insert your index finger, pad up, about 1¼ inches (3 cm) into the anterior vagina. Press the pad of your finger upward, and pull outward to milk the urethra. Note any pain or discharge.

LIFESPAN CONSIDERATIONS

As estrogen levels diminish after age 40, changes to the female genitalia begin to occur. You may observe a narrowing of the vaginal opening and changes in the vagina, including shortening and narrowing of the vaginal canal and a lack of moisture. If you are not planning to obtain a Papanicolaou (Pap) smear or take other samples for testing, use a water-based lubricant when performing a vaginal examination to decrease discomfort.

If you have received special training, perform a full internal pelvic examination.

NORMAL FINDINGS

- No tenderness with light or deep palpation
- Inguinal lymph nodes small (¼ to ½ inch [0.5 to 1.0 cm] in diameter), smooth, and mobile
- In a thin patient, palpable pulsatile mass at the midline of the upper abdomen, reflecting aortic pulsations
- In a male patient, testicles mobile and tender under pressure (If your patient is older, the testes may be softer and smaller in size. Your fingers should meet when palpating the skin at the root of the scrotum.)
- Epididymis firm and rubbery
- Spermatic cord round, cordlike, smooth, and firm with resilience
- Inguinal ring that exerts a slight pulsation against your finger
- In the female patient, labia free of nodules or masses
- Bartholin's glands nonpalpable
- Urethra producing no pain or discharge (See ▓ *What to Expect When Examining the Abdomen.*)

NORMAL FINDINGS

WHAT TO EXPECT WHEN EXAMINING THE ABDOMEN

Inspection
- Smooth, unbroken skin, relatively pale, with fine venous network
- No skin lesions or nodules
- Flat, round, or concave abdominal contour that is symmetrical
- Striae from pregnancy or weight gain
- Smooth, even abdominal movement in males, and costal movement in females, during breathing
- No peristalsis; thin patients may show slight motion

- Pulsations of the aorta visible in thin patients

Palpation
- No masses
- No tenderness

Auscultation
- High-pitched bowel sounds at least every 15 seconds

ABNORMAL FINDINGS

- Rebound tenderness, indicating peritoneal inflammation
- Voluntary rigidity of abdominal muscles during palpation, possibly resulting from peritoneal irritation or anxiety
- Involuntary contraction of the abdominal wall (commonly described as a *boardlike abdomen*), indicating peritonitis
- Abdominal tenderness elicited by heel jarring, indicating peritoneal inflammation
- Suprapubic mass, possibly resulting from bladder distention (In a female patient, it may result from an ovarian cyst or a uterine fibroid.)

- Decreased or absent femoral pulse, possibly indicating coarctation of the aorta, thrombosis of the iliac artery, or dissecting aortic aneurysm
- In the male patient, a scrotal mass (If an abdominal mass protrudes into the scrotal sac, your fingers will not be able to approximate above it.)
- Discharge from the penile meatus, indicating infection
- Fibrotic thickening, indurations, or protrusions of the penis, possibly indicating venereal disease, such as condyloma
- Small, palpable nodules in the midline ventral surface of the penis (possibly occluded periurethral glands)
- Small, yellowish, palpable nodules on the scrotal skin (sebaceous cysts caused by blocked sebaceous glands)
- Dilated, tortuous testicular veins, possibly indicating benign, pain-producing varicosities or metastatic cellular proliferation
- A spindlelike mass on the spermatic cord, possibly indicating hydrocele of the cord
- A hard, nodular, elongated spermatic cord, possibly indicating varicoceles, varices, or varicose veins
- The sensation of sliding or bulging during the inguinal ring examination, indicating a hernia
- In the female patient, reddened or excoriated perineal skin, indicating chronic incontinence, poor hygiene, or recurrent infections (e.g., vaginal yeast infections)
- Reddened and inflamed hair follicles, with or without pustules, indicating folliculitis (inflamed hair follicles) or shaving against the direction of hair growth
- Swollen labia (unilaterally or bilaterally), possibly resulting from injury, inflammation, or infection of the Bartholin's gland (The swollen area may be tender and warm.)
- Vaginal discharge that is white, green, or yellow and thin, thick, creamy, or of a consistency like cottage cheese, often indicating vaginal infection
- Lesions on or around the labia (If they are painful, raised, reddened, and filled with fluid, they may be herpetic vesicles. If they appear as painless, rubbery skin tags, they are probably condylomas. If they appear as discrete ulcers or nontender chancres, they may have been caused by syphilis.)
- Bulging of the vaginal wall, probably resulting from internal muscle weakness that may be seen through the vaginal opening (If the bulging occurs anteriorly, it may be the result of a cystocele, or bladder prolapse. A posterior bulging may be related to a rectocele, or prolapse of the rectal wall.)

EXPLORING CHIEF COMPLAINTS

In the abdominal region, chief complaints can take many forms and involve a large variety of organs and structures. To explore your patient's chief complaint accurately and quickly, refer to your patient's medical history, family history, previous surgeries (especially abdominal surgeries), previous traumatic injuries to the abdomen, and current medications for clues to the patient's problem. For a female patient, make sure you know the date of her last menses, her typical pattern of menstruation, number of previous pregnancies, and past gynecologic infections.

NAUSEA AND VOMITING

If your patient complains of nausea and vomiting, investigate further by asking the following questions:

- Did you experience pain or nausea before or after vomiting?
- Did you vomit once or several times?
- Will you describe the episode of vomiting? Did it come out in a forceful stream? Did you retch without actually vomiting? Did you regurgitate burning fluid? Did you regurgitate food?
- Was there blood in your vomit?
- Did you vomit after you ate? What had you eaten?
- What characteristics did the vomit display?
- What have you eaten in the last 24 hours?
- When was your last bowel movement?
- Have you lost weight recently?
- What medications are you currently taking?

Focusing Your Assessment

When you examine a patient who complains of nausea and vomiting, focus your assessment as follows:

- Inspect the patient's skin turgor. Poor turgor indicates dehydration, probably as a result of vomiting.
- Check vital signs. Increased heart rate and low blood pressure are signs of dehydration. Fever is a sign of infection, as in gastroenteritis or pelvic inflammatory disease.
- Inspect the abdomen for distention or visible peristaltic waves. Abdominal distention may suggest intestinal obstruction, paralytic ileus, or constipation. Visible peristaltic waves may occur early in intestinal obstruction and gastroenteritis.
- Auscultate for bowel sounds, listening for changes in their normal frequency and pitch (see ▓ *Assessing Bowel Sounds*).

INTERPRETING ABNORMAL FINDINGS

ASSESSING BOWEL SOUNDS

Bowel sounds reflect the activity of underlying intestines and offer information about intestinal health and function. Normally the bowel produces soft clicks and gurgles every 5 to 15 seconds. Because bowel sounds are usually irregular, listen for 1 full minute in all four quadrants using the diaphragm of your stethoscope. Changes in the frequency and pitch of your patient's bowel sounds may indicate a problem. Use this table to help pinpoint the cause of abnormal bowel sounds.

Bowel Sound	Probable Mechanism	Probable Causes
• Hyperactive sounds not related to hunger	• Abnormally rapid passage of air and fluid through the intestine	• Diarrhea • Early intestinal obstruction

continued

INTERPRETING ABNORMAL FINDINGS—cont'd

Bowel Sound	Probable Mechanism	Probable Causes
• Hypoactive or absent sounds	• Inactivity of smooth muscle in the bowel	• Paralytic ileus • Peritonitis • Decreased bowel motility
• High-pitched rushing sounds	• Intestinal straining to push fluid and air past an obstruction	• Intestinal obstruction
• High-pitched tinkling sounds	• Intestinal fluid and air under tension	• Dilated bowel loops • Fecal impaction

- Assess for abdominal pain. Right lower quadrant pain may indicate appendicitis. Diffuse lower abdominal pain may accompany bowel obstruction or pelvic inflammatory disease.

Possible Causes
- *Small intestine obstruction.* Colicky pain, nausea, vomiting, constipation, and abdominal distention characterize this condition. The vomitus begins as gastric juice and bile. Eventually, it contains ileal fecal contents.
- *Gastroenteritis.* This condition is characterized by nausea and vomiting accompanied by diarrhea and abdominal discomfort. Other signs include fever, malaise, and hyperactive bowel sounds.
- *Peptic ulcer disease.* Ulcers in the stomach and duodenum may result in bloody vomitus.
- *Esophageal varices.* A large volume of bright-red blood in the vomit may result from ruptured esophageal varices and constitutes a life-threatening medical emergency (see ◰ *Responding to Gastrointestinal Bleeding*).

ACTION STAT

RESPONDING TO GASTROINTESTINAL BLEEDING
Gastrointestinal (GI) bleeding, which you will usually observe coming from a patient's mouth, anus, or both, can result from various conditions. Blood that appears in vomitus could signal a gastric ulcer, life-threatening esophageal varices, or other upper GI problems. Blood that exits the anus may be bright red or tarry black and can warn of a disorder as simple as hemorrhoids or as serious as gastric or colon cancer.

All cases of GI bleeding deserve prompt attention. However, bleeding that occurs unchecked and in large amounts requires immediate intervention to protect the patient against hypovolemic shock, ischemia, and possible death.

What to look for
Clinical findings vary, depending on the location of the bleeding, but may include the following:
- Vomiting of bright-red blood or brownish-black granular material that looks like

continued

coffee grounds, indicating old blood and gastric juices from a slow bleed
- Passing of bright-red blood via the anus, indicating lower GI bleeding
- Passing of black, tarry stools, indicating upper GI bleeding
- Pale, cool skin with delayed capillary refill
- Narrow pulse pressure
- Tachycardia
- Hyperactive bowel sounds
- Positive tilt test (increase in heart rate of more than 20 beats per minute [bpm] or decrease in blood pressure of more than 10 mm Hg when the patient rises from a lying to a sitting position, suggesting hypovolemic shock)

What to do immediately

If you suspect your patient has acute GI bleeding, notify the physician, then proceed as follows:
- Maintain nothing by mouth status and administer intravenous (IV) fluids (lactated Ringer's or isotonic saline solutions) by large-bore IV catheter, as ordered, to maintain circulatory volume.
- Expect to insert a nasogastric (NG) tube to administer saline lavages to clear blood from the stomach. In cases of uncontrolled upper GI bleeding, norepinephrine may be added to the saline to constrict the blood vessels.
- If the physician suspects esophageal bleeding or a Mallory-Weiss tear (an esophageal tear associated with prolonged vomiting or retching), an NG tube usually is not inserted because it could worsen the bleeding. Instead, a chambered-balloon tube (Sengstaken-Blakemore) may be inserted to apply pressure to the bleeding areas.

- Assess vital signs frequently. Monitor the patient for signs of shock, including increased pulse rate, hypotension, and pallor.
- Administer blood transfusions, as ordered, to replace volume. Monitor hemoglobin and hematocrit to assess blood loss and recovery.
- Administer prescribed medications, such as H_2-blockers (cimetidine) or proton-pump inhibitors (omeprazole), to decrease gastric acidity. Antacid agents may be ordered by mouth or NG tube to neutralize stomach acids. If bleeding results from a peptic ulcer and *Helicobacter pylori* is the cause, antibiotic agents may be prescribed.
- If the bleeding cannot be controlled by saline lavage or medications, prepare the patient for possible surgery, depending on the site and cause of the bleeding. The patient may have a Billroth procedure, for example, or a rectal resection.
- Expect to insert an indwelling urinary catheter to monitor urinary output.

What to do next

Once the patient has been stabilized, you will need to do the following:
- Maintain and monitor fluid intake and output. Include all vomitus and drainage in your calculation of output. If ice chips are allowed, make sure you include them as intake.
- Continue monitoring hemoglobin and hematocrit. Look for signs of decreased hemoglobin, such as pale mucous membranes and conjunctivae.
- Administer transfusions, as ordered, and watch for signs of adverse transfusion reactions, such as fever, chills, and lower back pain.
- Begin a clear liquid diet when ordered. Watch for any signs of vomiting.

- *Paralytic ileus.* A physiologic intestinal obstruction usually affecting the small bowel and occurring most often after abdominal surgery or use of anticholinergic medications. Signs include severe abdominal distention and vomiting.
- *Constipation.* This condition may occur with narcotic use, poor dietary habits, or sluggish bowel function. Nausea and vomiting begin after several days.

- *Pregnancy.* From early in pregnancy until about the sixteenth week, nausea and vomiting may occur, most often in the morning (morning sickness).

ABDOMINAL PAIN

If the patient complains of abdominal pain, investigate further by asking the following questions:

- Where is the pain located?
- Does the pain radiate or extend to another part of your body?
- Did it begin gradually or suddenly?
- Can you describe the pain?
- How often have you experienced the pain, and how long has the pain lasted? What is the timing and pattern of your pain?
- Which activities make the pain worse? What makes it better?
- What are you doing when the pain begins? Does it wake you from sleep?
- Are you (female patient) possibly pregnant?
- Where are you (female patient) in your monthly cycle?
- Have you (female patient) noticed any vaginal discharge?

Focusing Your Assessment

When examining a patient who complains of abdominal pain, focus your assessment as follows:

- Identify the type of pain involved. The three major types include (1) visceral, (2) somatic (also called *parietal*), and (3) referred. Visceral pain results from stretching or distention of an abdominal organ (viscus) and is usually described as diffuse, poorly localized, and cramping or gnawing. Somatic pain emanates from the abdominal wall, peritoneum, mesentery, or diaphragm. It is more intense and localized. Referred pain is experienced at a site removed from the actual source of pain. Usually it is sharp, well localized, and resembles somatic pain (see *Telltale Signs of Peritonitis*).

TELLTALE SIGNS OF PERITONITIS

An acute localized or generalized inflammation of the peritoneal layer of the abdominal cavity, peritonitis results from bacterial contamination after perforation of an abdominal organ, such as the large bowel, or the release of irritating chemicals, such as pancreatic enzymes.

If you suspect your patient has peritonitis, notify the physician immediately. Peritonitis requires rapid intervention, including administration of antibiotics and surgery.

Clinical findings associated with peritonitis can vary, depending on the severity of the infection, but may include the following:

- Acute, diffuse, abdominal pain with rebound tenderness and abdominal rigidity
- Pain that eventually localizes to the source of infection
- Referred pain to the shoulder, at times accompanied by hiccups caused by diaphragmatic irritation
- Elevated temperature, often as high as 103° F (39.4° C), along with chills, nausea, and vomiting
- Abdominal distention
- Diminished or absent bowel sounds
- Elevated white blood cell counts with high neutrophil count

- Identify the area of the abdomen where the pain is occurring. Knowing where your patient's pain is located and where the pain is referred can help you identify the organ involved (see ▦ *Acute Abdominal Pain*).

INTERPRETING ABNORMAL FINDINGS

ACUTE ABDOMINAL PAIN

Acute abdominal pain is a common complaint that can have many causes. When thinking of the source of the pain, it helps to mentally divide the abdomen into four quadrants: upper and lower right and upper and lower left. Then remember the organs that lie within these quadrants. As you proceed with the physical examination, watch the patient's facial expression for grimacing and other signs of pain. Prepare to intervene quickly if the cause is one of the serious disorders listed in this chart.

Characteristics	Location	Possible Findings	Probable Cause
• Sudden and severe • Colicky	• Generalized • May refer to shoulder	• Nausea and vomiting • Constipation • Abdominal distention • Visible peristalsis • High-pitched, hyperactive bowel sounds or absent lower-bowel sounds • Hiccups • Signs of shock, such as hypotension, with bowel ischemia or infarction	• Intestinal obstruction
• Severe and acute • Rebound tenderness	• Diffuse, may localize to the source of infection • Referred to shoulder	• Fever • Nausea, vomiting, anorexia • Guarding, boardlike abdomen, abdominal distention • Diminished or absent bowel sounds • Leukocytosis	• Peritonitis
• Steady, with episodes of severe, extreme pain	• Epigastric, close to umbilicus	• Vomiting	• Pancreatitis

continued

Characteristics	Location	Possible Findings	Probable Cause
	• May involve flanks and left upper quadrant • Radiates to area between tenth thoracic and sixth lumbar vertebrae, left shoulder, groin	• Abdominal tenderness and rigidity • Cullen's sign (periumbilical ecchymosis) • Grey Turner's sign (ecchymosis of flanks) • Elevated lipase and amylase levels • Leukocytosis	
• Sharp or colicky	• Periumbilical and generalized • Localized in right lower quadrant or McBurney's point	• Fever • Nausea, vomiting, anorexia • Guarding, boardlike abdomen • Pain with flexion of the right leg at the knee and hip to 90 degrees • Rebound tenderness • Diarrhea • Leukocytosis	• Appendicitis
• Severe and acute • Often nocturnal and precipitated by rich foods	• Right upper quadrant or epigastric • May radiate to the back in the subscapular area	• Flatulence • Diaphoresis • Nausea and vomiting • Jaundice or clay-colored stool (with biliary obstruction)	• Cholecystitis
• Colicky	• Usually left lower quadrant or epigastric radiating to left side or back	• Abdominal tenderness • Low-grade fever • Alternating constipation and diarrhea • Flatulence • Nausea • High-pitched, hyperactive bowel sounds	• Diverticulitis

continued

INTERPRETING ABNORMAL FINDINGS—cont'd

Characteristics	Location	Possible Findings	Probable Cause
• Severe and sudden	• Lower quadrants • Referred to shoulder (especially left shoulder)	• Symptoms of pregnancy, including amenorrhea or irregular menstruation • Abdominal tenderness and distention • Palpable mass • Signs of shock, such as hypotension	• Ruptured ectopic pregnancy
• Progressively severe	• Lower quadrant	• Cervical and adnexal tenderness • Abdominal guarding and rebound tenderness • Vaginal discharge, often purulent • Fever • Dyspareunia	• Pelvic inflammatory disease
• Deep, boreing • Steady, occasional, relieved by position change	• Lower quadrants • Lumbosacral region	• Wide aortic pulsation • Abdominal bruit • Nausea and vomiting • Possible tenderness • Signs of shock and loss of distal pulses with rupture	• Abdominal aortic aneurysm
• Severe, may worsen with feet elevation	• Left upper quadrant • Radiates to left shoulder	• Hypothermia • Signs of shock, such as hypotension • Abdominal trauma • Mononucleosis	• Ruptured spleen

- Inspect the abdomen for distention, a sign of intestinal obstruction.
- Inspect the perineal area of a female patient for vaginal discharge.
- Check your patient's temperature. Abdominal pain with a fever may indicate appendicitis or gastroenteritis.
- Auscultate for vascular sounds. A bruit heard over the abdominal aorta may indicate an abdominal aortic aneurysm.
- Auscultate for bowel sounds. Absent or hypoactive bowel sounds may indicate peritonitis. Hyperactive bowel sounds may suggest Crohn's disease or ulcerative colitis.
- Check for rebound tenderness and heel-jarring tenderness, signs of appendicitis and peritonitis.

Possible Causes

- *Peritonitis.* Sudden, diffuse abdominal pain usually is most intense over the area of the underlying problem. The patient will also have weakness, pallor, sweating, and cold skin from loss of fluids and electrolytes. As bacterial toxins invade the intestinal muscles, intestinal motility decreases, and paralytic ileus develops.

- *Intestinal obstruction.* Colicky pain, nausea, vomiting, constipation, and abdominal distention characterize this condition. The patient may also complain of drowsiness, intense thirst, malaise, and aching. Bowel sounds are hyperactive with a rushing sound.

- *Pancreatitis.* Steady epigastric pain centers close to the umbilicus and radiates between the tenth thoracic and sixth lumbar vertebrae. The pain is unrelieved by vomiting. Severe attacks produce extreme pain, persistent vomiting, and abdominal rigidity.

- *Diverticulitis.* Recurrent left lower quadrant pain is accompanied by alternating constipation and diarrhea. The pain usually abates after defecation or passage of flatus. The patient may have mild nausea and a low-grade fever.

- *Peptic ulcer.* This condition is characterized by localized midepigastric pain with heartburn that develops 2 hours or more after meals, when the stomach is empty. Eating may relieve the pain. Acidic liquids, such as orange juice or coffee, may aggravate the pain (see 🔍 *Peptic Ulcer Disease*).

DISORDER CLOSE-UP

PEPTIC ULCER DISEASE

A common and potentially serious problem, peptic ulcer disease, affects about 1 in 10 Americans. A peptic ulcer can develop in any area of the gastrointestinal (GI) tract exposed to acid-pepsin secretions, including the esophagus, stomach, and duodenum. A defect develops in the GI mucosa when the mucosal barrier fails to protect the mucosa from damage by hydrochloric acid and pepsin, the gastric digestive juices.

For many years, most experts believed this failure resulted from the patient's lifestyle and stress level. Now it is known that the bacterium *Helicobacter pylori* plays a major role in the formation of duodenal ulcers, and the incidence is falling because recent treatment has targeted the bacterium. The organism most likely damages the mucosa by producing urease, an enzyme that splits urea into ammonia,

carbon dioxide, and bicarbonate. The ammonia erodes the mucosa.

Nonsteroidal antiinflammatory drug use is a common cause of gastric ulcers. Other factors can aggravate the problem, including smoking and excessive alcohol use.

Another cause of peptic ulcer disease is increased production of, or susceptibility to, gastric acid. With duodenal ulcers, increased hydrochloric acid production by the stomach's parietal cells and faster emptying of stomach contents means the duodenum receives more acid more quickly. Gastric ulcers are accompanied by normal or reduced acid secretion. However, the mucosa seems more permeable to damaging acid backflow.

Characteristic findings

Expect health history information and physical examination findings to vary among patients

continued

DISORDER CLOSE-UP—cont'd

with peptic ulcer disease, depending on the extent and severity of the disease. Use the information that follows to help distinguish between expected and unexpected findings.

Health History
- Gnawing or burning epigastric pain
- Pain occurring 2 hours or so after meals and at night, usually relieved by food (duodenal ulcer)
- Pain of varying pattern that may be relieved or aggravated by food (gastric ulcer)
- History of analgesic use, especially aspirin, ibuprofen, or naproxen
- History of smoking
- Recent loss of weight or appetite (gastric ulcer)
- Feelings of fullness or distention

Inspection
- Pallor (if anemic from blood loss)

Auscultation
- Hyperactive bowel sounds (possible)

Palpation
- Epigastric tenderness

Complications
- GI hemorrhage
- Hypovolemic shock
- Perforation
- Obstruction
- Intestinal infarction
- Penetration to adjacent structures, such as the pancreas, biliary tract, liver, or gastrohepatic omentum

- *Crohn's disease.* This condition produces steady, colicky pain in the right lower quadrant, with cramping, tenderness, flatulence, nausea, fever, and diarrhea. The patient may have bloody stools and complain of weight loss, weakness, and fatigue.
- *Appendicitis.* Beginning as epigastric or periumbilical abdominal pain, the pain later localizes in the right lower quadrant. Palpation reveals a rigid, boardlike abdominal wall and rebound tenderness. Diarrhea, fever, and tachycardia develop later.
- *Cholecystitis.* This condition produces acute abdominal pain in the right upper quadrant, occasionally radiating to the back. The pain usually develops after a meal rich in fats. It may occur at night, awakening the patient from sleep. The patient also may complain of belching, gassiness, sweating, vomiting, and clay-colored stools (if a stone obstructs the common bile duct). Jaundice will occur if the bile duct is blocked (see ▧ *Cholecystitis*).

DISORDER CLOSE-UP

CHOLECYSTITIS

An inflammation of the gallbladder, cholecystitis usually results from the obstructing presence of gallstones in the cystic or common bile ducts.

Gallstones develop in the gallbladder when such factors as age, obesity, and estrogen imbalance cause the liver to secrete bile abnormally high in cholesterol or lacking in the proper concentration of bile salts. Excessive water and bile salts are reabsorbed, making the bile less soluble. Cholesterol, calcium, and bilirubin then precipitate into gallstones.

continued

DISORDER CLOSE-UP—cont'd

Usually cholecystitis develops after a high-fat meal. Fat entering the duodenum causes the intestinal mucosa to secrete cholecystokinin, a hormone that prompts the gallbladder to contract and empty its bile. If the gallbladder contains stones, this strong contraction can force one or more of them to lodge in the cystic duct, the common bile duct, or other locations. The obstruction prevents bile from flowing into the duodenum and causes bilirubin to be absorbed into the blood.

Biliary stasis and ischemia of tissues around the calculus may irritate and inflame the common bile duct. This inflammation can progress up the biliary tree and lead to infection of any of the bile ducts, causing scar tissue, edema, cirrhosis, portal hypertension, and variceal hemorrhage.

Characteristic findings

Expect health history information and physical examination findings to vary among patients with cholecystitis, depending on the extent and severity of the disease. Use the information that follows to help distinguish between expected and unexpected findings.

Health history

- Asymptomatic
- Sudden onset of severe, steady or aching pain in the midepigastric region or right upper abdominal quadrant that radiates to the back, between the shoulder blades, or over the right shoulder or shoulder blade
- Recent ingestion of a large or fatty meal, especially after fasting
- Nausea and vomiting
- Chills
- History of mild upper gastrointestinal (GI) symptoms, such as indigestion, vague abdominal discomfort, belching, and flatulence after high-fat meals or snacks

Inspection

- Pallor
- Diaphoresis
- Exhaustion
- Abdominal muscle guarding
- Jaundice of sclerae and mucous membranes (chronic)
- Dark-colored urine (chronic)
- Clay-colored stools (chronic)

Palpation

- Rebound tenderness over gallbladder area, increasing with inspiration
- Abdominal rigidity, with peritoneal involvement
- Painless, sausagelike mass in the abdomen (calculus-filled gallbladder without obstruction)

Auscultation

- Hypoactive bowel sounds

Vital signs

- Fever
- Tachycardia

Complications

- Empyema, mucocele, or gangrene of gallbladder
- Perforation
- Peritonitis
- Fistula formation
- Pancreatitis
- Chronic cholecystitis
- Cholangitis

- *Renal calculi.* A calculus traveling down the ureter may cause severe abdominal and flank pain. Nausea and vomiting usually are also present.
- *Pyelonephritis.* Resulting from an infection (usually with *Escherichia coli*), this condition affects the renal pelvis and parenchyma. The patient will complain of severe flank pain. Other symptoms include shaking chills, elevated temperature, tachycardia, hematuria, nausea, vomiting, and costovertebral angle tenderness.

- *Pelvic inflammatory disease.* This condition affects female subjects and results from infection by anaerobic or aerobic organisms, most commonly *Neisseria gonorrhoeae* and *Chlamydia trachomatis.* Fever and a purulent vaginal discharge usually are present.
- *Ruptured ectopic pregnancy.* This condition is characterized by a rapid onset of sharp, lower abdominal pain, occasionally radiating to the shoulders and neck. Commonly, the pain begins after an activity that increases abdominal pressure, such as a bowel movement. Vaginal bleeding may or may not be present.
- *Endometriosis.* Characterized by constant pain in the lower abdomen, vagina, posterior pelvis, and back, this condition usually begins 5 to 7 days before menses peaks and lasts for 2 to 3 days.

ABDOMINAL DISTENTION

If the patient complains of abdominal distention, investigate further by asking the following questions:

- When did you first notice an increase in the size of your abdomen?
- Are you having any difficulty breathing?
- Do you have a feeling of fullness or pressure?
- When was your last bowel movement?
- Have you noticed any change in your bowel or bladder habits?
- Could you (female patient) possibly be pregnant?
- What medications are you currently taking?

Focusing Your Assessment

When examining a patient who complains of abdominal distention, focus your assessment as follows:

- Examine your patient's sclerae and mucous membranes for signs of jaundice. Jaundice and abdominal distention caused by ascitic fluid are signs of liver disease.
- Inspect the abdomen for signs of asymmetry. Asymmetrical distention may result from tumor, cysts, or bowel obstruction. A lump in the abdominal wall may be a section of herniated intestine. In a female patient with distention that appears between the umbilicus and symphysis pubis, consider bladder distention, pregnancy, or ovarian tumor. Distention of the upper half of the abdomen may indicate gastric dilation or a pancreatic cyst or tumor. Ascites appears as a single curve from the xiphoid process to the pubic symphysis when viewed from the side. In the supine position, a patient with ascites will appear to have bulging flanks.
- Inspect the umbilicus to determine if it is inverted or everted. Symmetrical distention with an inverted umbilicus suggests obesity or recent fluid or gas pressure within the hollow intestines. An everted umbilicus suggests ascites or an underlying tumor.
- Inspect the abdominal wall for enlarged superficial abdominal veins, a sign of portal congestion.
- Auscultate the abdomen for bowel sounds or venous hum. Absent or hypoactive bowel sounds may indicate a paralytic ileus. Hyperactive bowel

sounds may indicate an intestinal obstruction. A venous hum may indicate portal congestion from liver disease.

- Palpate the abdomen for an enlarged liver (a sign of cirrhosis) or palpable feces (a sign of fecal impaction or large bowel obstruction).
- Assess the abdomen for a fluid wave, which indicates ascites. Ascites is found in cirrhosis, peritonitis, metastatic carcinoma, ovarian carcinoma, and pancreatitis.

Possible Causes

- *Cirrhosis.* Ascites from portal congestion may cause abdominal distention severe enough to impair breathing. A late symptom, abdominal distention accompanies jaundice, lethargy, mental status changes, asterixis, coagulopathies, pruritus, dependent edema, and enlarged superficial abdominal veins.
- *Ovarian cancer.* Abdominal distention from ascites occurs in advanced disease. Other symptoms are dyspepsia, urinary frequency, constipation, pelvic discomfort, and weight loss.
- *Pregnancy.* Abdominal distention and weight gain typically begin in the thirteenth week of pregnancy. Consider pregnancy in a woman of childbearing age who reports irregularities in menses. Other early signs include urinary frequency, nausea and vomiting in the morning, and breast swelling and tenderness.
- *Intestinal obstruction.* Abdominal distention is accompanied by hyperactive bowel sounds. The patient also may complain of nausea, vomiting, or diarrhea (see ◹ *Responding to Acute Intestinal Obstruction*).

ACTION STAT

RESPONDING TO ACUTE INTESTINAL OBSTRUCTION

Abdominal distention is a hallmark of acute intestinal obstruction, a common but potentially life-threatening disorder. When left untreated, an intestinal obstruction can lead to peritonitis, septicemia, bowel ischemia, perforation, or necrosis. These conditions, in turn, may lead to septic or hypovolemic shock and eventually death.

If you discover abdominal distention during your inspection, quickly assess your patient for a possible intestinal obstruction.

What to look for
Clinical findings vary, depending on the location of the obstruction, but may include the following:
- Sudden, severe, colicky epigastric or periumbilical pain
- Vomiting
- Visible peristalsis
- Hiccups
- Localized tenderness
- Minimal rigidity and rebound tenderness
- Absent bowel sounds (nonmechanical obstruction, such as paralytic ileus)
- Hyperactive, high-pitched borborygmi, with rushes coinciding with cramps (e.g., from mechanical obstruction caused by fecal impaction or tumor)

What to do immediately
If you suspect that your patient has an acute intestinal obstruction, notify the physician and follow these measures:
- Maintain nothing by mouth status until bowel sounds return or the obstruction is

continued

ACTION STAT—cont'd

resolved through decompression or surgical intervention.

- Administer intravenous (IV) fluids (lactated Ringer's or isotonic saline solutions), as prescribed, to maintain fluid and electrolyte balance.
- Expect to insert a nasogastric (NG) tube and attach it to low, intermittent suction to help remove fluids from the gastrointestinal (GI) system, relieve abdominal distention, and stop the vomiting.
- If a long intestinal tube (e.g., a Cantor, Harris, or Miller-Abbott) is indicated, assist with insertion. After insertion, reposition the patient from side to side to help advance the tube. Check the tube periodically to make sure it is advancing.
- Assess vital signs frequently. If you suspect a strangulating obstruction, monitor the patient for signs of shock (increased pulse rate, hypotension, and pallor).
- Administer prescribed medications, such as analgesic agents, antiemetic agents, and broad-spectrum antibiotic agents. Analgesic agents may be withheld until a diagnosis is confirmed because they can mask other signs and symptoms and decrease intestinal motility. Broad-spectrum antibiotic

agents may be prescribed if the patient has a strangulating obstruction.
- Expect to insert a catheter to monitor urinary output.

What to do next

Once your patient has been stabilized, you will need to do the following:

- Maintain and monitor fluid intake and output. Include all vomitus and tube drainage as output. If ice chips are allowed, make sure you include them as intake.
- Monitor fluid and electrolyte status. Monitor serum electrolyte, blood urea nitrogen, and creatinine levels. Look for signs of dehydration, such as poor skin turgor, dry skin, parched tongue, dry mucous membranes, and decreased urinary output. Monitor daily weights.
- Administer rectal enemas, as prescribed, to relieve partial obstruction.
- Keep the patient in semi-Fowler's or Fowler's position to alleviate respiratory distress from abdominal distention and to promote optimal pulmonary ventilation.
- Measure abdominal girth every 8 hours to monitor the patient's condition.

- *Paralytic ileus.* Abdominal distention is accompanied by absent or hypoactive bowel sounds. Symptoms occasionally include nausea and vomiting.
- *Fecal impaction.* Abdominal distention is accompanied by high-pitched tinkling bowel sounds. Diarrhea may develop from liquid stool being forced around the fecal blockage.
- *Hernia.* A protrusion of intestine through the abdominal wall, a hernia may disappear momentarily when pressed back into the abdominal wall. If the section of intestine becomes strangulated, the patient will complain of pain and may experience anorexia and vomiting.
- *Obesity.* A uniformly rounded abdomen is accompanied by an umbilicus buried deeply in the abdominal wall and excessive fat in other body areas.
- *Aerophagia.* Swallowing air can cause an excess of air in the GI tract (tympanites), resulting in abdominal distention. Some patients swallow air when they are anxious, in pain, or nauseated. Ingestion of gas-forming foods, such as cabbage, turnips, and onions, and drinking fluids through a straw

are other possible causes. The patient will have a large area of tympany on percussion, with voluntary or involuntary muscle spasm of the abdominal wall.

FECAL INCONTINENCE

If the patient complains of fecal incontinence, investigate further by asking the following questions:

- When does the fecal incontinence occur?
- Is it associated with activity, such as exercise or walking, or does it occur during periods of rest?
- Does it occur in the morning?
- How long has it been occurring?
- What is your normal pattern of bowel elimination?
- Do you ever find fecal matter on your underwear?
- Do you ever engage in anal sex?

Focusing Your Assessment

When examining a patient who complains of fecal incontinence, focus your assessment as follows:

- Use a gloved and lubricated index finger to assess anal sphincter tone, and inspect any stool found in the rectum. Blood or mucus in the stool or rectum could indicate colorectal cancer. Poor sphincter tone may be the result of sphincter trauma.
- Inspect the anus for rectal prolapse or signs of trauma.
- Assess lower extremity strength. Lower extremity weakness may be a sign of spinal cord compression.

Possible Causes

- *Colorectal cancer.* Signs include loss of sphincter control or an urgent need to defecate on arising in the morning, blood or mucus in the stool, and a sense of incomplete evacuation.
- *Sphincter trauma.* Injury can cause loss of sphincter control and lead to incontinence.
- *Rectal prolapse.* This condition is evidenced by protrusion of the rectal mucosa through the anus. The patient may also complain of a persistent sensation of rectal fullness, bloody diarrhea, and pain in the lower abdomen from ulceration.
- *Spinal cord compression.* Compression affecting the lumbar or sacral area may cause loss of bowel control.

URINARY INCONTINENCE

If the patient complains of urinary incontinence, investigate further by asking the following questions:

- When does the urinary incontinence occur?
- Is it associated with activity, such as exercise, lifting, coughing, or laughing? Does it occur during periods of rest?
- How long has this been occurring? Did it start gradually or suddenly?

- What is your normal pattern of bladder elimination?
- Have you noticed any changes in the color or odor of your urine?
- Do you have urinary hesitancy or urgency?
- Can you describe your fluid intake during a typical day?
- What medications are you currently taking?
- Might you (female patient) be pregnant?

Focusing Your Assessment

When examining a patient who complains of urinary incontinence, focus your assessment as follows:

- Inspect the abdomen for distention. Abdominal distention may indicate urinary retention or pregnancy.
- Ask your patient to void into a specimen cup, and inspect the urine. Cloudy or foul-smelling urine suggests infection.
- Inspect the vulva or penis for purulent discharge or redness and swelling, signs of gonorrhea.

Possible Causes

- *Muscle weakness.* Urine leakage results from physical strain, such as sneezing, coughing, or quick movements (stress incontinence). Older female patients and female patients who have given birth vaginally are candidates for this type of incontinence.
- *Pregnancy.* Incontinence in pregnancy is a form of stress incontinence arising from pressure on the bladder by the enlarging uterus.
- *Urinary retention.* Retention causes dribbling because the distended bladder cannot contract strongly enough to force a urine stream (overflow incontinence). The bladder will be distended on palpation.
- *Diuretic medications.* These medications can cause bladder distention, which may result in incontinence from overflow or from weak muscles unaccustomed to a full bladder.
- *Gonorrhea.* Urinary incontinence accompanies purulent vaginal or penile discharge and dysuria.
- *Cognitive impairment.* Your patient may be unaware of the need to urinate.

CONSTIPATION

If the patient complains of constipation, investigate further by asking the following questions:

- What is your usual pattern of bowel movement?
- Do you take anything on a regular basis to assist with bowel movement?
- When was your last bowel movement?
- How is your appetite? Do you feel full more easily than you did in the past?
- Have you changed your diet recently?
- Have you lost weight recently?
- Has the shape, color, or consistency of your stool changed recently?
- What medications are you currently taking?

Focusing Your Assessment

When examining a patient who complains of constipation, focus your assessment as follows:

• Inspect the abdomen for distention.
• Assess the abdomen for symmetry. An asymmetrical contour may indicate tumor, hernia, or bowel obstruction.
• Auscultate for bowel sounds. Absence of bowel sounds may indicate a paralytic ileus.
• Palpate the abdomen. Masses may be tumors or distended sections of intestine. A palpable colon may be a sign of inactive colon or large bowel obstruction.
• Use a gloved and lubricated index finger to examine rectal contents. Stool is found in the lower portion of the rectum with inactive colon.

Possible Causes

• *Large intestine obstruction.* Constipation may be the only early sign. After several days, your patient may complain of colicky abdominal pain with spasms. The abdomen will be distended, and loops of large bowel may become visible on the abdominal wall.
• *Colorectal cancer.* A tumor can occlude the lumen of the descending colon. If so, your patient probably will report a history of pencil-shaped or ribbon-shaped stools.
• *Narcotic use.* Narcotic agents slow bowel motility, possibly causing fecal material to block the large intestine.
• *Inactive colon.* This condition is characterized by chronic constipation. Causes include low dietary fiber, chronic laxative or enema use, poor hydration, and a sedentary lifestyle. Your patient will complain of mild abdominal discomfort and of having to strain to produce hard, dry stool.

LIFESPAN CONSIDERATIONS

Constipation and fecal impaction occur more commonly in older adults because intestinal motility declines with age.

DIARRHEA

If the patient complains of diarrhea, investigate further by asking the following questions:

• How long have you had the diarrhea? (If less than 3 weeks, it is considered an acute episode. If more than 3 weeks, it is considered chronic.)
• How often do you have episodes of diarrhea?
• What are the consistency and volume of your stool?
• What color is the stool?
• Is eating meals followed by diarrhea?
• Do you have any abdominal pain?
• Have you traveled recently out of the state or out of the country?

- What prescription and over-the-counter medications are you currently taking?
- Have you participated recently in anal sex?

Focusing Your Assessment

When examining a patient who complains of diarrhea, focus your assessment as follows:

- Assess hydration by checking your patient's skin turgor and mucous membrane moisture. Diarrhea can lead to dehydration.
- Check vital signs. Low blood pressure is a sign of dehydration.
- Inspect the abdomen for distention or peristaltic waves, which may indicate bowel obstruction or fecal impaction.
- Auscultate for bowel sounds. Hyperactive sounds may indicate gastroenteritis.
- Assess the color, amount, and odor of any stools passed.

Possible Causes

- *Gastroenteritis.* This condition is characterized by diarrhea with nausea, vomiting, and abdominal discomfort. Other symptoms include fever, malaise, and hyperactive bowel sounds.
- *Ulcerative colitis.* This condition is characterized by recurrent bloody diarrhea that commonly contains mucus. Patients with ulcerative colitis experience intermittent asymptomatic remissions. The intensity of the attacks varies with the extent of the inflammation. Other symptoms include spastic rectum and anus, abdominal pain, irritability, weight loss, weakness, anorexia, nausea, and vomiting.
- *Acquired immunodeficiency syndrome (AIDS) or its treatment.* A common problem for AIDS patients, diarrhea may result from opportunistic infection in the GI tract, Kaposi's sarcoma (KS), drug therapy, chemotherapy, or radiation therapy (see 🔍 *Acquired Immunodeficiency Syndrome*).

🔍 **DISORDER CLOSE-UP**

ACQUIRED IMMUNODEFICIENCY SYNDROME

An infectious disease syndrome that destroys the body's immune system, acquired immunodeficiency syndrome (AIDS) can result in death by overwhelming opportunistic infection. The syndrome originates with infection by the human immunodeficiency virus (HIV).

HIV spreads through contact with infected blood or body fluids. Most often, transmission occurs from blood or blood products transfusion, sexual contact, needle sharing among intravenous (IV) drug users, perinatal exposure (including through breast milk), and occupational exposure (e.g., through needle-stick injuries). The virus is not spread by casual contact or by insects.

A retrovirus that carries its genetic material in ribonucleic acid (RNA) rather than deoxyribonucleic acid (DNA), HIV cannot replicate until it invades host cells. The invasion process begins when the virus attaches to CD4+

continued

DISORDER CLOSE-UP

receptors on the surface of cells, including the following:

- Lymphocytes
- Macrophages
- Colorectal cells
- Glial cells (central nervous system)
- Langerhans' cells
- Follicular dendritic cells

Because of this variety in host cells, the virus can express itself in many ways, producing a wide variety of symptoms that mimic other diseases.

Once HIV binds to a CD4+ receptor site, it enters the cell and injects its genetic material into the host cell's cytoplasm. There, reverse transcriptase (an enzyme) transcribes DNA from viral RNA. Because this transcription process is faulty, mutations occur that prevent antiviral drugs from having a consistent and long-term effect.

This newly formed DNA invades the host cell's nucleus and is transcribed back into RNA. Now, every time the cell divides, it spreads the HIV infection. Transcribed RNA is translated into long protein chains and enzymes. A viral enzyme called *protease* cuts the long chains and incorporates them into new virus particles. New HIV particles can then bud away to infect other cells.

The body's immune system produces antibodies in an attempt to fight the HIV infection. However, by selectively infecting immune system cells, and by mutating regularly, the virus ultimately destroys the body's defense against infection, leaving the person vulnerable to opportunistic infections. These opportunistic infections account for 90% of AIDS-related deaths.

Characteristic findings

Expect health history information and physical findings to vary among patients with AIDS, depending on the extent and severity of the disease, the stage of the disease, and the AIDS-related conditions present. Use the information that follows to help distinguish between expected and unexpected findings.

Health history

- Exposure to HIV-infected blood or body fluids
- History of flulike symptoms, including fever, sweats, sore throat, malaise, myalgia, arthralgia, photophobia, diarrhea, anorexia, nausea, vomiting, or headache
- Weight loss
- Increasing incidence and severity of infections
- Chest pain, as in *Pneumocystis carinii* pneumonia (PCP)
- Cough and increased sputum production (PCP)
- Mood, motor, behavioral, or cognitive changes (AIDS dementia)
- Visual changes, such as blurring or loss of vision
- Stiff neck (cryptococcal meningitis)

Inspection

- Diaphoresis
- Transient maculopapular rashes on chest and extremities
- Hairy leukoplakia of the oral mucosa
- Pink, red, or purple nodules or plaques, as in Kaposi's sarcoma (KS)
- Tachypnea (PCP)
- Flat affect and apathy (AIDS dementia)
- Unsteady gait and incoordination
- Confusion, staring, disorientation, and delirium (advanced stages)
- Retinitis, as in cytomegalovirus (CMV), with granular areas, perivascular exudates, and hemorrhages at the optic fundus
- Candidiasis of mouth, esophagus, or vagina
- Loss of more than 10 pounds or 10% of body weight

Palpation

- Firm, nontender nodules or plaques on the skin (KS)
- Generalized lymphadenopathy (lymph nodes larger than ½ inch [1 cm] in diameter in two or more extrainguinal sites for more than 3 months)

continued

DISORDER CLOSE-UP—cont'd

- Hepatomegaly
- Splenomegaly

Auscultation
- Hyperactive bowel sounds (cryptosporidiosis)
- Normal breath sounds or coarse breath sounds (PCP)

Vital signs
- Fever
- Increased respiratory rate

Complications
- Repeated overwhelming opportunistic infections of the respiratory and gastrointestinal (GI) tracts, central nervous system involvement, and KS
- Gingival erosion and loss of teeth from oral candidiasis
- Night blindness and loss of peripheral vision from CMV retinitis
- Anemia and neutropenia
- Dermatologic problems, such as folliculitis, molluscum contagiosum, and dermatitis
- Neuropathy
- Wasting syndrome
- Respiratory failure, typically related to PCP

Categories of HIV infection
Experts at the Centers for Disease Control and Prevention have identified three category systems of HIV infection based on clinical symptoms (A, B, and C) and three categories based on CD4+ cell count (1, 2, and 3).

Clinical symptoms
A = The patient is infected with HIV but has no symptoms other than those produced by the initial seroconversion. These flu-like symptoms and persistent generalized lymphadenopathy can last up to 3 months. Symptoms then resolve, and the infection becomes latent, sometimes for 10 years or more.

B = The patient has symptoms of impaired cell-mediated immunity but no AIDS indicator conditions. Symptoms can include weight loss, thrush, cervical dysplasia, fever, diarrhea lasting more than a month, peripheral neuropathy, and pelvic inflammatory disease.

C = The patient has one or more AIDS indicator conditions. AIDS indicator conditions are characterized by the development of tumors and opportunistic infections, such as PCP, cryptococcal meningitis, toxoplasmosis, cryptosporidiosis, herpes simplex infection, CMV, tuberculosis, HIV-related encephalopathy, *Mycobacterium avium* complex (MAC), KS, and non-Hodgkin's lymphoma.

CD4+ cell count categories
Normal CD4+ cell count is 800 to 1500/mm^3, depending on the laboratory values used.

1 = Greater than 500 mm^3
2 = 200 to 499/mm^3
3 = Less than 200 mm^3

Combining both systems, the CDC uses nine separate categories to further define the progression of the disease. Keep in mind that patients in categories A3, B3, and C1 to C3 are categorized as having AIDS. The categories are as follows:

Host sites for HIV infection

CD4+ Cell Count Categories	Clinical Categories		
	A	B	C
1	A1	B1	C1
2	A2	B2	C2
3	A3	B3	C3

continued

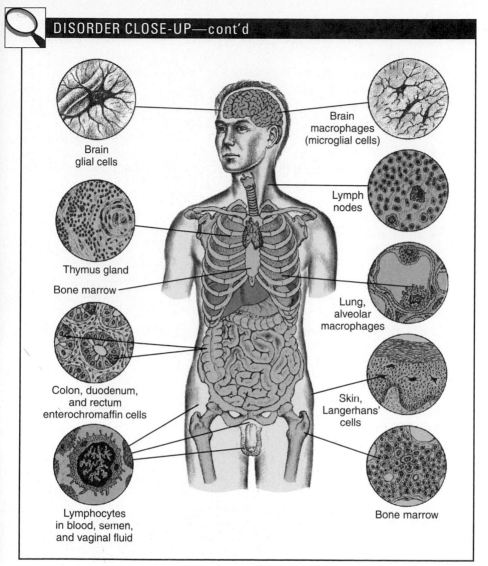

Brain
glial cells

Brain
macrophages
(microglial cells)

Lymph
nodes

Thymus gland

Bone marrow

Lung,
alveolar
macrophages

Colon, duodenum,
and rectum
enterochromaffin cells

Skin,
Langerhans'
cells

Lymphocytes
in blood, semen,
and vaginal fluid

Bone marrow

From McCance K, Huether S: *Pathophysiology: the biologic basis for disease of adults & children*, ed 5, St Louis, 2006, Mosby.

- *Crohn's disease.* This condition is characterized by diarrhea accompanied by colicky abdominal pain in the right lower quadrant, cramping, tenderness, flatulence, and fever.
- *Fecal impaction.* Diarrhea may result from liquid stool being forced around a fecal blockage. The patient may have high-pitched, tinkling bowel sounds and a distended abdomen.
- *Partial or early small bowel obstruction.* Diarrhea results from hypermotility of the intestinal tract as it attempts to move material past the obstruction.

FREQUENT URINATION

If the patient complains of urinary frequency, investigate further by asking the following questions:

- Have you recently increased the amount of fluid you drink?
- Have you been outside in the heat recently?
- How many cups of coffee or tea do you drink a day?
- Have you recently had an episode of vomiting, diarrhea, or nausea?
- Do you have diabetes? Does anyone in your immediate family have diabetes?
- Do you wake up in the night to urinate? Is that your usual pattern or something new?
- What medications do you take?
- Is your urine dark or light?
- What volume of urine do you pass each time?
- Do you have any pain during or after urination?

Focusing Your Assessment

When examining a patient who complains of frequent urination, focus your assessment as follows:

- Assess skin turgor. Dehydration may accompany urinary frequency caused by diabetes mellitus or diuretic use.
- Palpate the abdomen. Bladder distention may be present with urethral obstruction or urinary retention.
- Ask the patient to void in a specimen cup, and inspect the urine for color and odor. Cloudy or hazy urine or urine with a foul odor may indicate an infection of the urinary tract or prostate.
- For a male patient, perform a digital rectal examination and palpate the prostate. A tender, indurated, swollen, firm prostate is a sign of prostatitis.

Possible Causes

- *Urinary tract infection.* Infection increases urinary frequency and decreases the amount voided each time. Other symptoms include dysuria, cramps or spasm of the bladder, nocturia, and a feeling of warmth during urination. Urine typically will be cloudy or may have a foul odor. In older people, confusion may be the first sign of a urinary tract infection.
- *Urinary tract obstruction.* Obstruction increases urinary frequency and decreases the amount voided each time.
- *Prostatitis.* This condition causes frequent, urgent urination. Other symptoms include dysuria, nocturia, fever, chills, low-back pain, and myalgia.
- *Urinary retention with incomplete emptying of the bladder.* A high residual volume in the bladder does not require much extra volume to produce the urge to urinate.
- *Excessive fluid intake.* Consider diabetes in patients who have high fluid intake and complain of thirst.
- *Alcohol or caffeine consumption.* These substances may cause polyuria.
- *Diabetes mellitus.* Diabetes usually increases urine excretion. Glucose spilling into the urine acts as an osmotic diuretic.

- *Diabetes insipidus.* This form of diabetes results from inadequate antidiuretic hormone and can be caused by a neurologic disorder or a primary renal disorder.
- *Bladder calculi and bladder cancer.* Typically pain is experienced when the bladder is full, so the patient urinates more often to avoid the pain.

DIFFICULT OR PAINFUL URINATION

If the patient complains of difficult or painful urination (dysuria), investigate further by asking the following questions:
- Do you have difficulty starting the urine stream (hesitancy)?
- Do you have difficulty maintaining the urine stream?
- Does pain occur with urination or after urination?
- What is your normal daily fluid intake?

Focusing Your Assessment

When examining a patient who complains of difficult or painful urination, focus your assessment as follows:
- Ask the patient to void in a specimen cup, and inspect the urine. Cloudy, hazy, or foul-smelling urine is a sign of infection.
- Palpate the abdomen for bladder distention, a sign of urethral obstruction.
- For a male patient, perform a digital rectal examination and palpate the prostate. A tender, indurated, swollen, and firm prostate is a sign of prostatitis.

Possible Causes

- *Urinary tract infection.* Infection produces pain during urination. Other signs include fever, urinary frequency, and cloudy, hazy, or foul-smelling urine. In older adults, confusion (linked to the effects of infection) may be the first sign of a urinary tract infection.
- *Urethral obstruction.* Obstruction may cause pain during urination. The bladder may be distended.
- *Bladder calculi.* Pain occurs after urination because stones in the bladder cause pain when the bladder is empty. Causes of calculi include dehydration, infection, and urinary stasis.
- *Prostatitis.* This condition causes dysuria and urinary frequency and urgency. Other symptoms include fever, malaise, chills, low-back pain, and myalgia.
- *Benign prostatic hyperplasia.* Symptoms include urinary frequency and hesitancy with postvoid dribbling, a diminished force of urinary stream, urgency, dysuria, and nocturia. On palpation, the prostate gland feels symmetrically enlarged but smooth and somewhat rubbery.

LIFESPAN CONSIDERATIONS

Benign prostatic hyperplasia commonly begins after age 50, and nearly 80% of males have the disorder by age 80. This disorder occurs because of gradual, progressive enlargement of the prostate gland.

HEMATURIA

If the patient complains of frank blood in the urine or tea-colored urine, investigate further by asking the following questions:

- Does the blood appear at the beginning, at the end, or throughout urination?
- Have you noticed any new bruises or bleeding from your gums?
- What medications are you currently taking?
- Do you smoke cigarettes?
- What is your exercise pattern?
- Have you had any recent abdominal trauma?
- Have you had a recent infection or sore throat?

Focusing Your Assessment

When examining a patient who complains of hematuria, focus your assessment as follows:

- Assess the skin for signs of bruising or petechiae.
- Assess the abdominal wall for signs of recent trauma.
- Palpate the abdomen for an abdominal mass. Hematuria may be the first sign of renal cell carcinoma.

Possible Causes

- *Renal cell carcinoma.* This condition accounts for 85% of all renal tumors. Your patient also may complain of colicky abdominal pain and have a palpable abdominal mass. Smoking increases the risk of renal cell carcinoma.
- *Trauma or injury to the kidneys.* Hematuria caused by bleeding from the kidneys is continuous during urination.
- *Thrombocytopenia.* Low platelet counts can cause bleeding from the kidney, bladder, or urethra. Bleeding usually is continuous during urination.
- *Bladder infection.* Infection can cause irritation and bleeding of the bladder wall. Bleeding occurs at the end of urination. Caffeine intake can contribute to bladder irritation.
- *Renal calculi.* Calculi cause bleeding by irritating the urethral wall. Bleeding usually occurs at the beginning of urination.
- *Glomerulonephritis.* Bleeding from glomerular damage usually is continuous during urination. A history of streptococcal infection or sore throat is usual.
- *Anticoagulation medications.* These medications can cause spontaneous bleeding in the urinary tract. However, many patients also have an underlying urinary problem.
- *Smoking.* Smoking may cause hematuria without any underlying pathologic condition.
- *Strenuous exercise.* Vigorous exercise may cause hematuria for unknown reasons.

ABNORMAL MENSES

If a female patient has irregular menses, dysmenorrhea (painful menstruation), menorrhagia (profuse menstruation), metrorrhagia (intermenstrual bleeding),

or amenorrhea (absence of menstruation), investigate further by asking the following questions:
- At what age did you begin your menstrual cycles?
- How often do you menstruate?
- Are your menstrual cycles regular?
- How many days does your menses usually last?
- How would you characterize your flow?
- Do you have pain at any time during your cycle? If so, when do you have it?
- What was the first day of your last cycle?
- Do you have any trouble tolerating heat or cold?
- Do you have any trouble sleeping?
- Have you gained or lost weight recently?
- Do you exercise excessively?
- Have you noticed any change in your sexual habits?

Focusing Your Assessment
When examining a patient who complains of abnormal menses, focus your assessment as follows:
- Assess your patient for abdominal pain. The pain of dysmenorrhea is sharp, intermittent, and cramping. It occurs in the lower abdomen and radiates to the back, thighs, groin, and vulva. The pain of endometriosis is constant. It usually begins 5 to 7 days before menses peaks and lasts for 2 to 3 days. Ectopic pregnancy is associated with sharp, lower abdominal pain that radiates to the shoulders and neck.
- Assess the skin for thinness, dryness, or flakiness (a sign of hypothyroidism).
- Palpate the neck for an enlarged thyroid gland (a sign of hyperthyroidism).

Possible Causes
- *Premenstrual syndrome.* For most patients, dysmenorrhea begins just before the menstrual flow and peaks within 24 hours. Other symptoms include urinary frequency, nausea, vomiting, diarrhea, headache, chills, abdominal bloating, painful breasts, and irritability.
- *Hypothyroidism.* This condition is associated with menorrhagia and amenorrhea. Symptoms include fatigue, cold sensitivity, weight gain, constipation, dry or flaky skin, a puffy face, and hoarseness.
- *Endometriosis.* Associated with menorrhagia and metrorrhagia, this condition produces constant pain in the lower abdomen.
- *Threatened abortion.* Your patient may experience a pink or scant brown discharge for several weeks before the onset of cramps and increased vaginal bleeding, signaling an abortion.
- *Ectopic pregnancy.* This condition is associated with amenorrhea or abnormal menstruation. Early symptoms mimic those of intrauterine pregnancy. As the pregnancy progresses, abdominal pain develops.
- *Neoplasms.* Tumors involving the uterus, cervix, or ovaries can cause abnormal menstruation.

- *Pelvic inflammatory disease.* This condition is characterized by bleeding between periods and a purulent vaginal discharge accompanied by abdominal pain, malaise, and fever.
- *Hypopituitarism.* This abnormality is associated with amenorrhea, lethargy, cold intolerance, anorexia, and abdominal pain.
- *Hyperthyroidism.* In addition to amenorrhea, this condition can cause an enlarged thyroid, nervousness, heat intolerance, weight loss with increased appetite, sweating, and diarrhea.
- *Anorexia nervosa.* Symptoms include amenorrhea, fear of being fat, anger, ritualistic behavior, loss of libido, fatigue, sleep alterations, and cold intolerance.
- *Female athletic triad.* If a young female athlete frequently misses a menstrual period or stops menstruating altogether, consider this condition. In addition to menstrual irregularities, the condition is also marked by abnormal eating habits, such as crash dieting, and excessive exercise. The patient may also develop osteoporosis.

PENILE OR VAGINAL DISCHARGE OR LESIONS

If the patient complains of a discharge from the penis or vagina, investigate by asking the following questions:

- What color is the discharge?
- Does the discharge have any odor?
- Do you have any pain or burning with urination?
- Do you (female patient) use vaginal spermicides or douches with intercourse?
- Do you (female patient) use birth control pills?
- Have you recently taken antibiotic agents?
- Do you wear tight underwear, or have you recently spent time in a wet bathing suit?
- Do your genitals itch or burn?
- Do you use douches, feminine hygiene sprays, bubble baths, talcum powder, or scented toilet paper?

Focusing your assessment

When examining a patient who complains of penile or vaginal discharge or lesions, focus your assessment as follows:

- Inspect the genital area for any open sores or other lesions. Syphilis produces an open chancre (a small, fluid-filled lesion).
- Inspect the genital area for redness or swelling, signs of gonorrhea.
- Check vital signs. Pelvic inflammatory disease typically causes fever.
- Inspect the genital area for the discharge. The color and consistency of the discharge provide clues to the causative organism (see ▨ *Assessing Vaginal Discharge*).
- Palpate the inguinal lymph nodes. Inflamed nodes are found with genital herpes.

INTERPRETING ABNORMAL FINDINGS

ASSESSING VAGINAL DISCHARGE

Does your patient have abnormal vaginal discharge? If so, the character and consistency of the discharge can give you clues to your patient's problem. Use this table to help guide your differential diagnosis.

Discharge Characteristics	Other Symptoms	Probable Causes
• White and thick, resembling cottage cheese • Odorless	• Severe itching • Dyspareunia • Patches on vaginal walls • Inflamed vaginal walls	• *Candida albicans* infection
• Gray-white color • Scant amount • Fishy or foul odor	• Itching • Normal mucosa	• *Gardnerella vaginalis* infection
• Green, yellow, or white • May be frothy • Foul smell	• Burning and itching • Dyspareunia • Strawberry spots on cervix	• *Trichomonas vaginalis* infection
• White or pink • Scant amount • Odorless	• Itching • Dyspareunia • Pale, thin, dry mucosa	• Atrophic vaginitis

Possible Causes
- *Syphilis.* Chancres develop on the genitalia and anus. The lesions are painless and have indurated, raised edges and clear bases. They usually disappear in 3 to 6 weeks.
- *Gonorrhea.* Purulent discharge from the penis or vagina is accompanied by dysuria. Redness or swelling may develop at the site of the infection. Your patient may complain of urinary frequency and incontinence. If the vulva is infected, the female patient will complain of burning and pain with occasional itching.
- *Chlamydia.* Mucopurulent discharge occurs with painful urination. Other symptoms include burning on urination and urinary frequency.
- *Genital herpes.* Fluid-filled vesicles with yellow, oozing centers, indicate this infection. Other symptoms include prodromal itching, tingling, redness, and pain at the site of the lesions, as well as tender inguinal lymph nodes.
- *Pelvic inflammatory disease.* Mucopurulent discharge occurs with severe abdominal pain and fever.
- *Urethritis.* This is an infection or inflammation of the urethra. Chemicals from vaginal spermicides or douches can cause urethritis in the female patient. Sexually transmitted diseases, such as gonorrhea and chlamydia, are other causes.
- *Vaginitis.* This inflammation of the vagina causes burning and itching of the labia and vulva. Overgrowth of *Candida albicans, Gardnerella vaginalis,* or *Trichomonas vaginalis* is commonly the cause. Use of antibiotics can cause an imbalance of vaginal microorganisms, allowing one to proliferate. Use of vaginal spermicides or douches can change the vaginal lining, allowing

bacterial invasion. Wearing underwear with a nylon crotch or wearing a wet bathing suit can create a moist, warm environment favorable for bacteria. Use of talcum powder, bubble baths, feminine hygiene sprays, or scented toilet paper can irritate the vaginal lining. Noninfectious vaginitis from chemical irritation has no discharge but does have intense itching and irritation.

ERECTILE DYSFUNCTION

If a male patient complains of erectile dysfunction, investigate further by asking the following questions:

- Are you experiencing stress in your job?
- Are you experiencing stress in any of your relationships?
- Are you afraid of having a heart attack during intercourse?
- How much alcohol do you consume?
- What medications or recreational drugs do you take?

Focusing Your Assessment

When examining a patient who complains of erectile dysfunction, focus your assessment as follows:

- Check for signs of decreased testosterone, including general muscle weakness, shrinkage of the testicles, softening of the testicular tissues, and decreased amounts of pubic, chest, and axillary hair.

Possible Causes

- *Stress.* A leading cause of erectile dysfunction, stress, can arise in the workplace, community, or family. Erectile dysfunction caused by stress is usually situational and temporary.
- *Psychogenic factors.* Along with stress, psychogenic factors include fear of intimacy, feelings of inadequacy, previous trauma, and lack of communication.
- *Alcohol use.* Excessive use can cause erectile dysfunction.
- *Medications.* Beta-blockers and steroids commonly cause erectile dysfunction. It usually resolves with discontinuation of the medication.
- *Decreased testosterone.* A result of hypopituitarism, decreased testosterone affects libido and causes erectile dysfunction.

RECTAL BLEEDING

If the patient complains of rectal bleeding, investigate further by asking the following questions:

- Is the blood a part of the stool, or does it appear on the toilet paper after the bowel movement?
- Do you have a strong urge to defecate in the morning?
- Do you have burning or itching in the anal area?
- Do you experience dizziness?
- Do you ever feel that you are not able to empty your rectum when defecating?
- Do you engage in anal intercourse?

Focusing Your Assessment

When examining a patient who complains of rectal bleeding, focus your assessment as follows:

- Inspect the anus for hemorrhoids, rectal prolapse, fissures, or drainage. Drainage may indicate an anorectal abscess.
- If possible, perform a digital rectal examination, and look for any acute bleeding or rectal polyps. Test any stool for occult blood. Positive stool findings may indicate colorectal cancer or high internal hemorrhoids.

Possible Causes

- *Hemorrhoids.* These structures cause intermittent bleeding with defecation. Bleeding from first-degree hemorrhoids appears on stool or toilet paper. Prolapsed, second-degree hemorrhoids usually return to the anal canal spontaneously after defecation. Third-degree hemorrhoids cause constant discomfort and prolapse in response to any increase in intraabdominal pressure.
- *Rectal prolapse.* This condition is characterized by bloody diarrhea and abdominal pain. Other symptoms include a persistent sensation of rectal fullness.
- *Anorectal abscesses or fissures.* Abscesses and fissures result from abrasions or tears in the lining of the anal canal and subsequent *Escherichia coli* infection. Abrasions may result from treatment of internal hemorrhoids, enema tips, puncture wounds from ingested eggshells or fish bones, anal sex, or insertion of foreign objects.
- *Lower GI bleeding.* This condition is characterized by blood in the stool. Frank blood indicates a lower GI source of bleeding. Black, tarry, guaiac-positive stools indicate a source of bleeding higher in the intestinal tract.
- *Anorectal stricture.* Excessive straining and the inability to completely evacuate the bowel characterize this condition. Pain, bleeding, and pruritus ani are other signs. Scarring after surgery, inflammation, or laxative abuse may cause anorectal strictures.
- *Rectal polyps.* Polyps high in the rectum leave a streak of blood on the stool. Low rectal polyps bleed freely.
- *Colorectal cancer.* Symptoms include the urgent need to defecate on arising and blood or mucus in the stool.

CHAPTER 9

Examining the Lower Extremities

The hips, legs, and feet function as a weight-bearing team to support ambulation and other body movements. When problems develop in the lower extremities, they can cause pain and discomfort, as well as disrupt the patient's ability to move at will. A variety of debilitating conditions can affect the lower extremities. These include arthritis, gout, thrombophlebitis, and chronic venous insufficiency. Therefore a skilled, thorough examination of the lower extremities based on an understanding of their anatomy is essential, especially if your patient has specific complaints involving them (see ▶ *Structures of the Lower Extremities*).

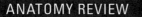

ANATOMY REVIEW

STRUCTURES OF THE LOWER EXTREMITIES

Skeletal Sctructure

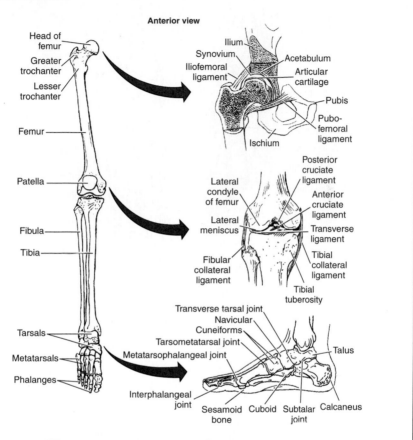

Anterior view

continued

ANATOMY REVIEW—cont'd

Muscles

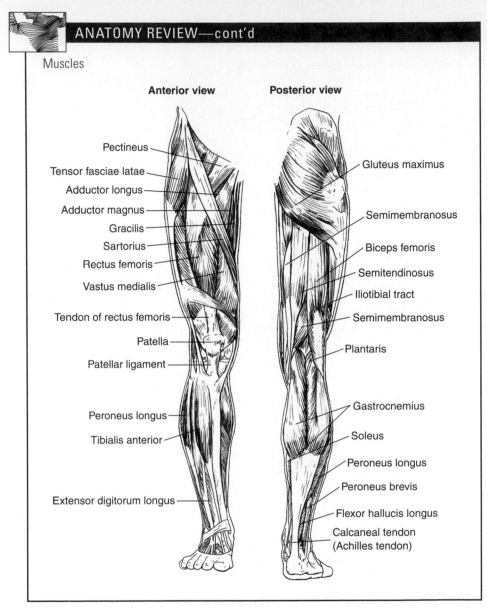

Anterior view

Pectineus
Tensor fasciae latae
Adductor longus
Adductor magnus
Gracilis
Sartorius
Rectus femoris
Vastus medialis
Tendon of rectus femoris
Patella
Patellar ligament
Peroneus longus
Tibialis anterior
Extensor digitorum longus

Posterior view

Gluteus maximus
Semimembranosus
Biceps femoris
Semitendinosus
Iliotibial tract
Semimembranosus
Plantaris
Gastrocnemius
Soleus
Peroneus longus
Peroneus brevis
Flexor hallucis longus
Calcaneal tendon
(Achilles tendon)

From Thibodeau G, Patton K: *Anatomy and physiology,* ed 5, St Louis, 2003, Mosby.

ANATOMY REVIEW—cont'd

Blood vessels

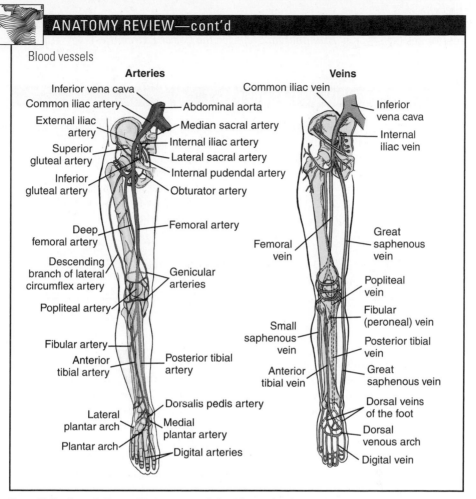

From Thibodeau G, Patton K: *Anatomy and physiology,* ed 5, St Louis, 2003, Mosby.

EXAMINATION STEPS AND FINDINGS

As always, review your patient's health history before beginning your examination. Note any important details in the history, and adjust your examination accordingly. For example, if your patient has had a recent hip replacement, you may need to alter some aspects of the typical lower extremity examination to avoid causing your patient discomfort.

Examining the lower extremities starts with the proper tools. Before starting your examination, gather the following equipment: tape measure, skin-marking pen, reflex hammer, cotton-tipped swab, and tuning fork.

For the lower extremities, you will rely primarily on inspection and palpation when conducting your examination. These two skills, typically used together for greater efficiency, also play a part in further testing for range of motion (ROM), muscle strength, deep tendon reflexes (DTRs), and sensory responses (see ▩ *Key Examination Steps for the Lower Extremities*).

EXPERT EXAMINATION CHECKLIST

KEY EXAMINATION STEPS FOR THE LOWER EXTREMITIES

Use this checklist to make sure you cover the most important steps when examining the lower extremities.

❏ Note their color.
❏ Look for any abnormalities.
❏ Feel skin temperature.

❏ Palpate femoral, popliteal, posterior tibial, and pedal pulses.
❏ Test joints and muscles for range of motion (ROM) and strength.
❏ Test deep tendon reflexes (DTRs) and sensory pathways for pain, touch, vibration, and position sense.

---

evolve Find PDF and PDA-downloadable versions of this Expert Exam Checklist online at http://evolve.elsevier.com/Mosby/expertexam/.

INSPECTION

Begin your examination by assessing skin color and integrity. Remember, whether your patient is standing, sitting, or lying down, inspection always depends on good lighting. Note any discoloration, such as erythema, jaundice, or ecchymoses. When assessing skin integrity, note any changes, such as rashes, abrasions, lacerations, ulcers, or hematomas. Check the toenails for color, shape, and thickness. Also look at hair distribution and quantity.

Now inspect the size and symmetry of your patient's legs, joints, and muscle groups. Look at the anterior and posterior aspects of the patient's legs in the standing position. Are the legs of equal length? Is the pelvis level? Do you see any muscle asymmetry or atrophy? Be sure to inspect each joint for erythema, swelling, and deformity. Remember to compare your findings bilaterally, especially if you think you have detected something abnormal.

With the patient still in the standing position, check the legs for varicosities or edema. The standing position accentuates varicosities not visible when your patient is lying down. One way to detect unilateral edema is by measuring the circumference of both legs and comparing your measurements. For example, you could measure both legs just above the ankle, at the widest circumference of the calf, and at midthigh for comparison.

NORMAL FINDINGS

- Skin color ranging from dark brown to light tan, with pink or yellow overtones (Skin color may be darker around the knees. Calloused areas on the feet may appear slightly yellow.)
- No obvious gross deformity

- Leg hair distributed evenly (Older patients may have normal variations, including skin that is thinner and drier, leg hair that is scarcer, and pigmentation that is somewhat altered.)
- Toenails equal in thickness (In older people, the nails thicken and are typically yellow.)
- Legs with no varicosities or only superficial varicosities (These are especially likely in patients who are now or were at one time overweight or pregnant.)
- No swelling or edema

ABNORMAL FINDINGS

- Brownish skin coloring and thickened skin, as with lymphedema and advanced venous insufficiency (You may also see brown discoloration around the ankles, with thickened skin and narrowed leg muscles as scarring develops. Skin temperature and pulses will be normal, but pulses will be difficult to palpate through the edema. Usually, the patient complains of little pain or aching pain when the legs are in a dependent position.)
- Skin ulcers, possibly indicating trauma, chronic arterial insufficiency, or chronic venous insufficiency (Ulcers develop most often on the toes or feet, but they may form on the shin or other areas of the lower leg after trauma. You may see gangrene if the patient's ulcers result from chronic arterial insufficiency. If you see scars above the patient's ankle from previous leg ulcers, the patient probably has chronic venous insufficiency [see Q *Chronic Venous Insufficiency*].)

DISORDER CLOSE-UP

CHRONIC VENOUS INSUFFICIENCY

Chronic venous insufficiency refers to stasis of blood in the lower extremities and resulting chronic lower leg edema. Over time the patient also develops dermatologic changes in the lower leg and foot from prolonged interruption in venous circulation.

These changes typically stem from thrombophlebitis and valvular incompetence. Many patients with chronic venous insufficiency also have varicose veins or tumorous obstructions in the pelvic veins.

When venous valves become incompetent, blood cannot progress efficiently from the legs back to the heart. Instead, it collects and stagnates in the lower legs. This increased collection of blood causes venous pressures to rise, distending the thin-walled veins. Unable to close completely, the incompetent veins allow blood to backflow. Over time the veins become weak, overstretched, and chronically distended from the excessive pressure.

As congestion increases in the lower extremities, peripheral circulation continues to slow down, thus interfering with the body's ability to provide sufficient oxygen and nutrients to the cells. Eventually cells begin to die. The result is formation of a venous stasis ulcer. Because impaired circulation prevents the body from sending extra nutrients and oxygen to the site to heal the ulcer, it tends to heal very slowly. In fact, it may enlarge and become chronic. Venous congestion also interferes with the normal inflammatory response, predisposing the patient to infection.

continued

DISORDER CLOSE-UP—cont'd

Characteristic findings
Expect health history information and physical examination findings to vary among patients with chronic venous insufficiency, depending on the extent and severity of the disease. The information that follows will help you distinguish between expected and unexpected findings.

Health history
• History of varicose veins
• History of deep vein thrombosis (DVT)
• Complaints of ankle swelling, legs feeling heavy
• Skin discoloration around the ankle
• Sore on the lower extremity that heals slowly

Inspection
• Prominent leg veins, possibly with ropelike and dilated appearance or purplish and spiderlike appearance
• Lower leg edema, possibly extending to the knee of the affected extremity
• Ulcer over the ankle, usually the medial aspect
• Shiny, atrophic, and cyanotic areas around the ulcer
• Brownish skin pigmentation
• Area easily traumatized
• Eczema or stasis dermatitis

Palpation
• Hard subcutaneous tissues
• Pitting edema of lower extremity
• Affected leg area hard and leathery to touch

Vital signs
• Fever, if ulcer is infected

Complications
• Wound infection
• Chronic stasis ulcers
• Amputation

• Skin color normal but cyanotic when the patient stands or sits
• Edema, possibly resulting from injury; inflammation, as seen with cellulitis; venous obstruction, as seen with thrombosis or thrombophlebitis; varicosities; congestive heart failure; or other conditions (Be sure to note whether the edema involves one or both legs.)
• Joint swelling, possibly resulting from gout, rheumatoid arthritis, or injury

PALPATION

This phase of the examination involves palpating the joints, bones, and surrounding muscles for tenderness, deformity, or crepitus. Have the patient lie supine, and start by palpating the hip joint. It is easily palpable by finding the major landmarks of the iliac crest and the greater trochanter of the femur. Then, with one hand on each lateral aspect of the iliac crest, gently rock the pelvis, testing for instability or tenderness.

After palpating the hips, move down to the knees. With your patient in either a sitting or supine position on the examination table, feel the major landmarks of each knee: tibial tuberosity, medial and lateral epicondyles, medial and lateral condyles, the adductor tubercle of the femur, and the patella. Also palpate the popliteal space and the tibiofemoral joint space. Palpation should be performed with the knee flexed and then extended.

While palpating, be sure to notice the temperature of the patient's legs, especially the feet. If they are cool, the patient could have a vascular problem; if they are warm, the patient could have an inflammatory problem.

Now palpate the major landmarks of each ankle, including the medial and lateral malleolus and Achilles tendon. Examine the metatarsal bones by compressing the forefoot between your thumb and forefingers, exerting pressure near the heads of the first and fifth metatarsals. Palpate each metatarsophalangeal joint individually by gently compressing it between your thumb and index finger.

If you noticed during inspection that your patient has dependent edema, be sure to palpate for pitting edema. Do so by pressing your thumb into the skin of the patient's lower leg for about 5 seconds. If the skin remains depressed after you remove your thumb, the patient has pitting edema.

If your patient has pitting edema, you can describe it in one of two ways. The first is to document it as *slight, moderate,* or *marked edema.* The second is to use a scale from +1 to +4. In this system, +1 signifies slight pitting edema of the foot or leg, +4 signifies deep pitting with loss of normal foot and leg contours, and +2 and +3 signify conditions in between.

Arterial Pulses

An important part of your assessment of the lower extremities, palpation of arterial pulses gives you information about the patient's vascular system. Comparing one side to the other, you will palpate the femoral, popliteal, posterior tibial, and pedal pulses. If necessary, you will also auscultate for abnormal vascular sounds or bruits (see ▧ *Palpating Difficult Pulses*).

EXAMINATION TIP

PALPATING DIFFICULT PULSES

If your patient has weak arterial pulses or is obese, you may have difficulty feeling the pulse. For the best results when palpating difficult arterial pulses, follow these examination tips.

- When checking each pulse site, make sure you and your patient are in a comfortable position. An awkward position may interfere with your tactile sensitivity.

continued

EXAMINATION TIP—cont'd

- Use the distal pads of your index and middle fingers, and apply firm pressure. Your fingertips are the most sensitive part of your hand for palpating pulses.
- To help find the pulse in a patient's leg, support and relax any nearby joint with your free hand while palpating with your examining hand. If you cannot find the pulse, move your fingers in and around the area, varying the pressure you exert with your finger pads.
- Once you locate the pulse, mark the spot with a felt-tipped pen so that you can find it easily the next time.
- Make sure you do not confuse your patient's pulse with your own pulsating finger pads. To make sure, palpate your own carotid pulse to determine your heart rate, and then compare it to your patient's. Usually the heart rates differ. Do not palpate with your thumb because it has strong pulsations easily confused with your patient's.
- Do not press too hard because you could occlude the artery and stop the pulse you are trying to find.
- If you are having difficulty palpating the femoral pulse in an obese patient, apply more pressure to feel through adipose tissue. Use both hands, placing one on top of the other, and apply downward pressure on the hand on the bottom.

When checking pulse points, keep in mind that an occlusion can affect any artery. The two most common causes of arterial occlusion are embolism (from the heart, aorta, or large arteries) and thrombus formation (from atherosclerosis or trauma). A diminished or absent peripheral pulse may indicate a partial or complete obstruction proximally. Typically, all pulses distal to the occlusion are affected.

To palpate the femoral pulse, place your patient in a supine position. Palpate in the groin crease halfway between the symphysis pubis and the anterior-superior (AS) iliac spine. After palpating each femoral pulse, gently place the bell of the stethoscope over the area just examined and listen for any abnormal vascular sounds.

To palpate the popliteal pulse, flex your patient's knee so the foot rests on the examination table. Place one hand on each side of the knee, with your thumbs near the front of the patella. Curl your fingers around the knee, and rest your fingertips in the popliteal fossa. Now gently press your fingers deep into the popliteal fossa. The pulse may be difficult to feel. If it is, then try straightening the patient's leg slightly to make the pulse more accessible.

To palpate the posterior tibial pulse, place your fingertips in the groove between the medial malleolus and the Achilles tendon, and feel for the pulse. Sometimes, passive dorsiflexion of the foot will make this pulse easier to palpate.

To palpate the dorsalis pedis pulse, place your fingers between the patient's great and first toes, and slowly move away from the toes between the extensor tendons until you feel the pulse. Plantar flexing the foot slightly makes the pedal pulse easier to palpate. Keep in mind that, in some patients, the pedal pulse may be congenitally absent or branch high up in the ankle.

Lymph Nodes

When assessing your patient's lower extremities, do not forget to palpate the superficial lymph nodes. They will give you important information about immune system activity in the area, such as the presence of a recent or active infection.

If you did not palpate the inguinal lymph nodes as part of the abdominal examination, you can easily do so now. You should be able to palpate horizontal and vertical chains of inguinal nodes in most patients. To palpate them, first locate the femoral pulse. Then gently press in that area to palpate the nodes. You may even be able to palpate popliteal nodes with the knee slightly flexed. Note the size, consistency, mobility, and any signs of tenderness of all nodes.

NORMAL FINDINGS

- No obvious deformity, tenderness, or swelling
- Extremities, especially feet, cool to warm with touch
- Extremities the same temperature bilaterally
- Skin texture smooth, with minimal moisture
- No edema or varicose veins
- Pulses equal and strong bilaterally
- Superficial inguinal nodes palpable at times but not tender

ABNORMAL FINDINGS

- Diminished or absent pulses, indicating a partial or complete arterial occlusion (All pulses distal to the occlusion are affected.)
- A decreased or absent femoral pulse, suggesting a pathologic condition of the aorta (A widened, exaggerated femoral pulse suggests a femoral aneurysm. If pulses are diminished, listen for a bruit to detect arterial narrowing. Remember that pedal pulses may be congenitally absent. However, if your patient has always had pedal pulses and now they are absent or diminished, consider arterial occlusive disease if popliteal and femoral pulses are normal. Sudden arterial occlusion causes intense leg pain distal to the occlusion, often with numbness and tingling. The limb becomes cold, pale, and pulseless.)
- Cold feet (especially unilateral), suggesting arterial insufficiency (Usually the foot is pale, especially on elevation, and dusky red after standing or sitting. Skin changes also occur with arterial insufficiency. The skin becomes shiny and thin. Hair becomes thin, and toenails thicken. Usually, the patient has no edema, and pulses are diminished or absent. The patient complains of intermittent calf pain that, if untreated, eventually progresses to pain at rest.)

Testing Range of Motion

Before testing ROM, be sure you are thoroughly familiar with the muscle groups involved in the lower extremities. Then check the patient's history to be sure ROM testing is safe. Once you are sure it is, test each major joint and related muscle group for active and passive ROM.

Start with hip flexion. With the patient's knees extended, raise one leg upward. The hip should be able to flex up to 90 degrees. With the knee flexed, raise the leg toward the patient's chest. The hip should be able to flex to 120 degrees.

Now move on to hip extension. With the patient standing or prone, swing the straightened leg out behind the body. The hip should be able to extend up to 30 degrees.

To test hip abduction, place the patient in a supine position with knees extended. Now swing the leg laterally. It should move out to 45 degrees. Then test hip adduction by swinging the leg medially. It should move to about 30 degrees. Lift the leg slightly to allow full movement during this phase of the examination.

To test internal rotation, ask the patient to remain in the supine position and flex the knee. Hold the patient's ankle and gently rotate the leg inward toward the other. The hip should rotate internally up to 40 degrees. To check the external rotation, hold the same ankle and gently rotate the leg outward toward you. External hip rotation should be up to 45 degrees.

Now check ROM in the patient's knees, with the patient either lying down or sitting up. Test knee flexion by asking him to bend the knee; it should have 130-degree flexion. Test knee extension by asking the patient to straighten the leg and stretch it; it should have full extension and up to 15 degrees of hyperextension.

One additional step you may consider is the ballottement test, which you should perform if the patient has excessive fluid or an effusion in the knee. With the knee extended, apply downward pressure on the suprapatellar pouch with the thumb and fingers of one hand. Then sharply push the patella upward against the femur with the fingers of your other hand. Sudden release of pressure on the patella may cause a tapping sensation against your fingers. This tapping suggests fluid on the knee.

The bulge test also can help you determine if fluid is present. With the patient's knee extended, milk the medial aspect of the knee upward a few times. Then tap the lateral side of the knee; if the patient has excess fluid, this may create a bulge of fluid moving to the medial aspect of the knee.

Test flexion of the tibiotalar joint by instructing your patient to bend the foot downward, a procedure called *plantar flexion.* The patient should have 45 to 50 degrees of flexion. In addition, test hyperextension or dorsiflexion by instructing your patient to bend the foot upward. He should have 20 degrees of flexion.

Inversion is accomplished by asking your patient to point the toes and turn the foot inward. Asking your patient to point the foot outward is called *eversion.* Both should reach 25 degrees.

Flexing and extending each toe assesses the ROM in that joint. Normally, both flexion and extension will reach 40 degrees.

NORMAL FINDINGS
- Joints with full ROM without pain
- Joints with equal ROM bilaterally

ABNORMAL FINDINGS
- Limited ROM, possibly resulting from swelling or pain caused by injury, a flare-up of gout, or arthritis

Testing Muscle Strength

When testing muscle strength, remember that strength varies normally with the patient's age, sex, and physical condition. Also remember that the dominant side typically is stronger than the nondominant side.

Test muscle strength by asking your patient to move actively against your resistance. Then issue a grade based on the 0 to 5 muscle strength rating system as follows:

0 Flaccid
1 Trace (slight contractility but no movement)
2 Weak (movement possible when gravity is eliminated)
3 Fair (movement against gravity but not against resistance)
4 Good (movement against gravity, with some resistance)
5 Normal (movement against gravity and resistance)

Tests to judge the strength of your patient's muscles include flexion, extension, adduction, and abduction. You will also perform the Thomas test.

Hip flexion assesses the iliopsoas muscle. Have the patient lie supine. Place your hand on your patient's anterior thigh, and ask him to raise the leg against your resisting hand.

Hip extension tests the gluteus maximus muscle. With your patient in the supine position, place your hand on the posterior thigh, and ask him to push the leg down against your hand as you offer resistance.

Next, test the adductor muscles. Place your hands between your patient's knees, and ask him to press the legs together as your hands offer resistance.

Now test abduction, which allows you to evaluate the gluteus medius and minimus. Place your hands on the outside of your patient's knees, and ask him to spread the legs against your resistance.

Finally, perform the Thomas test to assess for flexion contracture of the hip. With your patient in a supine position, ask him to fully extend one leg flat on the examination table while flexing the other leg so that the knee touches the chest. With a hip contracture, the extended leg will lift off the table.

Knee flexion helps you evaluate the hamstrings. With the patient's leg partially flexed, rest your hand on the knee and the other behind the lower leg. With your patient's foot planted on the bed, try to straighten the leg, pushing it down toward the examination table while the patient resists.

Knee extension tests the quadriceps. With the knee in partial flexion, place one hand behind the knee and the other on the anterior lower leg. Then, ask your patient to try to straighten the leg against your hands.

Plantar flexion and dorsiflexion assess the strength of the foot and ankle muscles. To assess plantar flexion, ask your patient to extend the foot against your hand; for dorsiflexion, ask your patient to pull the foot up against your hand.

NORMAL FINDINGS

- Legs symmetrical in length, circumference, and alignment
- Muscles symmetrical in size bilaterally
- Muscles with firm tone

ABNORMAL FINDINGS

- Muscle strength graded below 5 (Older patients may lose muscle bulk, but those muscles should retain strength. Older patients also may have a slight change in ROM, usually because of osteoarthritis.)

Testing Deep Tendon Reflexes

DTRs, also called *stretch reflexes,* depend on intact sensory and motor nerves, muscle fibers, and an intact spinal cord at the level of the reflex. You will use a reflex hammer to examine DTRs.

Have your patient sit on the side of the bed or on a chair with the legs dangling. If your patient cannot sit up, then he may remain supine, but you will need to raise and support the extremity you are testing with your hand to gently stretch the tendon (see 📷 *Testing Reflexes in the Lower Extremities*).

EXAMINATION TIP

TESTING REFLEXES IN THE LOWER EXTREMITIES

Here is how to accurately and thoroughly test deep tendon reflexes (DTRs) in the lower extremities.

Knee Reflex

To test the patellar tendon, which is mediated by the spinal cord at the level of L2, L3, and L4, flex the knee to 90 degrees. If your patient is sitting, make sure the upper leg is not resting against the edge of the examination table. Palpate the patellar tendon just below the patella. Then tap the pointed end of a reflex hammer briskly on the tendon, using a quick wrist motion. The normal response is contraction of the quadriceps muscles with knee extension.

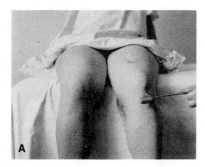

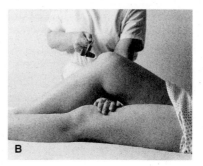

Testing the knee reflex in a patient sitting up.   Testing the knee reflex in a patient lying down.

Ankle Reflex

The Achilles reflex is mediated at spinal cord segments S1 and S2. It is usually tested with the foot slightly dorsiflexed and your patient in the sitting position. Alternatively, if your patient is supine, flex the leg at the hip and knee and rotate it externally, placing the foot on its side, resting on the shin of the opposite leg. Strike the Achilles tendon with the pointed end of the reflex hammer. The normal response is plantar flexion of the foot.

continued

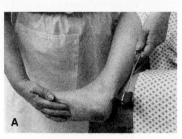

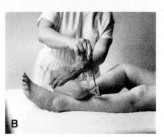

Testing the Achilles reflex in a patient sitting up.   Testing the Achilles reflex in a patient lying down.

Plantar Response

The plantar response, often called *Babinski's response,* is a superficial reflex mediated by spinal cord segments L5 and S1. Using the handle end of the reflex hammer, stroke the lateral aspect of the sole, from the heel to the ball of the foot. The toes should flex inward and downward. If you see dorsiflexion of the great toe, possibly accompanied by fanning of the other toes, Babinski's response may be present. This indicates an abnormality in the pyramidal tract in an adult but is a normal finding in a newborn. Because this finding sometimes is normal, document it by writing *"Babinski present,"* rather than using "negative" or "positive."

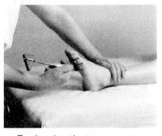

Testing the plantar response.

Ankle Clonus

Test ankle clonus if the other reflexes seem hyperactive. Supporting the knee in a slightly flexed position, plantar flex and dorsiflex the foot several times with your other hand. Then sharply dorsiflex the foot, maintaining that position. Look and feel for rhythmic oscillations. Normally, a few clonic oscillations may be seen and felt. But sustained clonus, where the foot plantar flexes and dorsiflexes in rapid succession, indicates upper motor neuron disease.

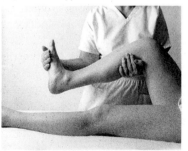

Testing for ankle clonus.

When performing these tests, keep in mind that the reflex action may be inhibited if the patient is not relaxed. Promote relaxation by having the patient focus on another task. For example, have him lock the fingers together and pull one hand against the other when you tap the patellar tendon.

For each reflex you test, compare sides and assign a grade on the following DTR scale:

   0 No response
   + Sluggish or diminished response
   ++ Normal (active or expected response)
  +++ More brisk than expected (slightly hyperactive but could be considered normal)
 ++++ Very brisk (hyperactive with clonus)

NORMAL FINDINGS

- Patellar, Achilles, and plantar (Babinski) reflexes equal bilaterally (Patellar testing causes extension of the lower leg. Achilles testing causes plantar flexion of the foot. Plantar testing causes the toes to flex or curl down.)
- A DTR rating (++) that indicates normal reflex responses (Normal variations in the older patient include diminished or absent ankle reflexes. All the reflexes may be slower.)

ABNORMAL FINDINGS

- Diminished DTRs and muscle weakness, possibly suggesting such lower motor neuron disorders as amyotrophic lateral sclerosis (ALS) or Guillain-Barré syndrome (Loss of muscle tone and sometimes muscle atrophy will occur.)
- Muscle spasticity and hyperactive reflexes, resulting from such upper motor neuron disorders as stroke and paralysis, if the disorder is extensive enough (Usually you will find little or no muscle atrophy, but muscle strength may be decreased.)

Sensory Testing

Sensory testing evaluates the integrity of sensory pathways in the spinal cord and brain responsible for such sensations as light touch, pain, temperature, position, and vibration. Sensory testing is especially important for patients who complain of numbness or tingling. Check a dermatome chart to determine the approximate areas innervated by the sensory portion of each spinal nerve.

When a patient complains of sensory changes, you can determine which spinal nerve might be involved by comparing the reactions to sensory testing in each of the extremities.

To test for light touch, use a wisp of cotton. Ask your patient to close the eyes and tell you when he feels your touch. Lightly touch the cotton to the feet, calves, and thighs, both medially and laterally. Proceed systematically, comparing sides and moving distally to proximally.

To test pain sensation, poke your patient lightly with a sharp object, such as the stick end of a cotton-tipped swab or the end of an unbent paper clip. Take care not to break the skin. Be sure to apply the same amount of pressure to each site while you compare pain sensations. If you believe the patient may have peripheral neuropathy, or if your patient is known to have diabetes mellitus, test for sensory loss in the feet using a monofilament device (see ▣ *Using a Monofilament Device to Test for Sensory Loss*).

EXAMINATION TIP

USING A MONOFILAMENT DEVICE TO TEST FOR SENSORY LOSS

To test for sensory loss with the monofilament device, follow these key steps. If your patient cannot feel the end of the device in any one spot, consider sensory loss. As you proceed with the examination, remember to avoid areas that have broken skin or calluses.

- Have your patient close the eyes during the entire examination.
- Place the device in the spots shown in the illustrations. Make sure to use the device on both the dorsal and the plantar surfaces of the foot.
- Apply enough pressure to make the filament bend, and keep it there for 1.5 seconds.
- Use a random pattern, and avoid touching a spot more than once.

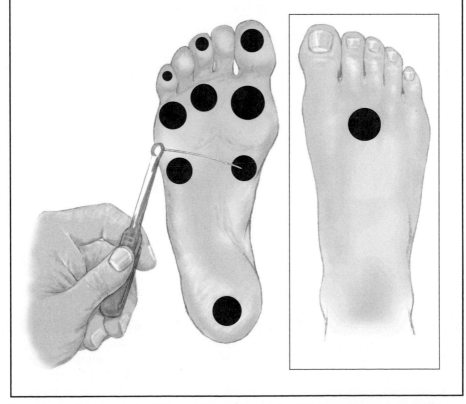

From Mosby: *Managing major diseases: diabetes mellitus and hypertension,* St Louis, 1999, Mosby.

Sensations of pain and temperature travel along the same spinothalamic tract in the spinal cord. When your patient responds normally to pain sensation, you probably do not need to test for temperature sensation. However, if you decide to check for temperature identification, then systematically touch cool and warm objects, such as test tubes filled with cold and warm water, to each leg, and check your patient's response.

To test vibration sensation, strike a tuning fork on the heel of your hand and place it firmly over the interphalangeal joint of the great toe. Ask if your patient can feel the vibration. If he can, no further vibratory testing is needed. If he cannot, then proceed to more proximal bony prominences, such as the medial malleolus, the patella, and the AS iliac spine.

Test position sense by telling your patient that you are going to move some of the toes so that they point up or down. Show the patient what you mean; then ask him to close his eyes. Grasping the great toe and holding it away from the others, move it up or down, and ask your patient to tell you its position. Repeat this several times on each side.

NORMAL FINDINGS
- Recognition of light touch and pain
- Vibratory sensation intact when testing the great toe (In older adults the vibratory sensation may be absent or diminished.)
- Accurate position sense (See 🧩 *What to Expect When Examining the Lower Extremities.*)

NORMAL FINDINGS

WHAT TO EXPECT WHEN EXAMINING THE LOWER EXTREMITIES

Use this quick review to confirm normal findings when examining the lower extremities.

Inspection
- Symmetrical extremities
- Uniform skin color, light variation
- No swelling or varicosities
- No gross deformities

Palpation
- Cool-to-warm skin temperature
- Smooth skin with minimal moisture

- Equal, easily palpated femoral, popliteal, pedal, and posterior tibial pulses
- No edema or varicose veins
- Full range of motion (ROM)
- Symmetrical muscle tone
- Muscle strength at 5 on a scale of 1 to 5
- Deep tendon reflexes (DTRs) ++ bilaterally at knee and ankle
- Plantar reflex negative
- No clonus
- Superficial touch and pain sensations bilaterally
- Intact vibratory and position senses

ABNORMAL FINDINGS
- Impaired sensory response, indicating a neurologic disorder (A loss of position sense may suggest a spinal cord lesion when associated with other neurologic complaints. Vibration is the first sense to be lost in peripheral neuropathies, such as diabetes mellitus. It also disappears in alcoholism, tertiary syphilis, and vitamin B_{12} deficiency.)

EXPLORING CHIEF COMPLAINTS

Complaints involving the lower extremities are common and wide ranging. If your patient has one of the following complaints, use this section of the chapter to quickly focus your assessment.

LIMB PAIN

Pain is perhaps the most common complaint involving the lower extremities. Most pain results from injury or inflammation, but it may also be caused by altered peripheral circulation or neurologic damage (see ▓ *Assessing Acute Leg Pain*).

INTERPRETING ABNORMAL FINDINGS

ASSESSING ACUTE LEG PAIN

Determining if leg pain is acute or chronic will guide you in your assessment. Chronic pain persists for 3 months or more, whereas acute pain usually is more sudden in onset and associated with hyperactivity of the sympathetic nervous system (tachycardia, increased respiratory rate and blood pressure, dilated pupils). The cause of acute limb pain is musculoskeletal, neurologic, or vascular. This chart reviews some commonly encountered causes of acute limb pain.

Type of Pain	Typical Findings	Associated Characteristics	Probable Cause
Musculoskeletal	History of recent trauma Refusal to bear weight or partial weight bearing Throbbing pain	Obvious deformity Swelling Crepitus Tenderness on palpation or movement Ecchymoses Paresthesias	Fracture or dislocation
	Usually involves only one joint Sudden pain Limited weight bearing Swelling Erythema Tenderness	Fever History of recent viral illness Movement decreases pain (except with rheumatoid arthritis)	Septic joint
Neurologic	Shooting pain radiating down one or both legs following distribution of sciatic nerve Often no complaint of back pain Pain is electrical, burning, aching Associated with paresthesias	Pain worsens with movement, such as walking, coughing, straining at stool Positive straight-leg raising test Decreased deep tendon reflexes (DTRs) Local muscle weakness and atrophy	Sciatica

continued

INTERPRETING ABNORMAL FINDINGS—cont'd

Type of Pain	Typical Findings	Associated Characteristics	Probable Cause
Vascular	Pain is distal to the occlusion Coldness Numbness Weakness Skin pallor Cyanosis	Diminished or absent pulses distally	Acute arterial occlusion
	Calf is common site May or may not be painful	Swelling of calf or ankle Calf tenderness and erythema Positive Homans' sign in some patients	Deep vein thrombosis (DVT)

If the patient complains of limb pain, investigate further by asking the following questions:

- Where is the pain? Is it localized or generalized? Can you point to where you feel the pain? Is it deep or superficial pain? Does it radiate to another location, such as your back?
- How bad is the pain? Where is it on a scale of 0 to 10, with 0 being no pain and 10 being the worst pain possible? Are you able to perform your usual daily tasks? Can you walk without pain?
- In what setting does the pain occur? Does it occur only after walking long distances or going up and down stairs? Does it occur after repetitive movements? Does it occur only at night?
- When did the pain first begin? Is it a new problem, or have you had it before? Did it begin suddenly or gradually? Is it intermittent or continuous? How long does the pain last?
- Can you describe the pain in your own words (burning, stabbing, dull, throbbing)?
- Is the pain associated with any other problems, such as swelling, redness, or tingling?
- Does anything make the pain worse?
- Does anything make the pain better?

Focusing Your Assessment
When examining a patient who complains of limb pain, focus your assessment as follows:

- Check to see if your patient can ambulate without difficulty and without assistance. Note whether the patient can bear weight on the affected leg. Also note whether the patient's legs are symmetrical.

- Determine whether the patient has pain with ROM. Check to see if ROM is restricted because of the pain. Remember to compare each side against the other.
- Palpate the patient's pulses to see if they are equal and strong bilaterally. Compare the lower extremities for color, temperature, and amount and distribution of hair growth. Also look for areas of skin breakdown or ulceration, possibly from incompetent veins.
- Be alert for patient reports of worsening calf pain if he dorsiflexes the foot when his knee is slightly flexed. Check for Homans' sign if your patient complains of lower leg pain with swelling and has risk factors for deep vein thrombosis (DVT), such as the use of oral contraceptives or prolonged immobility. This worsening of pain is Homans' sign, traditionally considered a sign of DVT and assessed for whenever DVT was suspected. Because there is a risk of dislodging a clot when the foot is dorsiflexed, and because a positive Homans' sign has been found in only 35% of patients with DVT, specifically checking for it is now in question. Homans' sign can also be positive with a herniated lumbar disc.
- Check for sciatic pain. This involves placing your patient in a supine position on the examination table and passively raising the extended leg, flexing it at the hip. If the patient complains of posterior leg pain when it is elevated between 30 and 60 degrees, this suggests sciatic pain.

Possible Causes

- *Soft tissue injury.* Pain can result from a fall or twisting injury, such as stepping the wrong way off a curb. The problem could affect muscles, tendons, or ligaments. Pain may be intense initially, improving with ice and rest. Gradual, progressive pain from activity or repetitive movements may also result from a sprain or strain. A sprain involves stretching or tearing a ligament; a strain involves stretching or tearing a muscle. An Achilles tear or a hamstring tear usually involves acute pain. Often the patient cannot bear weight.
- *Fracture.* Your patient almost certainly has a history of trauma or a fall that causes intense pain that is worse with movement. Your patient will not be able to bear weight on the painful extremity.
- *Tumor or metastasis.* This deep pain usually worsens at night.
- *Arterial embolism or thrombosis.* This sudden, severe pain is very localized. The affected limb will also become cold, pale, and pulseless.
- *Arterial or peripheral arterial disease.* Pain is gradual and intermittent in nature. If your patient has atherosclerotic disease in the peripheral arteries, he will likely complain of calf pain from exercise (intermittent claudication). The pain abates with rest. In cases of severe disease, the patient will complain of resting leg pain.
- *DVT.* Usually this condition causes gradual leg pain. It worsens with walking and dorsiflexion of the foot, and it commonly is associated with swelling and erythema of the affected extremity.

- *Sciatic pain.* Commonly caused by a herniated lumbar disk, this pain feels electrical to many patients and commonly is associated with a tingling or aching sensation that radiates down one or both legs. It worsens with activity and improves with rest. You can check for this condition with straight-leg testing.
- *Diabetic neuropathy.* This condition causes pain and paresthesias symmetrically in the feet and legs. Peripheral neuropathy is a syndrome involving sensory loss, muscle weakness and atrophy, pain, and vasomotor symptoms.
- *Peroneal nerve palsy.* This pain results from compression of the peroneal nerve against the lateral aspect of the head of the fibula. This cause of leg pain is common in bedridden patients and thin people who habitually cross their legs. If the problem is peroneal nerve compression, your patient will not be able to dorsiflex the great toe against resistance.

JOINT PAIN OR STIFFNESS

Patients often use the terms *joint pain* and *stiffness* interchangeably. Stiffness is difficult to assess, but it refers to a perception of tightness or resistance to movement. If the patient complains of joint pain or stiffness, investigate further by asking the following questions:

- Do you have other symptoms associated with the joint pain, such as swelling, tenderness, warmth, redness, or limited movement?
- Is the problem restricting any of your usual activities? Is walking difficult or painful? Can you use the stairs without pain? Do you have pain when rising from a sitting position?
- Does stiffness occur in the morning and, if so, how long does it last? (Stiffness associated with inflammatory arthritis usually lasts more than 60 minutes. Stiffness related to muscle soreness from strenuous exertion often peaks the second day after the exertion.)

Focusing Your Assessment

When examining a patient who complains of joint pain or stiffness, focus your assessment as follows:

- Inspect the joint, looking for erythema, swelling, or deformity.
- Check ROM in the lower extremities, comparing each side.
- Palpate the joint and surrounding tissues for tenderness while your patient flexes and extends the limb. Listen for crepitus, a crackling sound heard as the joints move.

Possible Causes

- *Fracture or dislocation.* Consider the possibility of a hip fracture in an older patient who complains of hip pain after a fall. Fractures commonly involve the femoral head or the pelvis. Dislocation of the hip joint is also common among older adults.
- *Gout.* This inflammatory reaction to uric acid crystals in joints, bones, and subcutaneous structures causes a pain that usually begins suddenly. It is associated with swelling, erythema, and warmth, and it usually affects only one joint, most often the great toe (see ◙ *Gout*).

DISORDER CLOSE-UP

GOUT

A metabolic disorder characterized by elevated serum uric acid concentration and deposits of urate crystals in synovial fluid and surrounding joint tissues, gout causes joint pain, usually in the great toe, ankles, and midfoot. Primary gout occurs most often in men and postmenopausal women. Secondary gout usually affects older people.

The exact cause of gout is unknown, although primary gout is believed to involve an inborn error of purine metabolism or a decrease in renal uric acid excretion. Secondary gout, marked by hyperuricemia, can result from a disorder or medication.

Normally, uric acid production is balanced through excretion, with about two thirds being excreted via the kidneys and the remainder in feces. When serum uric acid levels rise above 7 mg/dl, the serum is saturated and monosodium urate crystals may form. These crystals tend to form in the body's peripheral tissues, where lower temperatures reduce the solubility of the uric acid.

Other factors that can precipitate crystal formation and tissue deposition include a decrease in extracellular fluid pH and reduced plasma protein binding of urate crystals. Tissue trauma from a rapid change in uric acid levels also may lead to crystal deposits. Conversely, a rapid increase in uric acid may occur after tissue trauma and release of cellular components.

Unless treated, gout progresses in four stages: (1) asymptomatic hyperuricemia, (2) acute gouty arthritis (usually affecting a single joint), (3) an intercritical period (an asymptomatic period that can last up to 10 years), and (4) tophaceous or chronic gout. In this final stage, hyperuricemia continues untreated, with development of crystal deposits (tophi) in cartilage, synovial membranes, tendons, and soft tissues.

Characteristic findings

Expect health history information and physical examination findings to vary among patients with gout, depending on the extent and severity of the disease. The information that follows will help you distinguish between expected and unexpected findings.

Health history

- Sedentary lifestyle
- History of hypertension
- History of renal calculi
- Complaints of sudden onset of pain, often in great toe, initially moderate but increasing in intensity
- Difficulty bearing even the weight of bed sheets on the affected area
- Chills

Inspection

- Swollen, dusky-red or purple joint with limited movement
- Tophi, especially on outer ears, hands, and feet
- Ulceration of skin over tophi, with release of chalky white exudate or pus (in chronic stage)

Palpation

- Warmth and extreme tenderness over joint

Vital signs

- Fever
- Hypertension

continued

DISORDER CLOSE-UP—cont'd

Complications
- Renal calculi
- Atherosclerotic heart disease
- Cardiovascular lesions
- Cerebrovascular accident (CVA)
- Coronary thrombosis
- Hypertension
- Infection, with tophi rupture and nerve entrapment

- *Septic joint.* This condition is characterized by fever and joint pain, swelling, redness, and warmth. It must be evaluated and treated quickly to prevent osteomyelitis, joint destruction, or both.
- *Rheumatoid arthritis.* A chronic systemic disease with articular inflammation, rheumatoid arthritis is characterized by morning stiffness lasting more than 1 hour each day, pain in at least two joint groups, symmetrical joint swelling, and subcutaneous nodules. The pain can be constant or intermittent.
- *Osteoarthritis.* The "wear-and-tear joint arthritis" is the most common form of joint disease, with progressive destruction and loss of joint cartilage. Weight-bearing joints of overweight patients are often involved. Prolonged occupational or sports stress can lead to osteoarthritis.

SWELLING

Swelling is an excessive accumulation of interstitial fluid or edema. If the patient complains of swelling of the lower extremities, investigate further by asking the following questions:

- Where is the swelling located? Does it affect both legs? Does it involve the entire leg or just a certain area? How far up the leg does the swelling go? (See 🔍 *Thrombophlebitis*.)

DISORDER CLOSE-UP

THROMBOPHLEBITIS

Inflammation of a vein associated with thrombus formation, thrombophlebitis can result from vessel wall trauma; hypercoagulability of the blood; infection; chemical irritation; postoperative venous stasis; prolonged sitting, standing, or immobilization; or long periods of intravenous (IV) catheterization.

Both deep and superficial veins can be affected by thrombophlebitis. Deep vein thrombophlebitis usually involves the deep veins of the legs, primarily the calf. Superficial vein thrombophlebitis typically involves the veins of the upper extremities and is commonly associated with trauma (e.g., from insertion of catheters in the subclavian vein).

continued

Three pathologic factors, known as *Virchow's triad,* are associated with thrombophlebitis: (1) venous stasis, (2) increased blood coagulability, and (3) injury to the vessel wall. Two of these three factors must be present for thrombi to form in the vein.

Trauma to the endothelial venous lining brings subendothelial tissues in contact with platelets. These platelets aggregate, especially if the patient has venous stasis. Fibrin, leukocytes, and erythrocytes deposit into the platelet clump to cause a thrombus.

Initially a thrombus floats within a vein. Within 7 to 10 days, it adheres to the vein wall, but a portion may still float in the lumen of the vessel. Pieces of the tail may break loose and travel through the circulation as emboli. Fibroblasts eventually invade the thrombus, scarring the vein wall and destroying the venous valves.

Characteristic findings

Expect the health history and physical examination findings to vary among patients with thrombophlebitis, depending on the extent and severity of the disease. The information that follows will help you distinguish between expected and unexpected findings.

Health history

- Asymptomatic (early in the inflammatory process)
- Vague tightness or dull aching pain in affected extremity, especially on walking, increasing in severity
- Inability to walk without pain
- History of risk factors, including bed rest, use of IV catheters, immobilization, obesity, myocardial infarction (MI), heart failure, multiple sclerosis, oral contraceptive use, pregnancy and childbirth, altered coagulability states, and surgery in patients older than age 40
- Tenderness over affected area
- General malaise

Inspection

- Redness, cyanosis, and swelling of the affected extremity
- Marked redness along the course of the vein (superficial thrombophlebitis)
- Increased size of affected extremity

Palpation

- Warm and tender to the touch
- Palpable cordlike structure (superficial thrombophlebitis)
- Positive cuff sign
- Possible positive Homans' sign
- Diminished or absent pedal pulse on affected extremity
- Slowed capillary refill

Vital signs

- Possible fever

Complications

- Pulmonary embolism
- Chronic venous insufficiency

- Is the swelling slight, or is it marked? If the swelling has occurred before, is it more severe or less?
- When does the swelling occur? Does it occur on waking in the morning or at the end of the day? Is it constant or intermittent?
- When did you first notice the swelling? Was it gradual or sudden? Is it new or chronic? If intermittent, how long does it last?
- Do you have an imprint of a shoe or a sock line when you take your shoes and socks off (pitting edema)?
- Have you had surgery, or have you been injured recently? Do you have a history of heart or lung problems? Is the swelling associated with pain, warmth, or redness? Which medications do you take?
- Does anything make the swelling worse, such as sitting for long periods or eating salty foods?
- Does anything reduce the swelling, such as elevating your feet, using support hose, or putting ice on your feet?

Focusing Your Assessment
When examining a patient who complains of swelling, focus your assessment as follows:
- Inspect the skin for evidence of erythema, brawniness, skin breakdown, or ulceration.
- Palpate the swollen area for warmth and tenderness.
- Palpate for pitting or nonpitting edema.
- Note whether the swelling is unilateral or bilateral.
- Measure the swollen areas, and record their sizes.
- If you find joint swelling, assess ROM for each affected joint.

Possible Causes
- *Musculoskeletal problems.* Swelling from an injury, such as a fracture or sprain, commonly is associated with superficial bruising or hematomas. Swelling tends to occur a few hours after the initial injury. Localized joint swelling may indicate synovial inflammation, as in a septic joint or rheumatoid arthritis. On the other hand, you may notice an increase in synovial fluid around the joint after an injury.
- *Systemic sources of bilateral edema.* These conditions may include heart failure, which would be accompanied by shortness of breath; excessive renal retention of sodium and water, which may be accompanied by hypertension; and kidney failure, which most often would be accompanied by diminished urination or cirrhosis (you will be able to palpate a firm, smooth liver with a blunt edge).
- *Local causes of bilateral edema.* This condition could stem from sitting or standing for long periods, pregnancy, or menopause. You may find unilateral edema if your patient has cellulitis, in which you would find local erythema and tenderness; osteomyelitis, a bacterial bone infection associated with pain and tenderness in the affected area; venous obstruction from a thrombus, in which you would detect marked redness and a cordlike feeling along the course of the vein; or tumors that compress the vasculature.

CHANGES IN SENSATION

This problem may involve anesthesia, paresthesias, or dysesthesias. Anesthesia (numbness) is a loss of sensation to a body part. Paresthesias are abnormal tactile sensations not produced by stimulation and usually described as tingling or prickling. Dysesthesias are distorted, typically unpleasant sensations in response to a stimulus. They commonly last longer than the stimulus itself. A burning sensation that occurs in response to a simple pinprick is an example of dysesthesia. If the patient complains of changes in sensation, investigate further by asking the following questions:

- Where is the sensation? Is it in just one part of the leg, or does it involve the entire leg? Does it involve one or both legs?
- How intense is the sensation?
- When or where does it occur? Does it occur only when your legs are elevated? Does it occur when bending over?
- When did this problem begin? Was its onset sudden or gradual? Is this a new or chronic problem?
- Can you describe the type of sensation? Is it associated with other problems, such as weakness or pain? If so, how significant is the other problem? Have you experienced a recent injury?
- What worsens this sensory change? Do cold temperatures or sitting for long periods make it worse? Does it seem to occur in response to another stimulus, such as a pinprick?
- Does rest or leg elevation make the sensation better?

Focusing Your Assessment

When examining a patient who complains of changes in sensation, focus your assessment as follows:

- Evaluate the sensory system, including your patient's perception of pain, temperature, position, vibration, and light touch.
- Assess muscle tone and strength by testing each major muscle group against resistance. This procedure checks not only the musculoskeletal system but also the neurologic system that innervates the muscles.
- Test the DTRs.
- Assess circulation to the extremity by palpating pulses, feeling for coolness, and inspecting for pallor and blanching.
- Assess respiratory patterns. Note any increased or rapid respiratory rate, especially if the patient appears anxious and looks as though he may be hyperventilating.
- Gently palpate the spinal column, feeling for protrusions or masses that could indicate a herniated vertebral disk or a tumor.
- Ask the patient to bend forward and touch the toes; then ask if this movement made the sensation better or worse. In addition, while he is supine, raise the legs above heart level and see if this makes the symptoms worse.

Possible Causes

- *Fracture, tumor, or swelling.* These conditions place pressure on a nerve or compress the nerve, resulting in anesthesia or paresthesias. Bending forward and flexing the spine may produce or aggravate these abnormal symptoms.

- *Spinal cord injury.* This condition commonly produces dysesthesias or anesthesia below the level of the injury.
- *Occlusive vascular disease.* This condition produces a loss of sensation or a burning, prickling sensation in the extremities from diminished blood flow when the legs are elevated over the head. The extremities may pale and pulses diminish.
- *Neurologic disorder.* Vitamin B_6 deficiency or such neurologic disorders as multiple sclerosis and ALS can cause paresthesias. With ALS, your patient also may demonstrate increased DTRs and muscle weakness.
- *Hyperventilation.* This condition commonly causes a pins-and-needles sensation in the fingers and toes, along with a feeling of faintness.

CHANGES IN SKIN COLOR OR TEMPERATURE

Changes in skin color of the lower extremities, with or without temperature change, can suggest an inflammatory process or compromised vascular flow. If the patient complains of skin color or temperature change, investigate further by asking the following questions:

- Where on your legs did you notice the change in color or temperature?
- Did you notice a marked change to a bluish or reddish color or a feeling of coldness?
- Have you been doing anything in particular when you have noticed the change, such as crossing your legs, standing for a long period, or exerting yourself?
- Does the change occur at any particular time of day?
- How would you describe the skin discoloration (pale, bluish, reddened)?
- Do you have any other symptoms associated with the change in color or temperature?
- Are you aware of anything that aggravates the problem, such as smoking?
- Are you aware of anything that relieves the problem?

Focusing Your Assessment

When examining a patient who experiences changes in skin color or temperature, focus your assessment as follows:

- Inspect the area for erythema, pallor, swelling, and deformity.
- Palpate the pulses of the lower extremities (femoral, popliteal, dorsalis pedis, posterior tibial) for equality and strength. Note if any are absent.
- Palpate for warmth and tenderness. If you find a localized area of erythema, measure and document it for future comparison. Also outline the area with a felt-tipped marking pen.

Possible Causes

- *Anemia.* A common cause of pallor, this condition also causes fatigue.
- *Arterial insufficiency.* In this condition, the patient will have pain aggravated by exercise.

- *Respiratory conditions.* Chronic obstructive pulmonary disease (COPD) and other respiratory conditions can cause generalized cyanosis (especially in the distal digits) from hypoxemia.
- *Heart failure or congenital heart disease.* These conditions produce generalized cyanosis from hypoxemia. They are usually associated with edema and shortness of breath on exertion.
- *Venous obstruction.* In this case the area would be tender, edematous, and warm to the touch.
- *Arterial occlusion.* In this case the patient would have pain and skin that is cold to the touch (see ⊙ *Responding to Acute Arterial Occlusion*).
- *Anxiety or cold environment.* In these conditions the skin is usually cool to the touch.

ACTION STAT

RESPONDING TO ACUTE ARTERIAL OCCLUSION

An acute arterial occlusion of the leg can result in loss of the affected limb if not recognized and treated immediately. Most patients with peripheral vascular disease have a chronic condition with symptoms that develop over years. However, if your patient has an acute arterial occlusion, he will experience severe, unrelenting pain. Onset is sudden, and pain may involve the entire leg.

Occlusion of a major artery with acute loss of perfusion distal to it may result from a thrombus or an embolus that migrates to the point of occlusion. Diagnosis is based on a detailed examination, including history and Doppler studies. Prognosis varies. If the affected limb is in a confined space, such as with a cast, arterial occlusion can occur because of compartment syndrome. In this syndrome, tissue edema occludes arterial blood flow and presses on nearby nerves.

What to look for

Signs and symptoms of acute arterial occlusion vary, depending on the location of the obstruction. Typically the skin of the affected extremity is cold. You can also remember signs and symptoms by using the five Ps:

Pain that is diffuse and distal to the occlusion, not alleviated by position change
Pulselessness
Pallor, followed by proximal mottling and distal cyanosis
Paresthesias, with numbness, loss of light-touch sensation, and (in advanced ischemia) loss of pain or pressure sensation
Paralysis, or motor deficits, that arise after sensory deficits in advanced ischemia

What to do immediately

If you suspect an arterial occlusion, notify the physician immediately. Anticipate these orders:

- Insert an intravenous (IV) line for thrombolytic and anticoagulant agents. Also, if your patient needs surgery, he will need an IV catheter for administration of fluids during the procedure.
- Prepare your patient for ultrasound studies, such as lower extremity Doppler, to identify the extent and location of the blockage.
- Prepare your patient for surgery (e.g., femoral-popliteal bypass), percutaneous transluminal angioplasty of the affected artery, or thrombolytic therapy (e.g., recombinant tissue plasminogen activator or streptokinase).

continued

ACTION STAT—cont'd

- If compartment syndrome is the cause, prepare to take action to relieve pressure on the affected limb, such as cast removal or surgery.
- Maintain nothing by mouth status until you find out which of these interventions the patient will need.

What to do next
- Administer analgesic agents, as prescribed, to relieve limb pain.
- Continue to monitor circulation to the extremity, including its color, temperature, and the presence and strength of distal pulses.

- Prevent injury to the extremity because healing will be impaired in the compromised limb.
- If your patient requires anticoagulation therapy, monitor the activated partial thromboplastin time (PTT) if he is receiving heparin and prothrombin time (PT) if he is taking warfarin sodium (Coumadin).
- Teach the patient how to check the peripheral pulses and look for signs of worsened circulation, such as pallor and coolness. Also teach the patient how to care for and protect the extremity.

- *Inflammation, infection, or recent trauma.* These conditions typically redden the skin. Bacterial infection can cause a septic joint. The joint will be erythematous, swollen, tender, and warm. The patient will have a fever.
- *Cellulitis, first-degree (partial thickness) burns, and superficial thrombophlebitis.* In these cases skin usually is warm to the touch and tender.
- *Gout or a flare-up of rheumatoid arthritis.* These conditions cause erythema around a joint.

WEAKNESS OR PARALYSIS
If the patient complains of muscle weakness or decreased function related to paralysis, investigate further by asking the following questions:
- Is the weakness in only one or both legs? Can you move the leg at all, or do you have no control over movements?
- When did the problem first begin? Is it a new or chronic problem? How often does it happen? Is it there all the time or just sometimes? Do you have other symptoms or weakness elsewhere?
- How bad is the weakness? Does it affect your independence?
- What makes the muscle weakness worse? What makes it better?
- Do you stumble frequently or trip when walking? Do you have difficulty rising from a chair?

Focusing Your Assessment
When examining a patient who complains of weakness or paralysis, focus your assessment as follows:
- Assess the musculoskeletal and neurologic systems any time a patient has a change in leg function.
- Assess your patient's ambulation status. Is the patient's gait impaired?
- Look for muscle atrophy in the major muscle groups of the legs, comparing each side.

- Assess muscle tone and strength by testing each major muscle group against resistance. This procedure tests not only the musculoskeletal system but also the neurologic system that innervates the muscles. Absent or decreased muscle tone or strength may be caused by lower motor neuron disorders. Upper motor neuron disorders cause increased muscle tone and spasticity.
- Test DTRs. Absent or decreased DTRs occur with lower motor neuron disorders. Upper motor neuron disorders cause increased DTRs.

Possible Causes

- *Fatigue.* When a patient complains of weakness in the extremities, he may, in fact, be fatigued and have decreased activity tolerance. True muscle weakness is different from fatigue and can be caused by injury or by central or peripheral nerve degeneration.
- *Hypokalemia or hypothyroidism.* Chemical changes that occur in these conditions can result in generalized muscle weakness.
- *Upper and lower motor neuron disorders.* Upper motor neuron disorders include cerebrovascular accident (CVA) or central nervous system trauma. Lower motor neuron disorders include polio, ALS, and Guillain-Barré syndrome. With upper motor neuron disorders, increased or hyperactive DTRs accompany weakness. With lower motor neuron disorders, reflexes are diminished or absent.
- *Myopathies.* Caused by medications (e.g., corticosteroids) or diseases (e.g., muscular dystrophy), myopathies produce proximal muscle weakness (hips and thighs). Your patient will have difficulty rising from a seated position.
- *Neuropathies.* Seen in people with diabetes mellitus or lead poisoning, neuropathies cause weakness and loss of sensation in the feet and lower legs. Typically, the patient trips or stumbles while walking.
- *Paralysis.* An inability to voluntarily move a body part from loss of motor function, paralysis can occur in one, two, or all four limbs. Hemiplegia can be caused by a CVA or head injury. Paraplegia and quadriplegia can be caused by spinal cord injury.

MUSCLE SPASM OR CRAMPING

If the patient complains of muscle spasm or cramping, investigate further by asking the following questions:

- When did the spasm or cramping first begin? Is it a new or chronic problem? How often does it happen?
- How bad is the spasm or cramp? Does it affect your independence?
- When does the spasm or cramping occur? Does it occur only after strenuous activity or mostly at night? Is it constant or intermittent?
- What makes the muscle spasm worse? What makes it better?
- Do you take a diuretic, such as furosemide, or an immunosuppressive medication, such as cyclosporine?

Focusing Your Assessment

When examining a patient who complains of muscle spasm or cramping, focus your assessment as follows:

- Assess tone and strength by testing each major muscle group against resistance. This tests not only the musculoskeletal system but also the neurologic system that innervates the muscles.
- Test DTRs. Absent or decreased DTRs are observed in lower motor neuron disorders.
- Check the patient's serum electrolyte levels for imbalances.

Possible Causes

- *Muscle spasticity.* This term refers to increased muscle tone (hypertonia) and exaggerated DTRs. Upper motor neuron disorders are associated with spasticity, as seen in central nervous system trauma or a CVA.
- *Muscle spasms.* These painful muscular contractions usually involve the calf or foot. Commonly, they result from fatigue in the muscle and abate with rest or stretching of the muscle.
- *Electrolyte imbalances.* Painful, nocturnal leg cramps can result from impaired peripheral circulation and such electrolyte imbalances as hypokalemia, especially when induced by diuretic use. Other medications, such as cyclosporine, have the side effect of leg cramps.

Putting It All Together

For any nurse, accuracy represents the most important goal of physical assessment. Patients and the entire health care team rely on your ability to detect health problems and follow up with appropriate collaborative care. However, in this era of budget cuts and time demands, accuracy is not enough. You also must be fast. To help you stay focused and fast, this chapter presents no-nonsense instructions on how to perform a quick head-to-toe assessment and outlines essential normal findings for each body area. Based on the special *Normal Findings* features that appear in earlier chapters, these are the most crucial findings—findings you can investigate rapidly. Review them regularly to keep your assessments on target and on time.

Always keep in mind, however, that the nature and complexity of a physical examination depends on the patient's condition at the time of your encounter. If the patient is acutely ill with a specific health problem, a series of focused physical examinations to track and evaluate the chief complaint will be needed. This is why techniques for isolating your patient's chief complaint, performing a focused assessment, and pinpointing its probable cause have been given throughout the text.

On the other hand, imagine that your patient does not have a pressing complaint, or you do not know the medical diagnosis. Even in this situation, you can perform a rapid yet thorough assessment that includes all body systems if you follow the guidelines in this chapter.

The thing to remember is that, above all else, fast and accurate assessment requires readiness and repetition. This review chapter will help you gain both speed and accuracy in your physical examinations. By learning how to better organize and prioritize examination steps, you can gather pertinent patient information quickly and identify abnormalities before they turn into crises.

FIRST THINGS FIRST

Remember that physical examination begins the moment you encounter a patient, whether during admission, during a home or clinic visit, or during your shift. However, physical examination does not end with that single encounter. To provide quality ongoing health care, you need to perform physical examinations at regular intervals to assess expected and unexpected changes in a patient's condition.

To set yourself up for successful assessment, keep a few points in mind:

- Always review the patient's health history for important medical, surgical, and family details before you start your examination.
- If your patient has a chief complaint, be sure you have enough information about it. Ask the patient to explain the complaint fully. Investigate whether the problem is ongoing and whether it changes in character or severity. Also ask about any new problems or symptoms that may have developed since the history was taken.
- Think critically about the patient's chief complaint. Consider what might be causing it. Then, during the examination, look for related signs and symptoms that could confirm or disprove your suspicion. This focused approach will help you get to the root of your patient's problem more quickly.
- Make sure you have the proper equipment to perform your physical examination comfortably and completely: stethoscope, thermometer, sphygmomanometer, penlight, cotton-tipped swabs, latex or vinyl gloves, pupil gauge, tongue blade, scale (standing platform or bed), reflex hammer, and a pulse oximeter.
- Ensure an appropriate environment. For example, check to see if the room is warm enough and the lighting sufficient for you to observe your patient clearly. Take steps to ensure your patient's privacy by closing the door, for example, or drawing the curtain. If visitors or other health care providers are in the room, either ask them to leave or delay your examination until another time, unless your patient wants them present for the examination.
- Record your findings—both normal and abnormal—in note form as you go along. Doing so will keep you from forgetting important details that arise during your examination. Later, after the examination, you can enter the data onto a flow sheet or document your findings in the patient's medical record.

PERFORMING AN EXPERT RAPID EXAMINATION

Assess your patient informally at every opportunity to catch changes or problems as early as possible. This means you must be aware of your patient's condition any time you are in her presence, whether or not you are engaged in a formal physical examination. Consider the patient's condition and situation as you accomplish tasks that require you to be around her. Note whether anything seems awry. Look for obvious signs of distress or conditions that warrant immediate attention, such as bleeding or weakness.

If the patient is hospitalized, inspect all incisions and dressings for signs of bleeding, drainage, infection, dehiscence, and evisceration. Inspect the placement and function of drains and tubes, including postsurgical drainage or nasogastric tubes, and palpate intravenous (IV) insertion sites for infiltration or infection. Assess your patient's fluid balance by noting intake and output (intake includes oral and IV sources; output includes urine, nasogastric substances, and postsurgical drainage). In addition, if your patient is connected to a monitoring device, evaluate the information it provides. Finally, if your patient has a cardiac or respiratory condition, check the arterial oxygen saturation levels.

When you are ready to turn to a formal assessment, you will have to decide which areas of the patient's body you want to assess, based on individual needs. No matter what the specific complaint, you may want to start with a general survey.

TAKING A GENERAL SURVEY
The goal of a general survey is to assess your patient's vital signs and general condition. Afterward, you will be able to document a wide-ranging list of findings that offer a well-rounded view of your patient's condition (see ▨ *What to Expect When Conducting a General Survey*).

NORMAL FINDINGS

WHAT TO EXPECT WHEN CONDUCTING A GENERAL SURVEY
Use this review to confirm normal findings when conducting a general survey.
- Facial expression free of distress. If the patient is relatively content, she may smile, make eye contact, and have relaxed facial muscles. (Remember that facial expression reflects a patient's mood *and* physical condition.)
- Body temperature within the following ranges:
  Oral: 96.8° to 99.5° F (36° to 37.5° C)
  Rectal: 97.3° to 100.2° F (36.3° to 37.9° C)
  Tympanic (core): 97.2° to 100° F (36.2° to 37.8° C)
- Pulse rate between 60 and 100 beats per minute (bpm), with a regular rhythm, smooth upstroke and downstroke, and strong amplitude (Pulse rates less than 60 bpm are normal in athletes or people taking certain medications. Pulse rates greater than 100 bpm are normal when influenced by factors that stimulate the sympathetic nervous system.)
- Respiratory rate between 12 and 20 breaths per minute, with regular rhythm
- Breathing quiet, easy, and effortless
- Respiration producing pronounced abdominal movement and slight thoracic move-

ment in a patient in the supine position (In a patient in the sitting position, thoracic movement is more pronounced.)
- Systolic blood pressure ranging from 90 to 119 mm Hg
- Diastolic blood pressure 60 to 80 mm Hg
- Systolic blood pressure dropping by less than 20 mm Hg when the patient moves from a supine or sitting position
- Diastolic blood pressure rising only slightly when the patient moves from a supine or sitting position
- Blood pressure differing by no more than 10 mm Hg between the arms
- Body movements smooth, easily controlled, and coordinated
- Ambulation showing patient's ability to hold body and head erect, balance easily, and swing arms at sides (Turns are accomplished smoothly, with the shoulders and hips level during each stride.)
- Mechanisms intact for balance, coordination, and proprioception
- Level of consciousness (LOC) showing patient is awake, alert, and oriented (The patient should respond appropriately when addressed in a normal tone of voice, as well as participate in and pay attention during the conversation.)
- Speech fluid, articulate, and clear

To perform a general survey, follow these steps:
- Measure vital signs, temperature, pulse, respirations, and blood pressure for signs of abnormality.
- Assess height, weight, and body build. Note a weight gain or loss of more than 2 lb over 24 hours. Use a bed scale if the patient is bedridden or a chair scale if she is unsteady on her feet.
- Observe the patient's ability for self-care. Note personal hygiene and grooming. Also note the general condition of the patient's skin, hair, and nails. (see ▓ *What to Expect When Examining the Skin, Hair, and Nails*).

NORMAL FINDINGS

WHAT TO EXPECT WHEN EXAMINING THE SKIN, HAIR, AND NAILS

Use this review to confirm normal findings when examining the skin, hair, and nails.

- Skin color even throughout the body, except in dark-skinned people, in whom it is lighter on palms, soles, and nail beds
- Skin texture smooth and soft, except for such joints as elbows and knees
- Skin warm and dry
- Skin returning immediately to its normal position when pinched
- Hair thin, fine, and usually light in color over all areas except the scalp, axillae, eyebrows, pubic areas, palms, and soles
- Hair coarser, darker, and thicker on scalp, axillae, eyebrows, and pubic areas (In male subjects, the facial hair is also coarse and thick.)
- Hair texture and color that varies with race and age (The texture may be fine or coarse, straight or curly. The color is distributed evenly and ranges from light blond to black or gray.)
- Hair distribution even, except in cases of male-pattern thinning or baldness
- Nail plates smooth, round, and slightly convex, with angle of about 160 degrees between the nail and skin at the nail base
- Nail plates firmly attached to the nail beds
- Nail bed firm on palpation
- Capillary refill time less than 4 seconds
- Nail surface smooth, even, and hard, with smooth and rounded nail edges
- Periungual skin unbroken, smooth, and flat

- Observe the patient's posture. Look for signs of abnormal posture in the comatose patient by checking for unnatural positions. In addition, look for signs of pain in an alert patient.
- Observe general body movements, and look for tics, tremors, rigidity, or flaccidity.
- Observe the patient's gait. Assess balance, coordination, and position sense.
- Assess level of consciousness (LOC), attention, orientation, and speech patterns.

Remember that you may need to alter your methods for this general examination, depending on your patient's condition. Ideally, you will want her to stand and ambulate for important portions of the examination. However, if she is bedridden or comatose, you will have to do your best to perform the examination while she is in bed.

EXAMINING THE HEAD AND NECK

When examining your patient's head and neck, have her sit up, whether in a chair, on the side of the bed, or in the bed. When assessing jugular venous pressure, however, position your patient in bed with the head elevated 45 degrees. For your patient's comfort, you may wish to delay this part of the examination until she is supine (see ▨ *What to Expect When Examining the Head and Neck*).

NORMAL FINDINGS

WHAT TO EXPECT WHEN EXAMINING THE HEAD AND NECK

Use this review to confirm normal findings when examining the head and neck.

- Head round and symmetrical
- Scalp flesh colored, without scales, and covered with hair that is distributed evenly and is free from excess oils
- Skin firm, smooth, intact on head and neck; color distributed evenly
- Facial appearance symmetrical; palpebral fissures and distances between eyes and midline of nose are equal
- Eyes symmetrical, including placement, shape, and motility
- Eyelids free of drainage and edema, smooth and nontender to palpation (In older patients, ectropion or entropion can be a normal variant.)
- Lashes free of granulations or scales
- Lacrimal apparatus producing adequate tears, nontender, and free of discharge
- Conjunctiva clear and moist; sclera white and translucent; cornea smooth and transparent; iris flat and circular, with even bilateral pigmentation
- Pupils round, equal in size, and equally reactive to light and accommodation
- Nasal mucosa flat and slightly redder than oral mucosa; nasal septum midline
- Lips moist and free of cracks and fissures
- Symmetrical movement of uvula, tongue, and soft palate; positive gag reflex
- Auricles equal in height and size, symmetrically positioned, and able to move freely and painlessly (In the older patient, auricles may be more prominent and earlobes more pendulous.)
- External auditory canal patent and free of nodules, cysts, and drainage (A small amount of cerumen is normal.)
- Pulsation of the internal jugular vein visible and regular, changing with inspiration and expiration; no jugular distention
- Lymph nodes either nonpalpable or small, soft, and nontender
- Trachea midline without tugging
- Carotid pulse regular, full, and smooth

Assess your patient's head and neck by following these steps:

- Inspect and palpate the skin of the scalp and face for integrity. Look for any lesions or scars.
- Observe facial expressions for signs of distress or for the appearance of abnormal facies associated with disease. Observe the face for symmetry of structure and movement.
- Inspect the integrity of the mucous membranes of the nose and mouth.
- Inspect the placement and movement of the tongue, uvula, and soft palate. Check for the presence of a gag reflex.
- Inspect the neck for distention of the jugular vein, and estimate central venous pressure.

- Palpate for lymph node swelling in the preauricular and postauricular, submental and submandibular, and cervical chains located in and around the head and neck.
- Inspect and palpate the position and movement of the trachea.
- Auscultate for a carotid bruit and venous hum.
- Assess the symmetry and strength of neck and shoulder muscles.
- Inspect and palpate the eyes and associated structures for position, shape, and motility.
- Evaluate extraocular movements, observing for conjugate movement and any abnormal movements (e.g., nystagmus) in all six cardinal positions.
- Inspect pupil size, shape, and response to light and accommodation. After you use the penlight to test pupillary response, check the corneal reflections for bilateral symmetry.
- Inspect and palpate the external ear, noting skin color, texture, integrity, and any areas of tenderness. Note any drainage in the external ear canal.

EXAMINING THE CHEST AND BACK

During most of the chest and back examination, your patient should be sitting on the side of the bed or sitting up in bed. However, when auscultating heart sounds, ask your patient to lean forward or assume a left lateral recumbent position (see ▪ *What to Expect When Examining the Chest and Back*).

NORMAL FINDINGS

WHAT TO EXPECT WHEN EXAMINING THE CHEST AND BACK

Use this review to confirm normal findings when examining the chest and back.

- Anterior-posterior (AP) thorax diameter less than transverse diameter by nearly half
- Respirations even, regular, and unlabored, without use of accessory muscles
- Skin warm, dry, and free of lesions, masses, and areas of tenderness
- Spinal column straight, without obvious deformity
- Respiratory excursion equal bilaterally
- Point of maximum cardiac impulse felt for a radius of no more than 1 cm at the fifth intercostal space, midclavicular line
- Bronchial sounds over the trachea
- Bronchovesicular sounds over the mainstem bronchus posteriorly between scapulae
- Vesicular breath sounds throughout remaining lung fields
- S_1 heard loudest at apex of heart and S_2 heard loudest at base; splitting of S_2 on inspiration
- Costovertebral angle nontender

Assess your patient's chest and back by following these steps:

- Inspect skin integrity and color of the chest and back.
- Watch for the use of accessory muscles as the patient breathes.
- Assess anterior-posterior (AP) and lateral dimensions of the thorax to evaluate thoracic shape.
- Inspect the precordium for pulsations, and palpate the anterior chest for thrills. Locate the position and strength of the point of maximum impulse.
- Inspect the spinal column for curvature and obvious deformity.
- Evaluate respiratory excursion to observe equality of lung expansion.

- Auscultate the anterior chest for heart sounds.
- Auscultate the chest and back for the presence and quality of breath sounds.
- Palpate or use blunt percussion at the costovertebral angle to check for tenderness that may indicate pyelonephritis.

EXAMINING THE UPPER EXTREMITIES

When examining the upper extremities, have your patient sit up. However, if necessary, she can be supine (see ✂ *What to Expect When Examining the Upper Extremities*).

NORMAL FINDINGS

WHAT TO EXPECT WHEN EXAMINING THE UPPER EXTREMITIES

Use this review to confirm normal findings when examining the upper extremities.

- Skin warm and smooth, with minimal moisture
- Skin color matching rest of body, except normal areas of pigmentation, such as freckles (Skin color may be darker than on the torso if the upper extremities are routinely exposed to sunlight.)
- Upper extremities with no edema or obvious deformity. Radial, ulnar, and brachial pulses are easily palpated and bilaterally equal in strength and amplitude.
- Capillary refill brisk, less than 4 seconds
- Full range of motion (ROM) in all upper extremity joints without any pain
- Upper extremities and shoulder muscles with symmetrical strength bilaterally
- Handgrip strength equal bilaterally
- Deep tendon reflexes (DTRs) in brachioradialis, biceps, and triceps, measuring ++ bilaterally
- Infraclavicular and epitrochlear lymph nodes either nonpalpable or small, soft, mobile, and nontender

---

Assess your patient's upper extremities by following these steps:

- Inspect the upper extremities for color and any obvious deformity, such as shortening of one arm, edema, disruption of skin integrity, or muscle atrophy.
- Palpate the upper extremities for temperature, moisture, and lesions.
- Palpate the radial, ulnar, and brachial pulses for rate, rhythm, and contour.
- Check the capillary refill of nail beds.
- Assess the range of motion (ROM) and bilateral strength of the patient's shoulders, upper arms, elbows, wrists, and hands. Palpate the joints, and listen for crepitation as the extremity flexes and extends.
- Palpate the infraclavicular and epitrochlear lymph nodes.
- Test deep tendon reflexes (DTRs), including the brachioradialis, biceps, and triceps.

EXAMINING THE ABDOMINAL REGION

While you examine the patient's abdominal region, she should be lying down with the knees gently flexed to relax the abdominal muscles (see ✂ *What to Expect When Examining the Abdominal Region*).

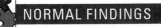

NORMAL FINDINGS

WHAT TO EXPECT WHEN EXAMINING THE ABDOMINAL REGION
Use this review to confirm normal findings when examining the abdominal region.
- Smooth, unbroken skin paler than other areas (if it has not been exposed to the sun); fine, visible venous network; no lesions or nodules (You may see striae from pregnancy or weight gain; they are usually pink or blue but over time become silvery white.)
- Symmetrical abdominal contour that is flat, rounded, or scaphoid (concave)
- Smooth, even movements during breathing (Abdominal movements during breathing are typically seen in males, whereas costal movements are seen in females.)
- Peristalsis not visible (A slight wavelike motion may be visible in thin patients.)
- Aortic pulsations (may be visible in thin patients)
- High-pitched bowel sounds at least every 15 seconds
- Palpation that reveals no masses or tenderness

Assess your patient's abdominal region by following these steps:
- Inspect the abdominal skin and surface for discoloration, scars, striae (stretch marks), lesions, nodules, or dilated veins. Inspect the umbilicus, noting its color, contour, and location. Look for signs of inflammation or herniation.
- Note abdominal contour, symmetry, and movement. Have the patient take a deep breath and hold it while you look for bulges or masses. Do the same as the patient raises the head off the mattress.
- Using the diaphragm of your stethoscope, auscultate for the presence and quality of bowel sounds.
- Using the bell of your stethoscope, listen over the umbilicus (aorta) and the renal arteries for bruits.
- Palpate the abdomen for tenderness and masses. First palpate lightly over all four quadrants. Then palpate deeply, using one or both hands (bimanual palpation). If you suspect peritoneal irritation, check for rebound tenderness.

EXAMINING THE LOWER EXTREMITIES
When examining the lower extremities, have your patient sit up on the side of the bed or in a chair (see ▧ *What to Expect When Examining the Lower Extremities*).

NORMAL FINDINGS

WHAT TO EXPECT WHEN EXAMINING THE LOWER EXTREMITIES
Use this review to confirm normal findings when examining the lower extremities.
- Skin warm and smooth, with minimal moisture
- Skin color matching the rest of the body, except for normal areas of pigmentation, such as freckles (Skin color may be darker than on the torso if the lower extremities are routinely exposed to sunlight.)
- Leg hair distributed symmetrically
- Lower extremities with no edema or obvious deformity

continued

NORMAL FINDINGS—cont'd

- Full range of motion (ROM) and painless in hip, knee, and ankle joints, as well as associated muscle groups
- Dorsalis pedis, posterior tibial, popliteal, and femoral pulses present and bilaterally equal in strength and amplitude
- Lower extremity muscles of equal strength bilaterally
- Deep tendon reflexes (DTRs) (patellar and Achilles) ++ bilaterally (A normal response for the plantar [Babinski] reflex is downward, with inward curling of toes.)
- Inguinal lymph nodes either nonpalpable or small, soft, mobile, and nontender

Assess your patient's lower extremities by following these steps:
- Observe for any obvious deformity, such as shortening of one leg, asymmetrical alignment, edema, disruption of skin integrity, or muscle atrophy. Note the skin temperature and color, as well as the quantity and distribution of hair.
- Palpate the femoral, popliteal, posterior tibial, and dorsalis pedis pulses.
- Palpate the inguinal lymph nodes for size, mobility, and tenderness.
- Test the hip, knee, and ankle joints and their associated muscle groups for ROM and strength.
- Test superficial reflexes and DTRs, including the plantar (Babinski), patellar, and Achilles.

KNOWING WHEN TO SHIFT GEARS

In performing a complete rapid physical examination, keep in mind that you may have to shift gears at any time, particularly if you discover an alarming abnormal finding.

Suppose, for example, you find that your patient's blood pressure is unusually low, say 80/40 mm Hg, and she begins to complain of feeling light-headed. No matter what else you are assessing, you will most likely want to focus your examination quickly on the possible causes of low blood pressure. You may want to examine your patient for signs of bleeding, dehydration, or cardiovascular compromise. Or, in some situations, your first step may be to call for help or notify the physician before proceeding with your examination.

You might also have to shift gears when it comes to your patient's comfort level. For example, if your patient is bedridden and has problems with mobility, you might want to assess the most accessible body parts (the front of the body) first before asking her to change positions. Whatever your approach, however, be sure it is systematic (head to toe and side to side), so you do not miss an important step.

Documenting Your Findings Accurately

Rapid changes in the health care environment have placed greater importance than ever before on documenting care. How crucial is nursing documentation? As an information-sharing tool and a link between disciplines in a health care facility, accurate, thorough, and timely documentation of a patient's history and your physical examination findings becomes the guide that all members of the health care team use when providing the patient's treatment and following his progress. Thorough, accurate documentation of the patient's physical, mental, and emotional condition is a fundamental nursing responsibility. Every time you document history and physical examination findings, interventions, or topics you have taught, you are helping to ensure the most effective treatment for your patient.

DOCUMENTING THE INITIAL ASSESSMENT

From a legal standpoint, documentation is the best protection the patient, health care team, and health care organization have. If you fail to record your health history and physical examination findings, interventions, and teaching, you are depriving other team members of information they need to treat patients effectively. In addition, you are putting yourself, your colleagues, and your employer in legal jeopardy. Remember, jurors rely heavily on what is documented in the medical records to determine if adequate care was provided. Most malpractice cases that involve nurses arise from possible failure to monitor a patient's condition or report changes in clinical status—situations that would not have arisen if the nurse had documented the patient's care properly.

ORGANIZING YOUR DATA

You no doubt recognize the importance of thoroughly documenting the health history and physical examination findings. However, it is not always easy to make documentation a priority. Time constraints may make other patient care activities seem more important, especially during a crisis. When you consider the amount of information you must record, you may be tempted to push documentation to the bottom of your must-do list.

You can make documentation less burdensome by organizing the information into these logical categories:

- What the patient tells you—information you obtain directly from the patient (or from indirect sources, if the patient is incapacitated)
- What you assess—physical examination findings (vital sign measurement, inspection, palpation, percussion, and auscultation)
- What you do and teach—interventions you perform in response to health history and physical examination findings, as well as instructions you give the patient and family

DOCUMENT WHAT THE PATIENT TELLS YOU

When obtaining the patient's health history, gather the following information:

- Current symptoms (chief complaint)
- Past health status
- Previous medical treatments
- Responses to those treatments

All these facts help the health care team identify successful interventions to incorporate into the treatment plan. Information you collect during the health history also serves as the basis of your teaching plan. By determining the patient's knowledge of his disorder, drugs, and health promotion measures, you can identify and prioritize appropriate teaching topics.

Identify the best information sources. Ideally, you should obtain information directly from the patient. In some situations (e.g., if your patient is unconscious), you will need to interview family members, refer to the patient's medical records, and consult other health care team members to find out what you need to know. Be sure to document as many details as you can, leaving no gaps or uncertainties that a retrospective review might reveal. If you are unable to obtain part of the health history, document the reason, such as the inability to communicate with the patient and the absence of family members.

Quote the patient directly. Record the patient's exact words, placing quotes around them. This helps others clearly differentiate his words from yours.

If your patient has allergies, document his description of the any allergic responses. (Keep in mind that what a patient reports as an allergy may be an expected or adverse effect of a drug.) Be sure to record information regarding patient allergies in as many places as possible and according to your facility's policies and procedures. At the very least, it should appear on the initial history and physical examination findings form, the medication administration record, the nursing plan of care, the front of the patient's chart, and the patient's identification band.

DOCUMENT WHAT YOU ASSESS

Next, document your findings from vital sign measurement, inspection, palpation, percussion, and auscultation. Describe abnormal findings in detail, paying special attention to those that relate to the patient's current condition. Also document findings related to symptoms the patient has denied. These pertinent negatives can be as useful as other data in determining the underlying problem.

Be objective and specific. Use objective language and avoid making judgments when documenting health history and physical examination data. For instance, if you write, "The patient's heart rate was only 60," this suggests that you think his heart rate is low.

Whenever possible, quantify your findings by citing specific numbers or ranges. Instead of "Mrs. Jones says she gets up a lot during the night to urinate," for example, write, "Mrs. Jones states she gets up seven or eight times during the night to urinate." Try to avoid phrases like *a little* and *a lot* because they are open to wide interpretation.

Be concrete. Describe only what you see, hear, feel, and smell during your history and physical examination. Do not document your interpretation of the patient's behavior. Instead of "Patient was crying because of his depression," for example, write, "Patient was crying during the physical examination." In addition, objectively document the patient's age, growth, physical abilities and limitations, and cognitive abilities (see 📖 *Documenting Growth and Developmental Information: What The Joint Commission Requires*).

LIFESPAN CONSIDERATIONS

DOCUMENTING GROWTH AND DEVELOPMENTAL INFORMATION: WHAT THE JOINT COMMISSION REQUIRES

The Joint Commission (formerly known as JCAHO) requires health care professionals to assess each hospitalized patient's physical, psychologic, and social status. In addition, The Joint Commission requires assessment of the patient's growth and development and the provision of age-appropriate care.

In most cases you will document growth and developmental needs as part of the admission assessment. The following examples show how you might document such needs for patients of various ages.

- Male, age 70—Mr. Harris talks about the recent loss of two close friends.
- Female, age 58, who has sustained a hip fracture—Ms. Robinson is concerned about her older uncle. She is the sole caregiver for the 88-year-old man and does not know how she will care for him now.
- Male, age 17, who has paraplegia—Billy describes his frustration with being dependent on his mother. He wants to attend a school on the West Coast and live in a dormitory.
- Male, age 2, with respiratory syncytial virus—Ryan cries for his mother and refuses to drink liquids.

DOCUMENT WHAT YOU DO AND TEACH

Your documentation should show that you took appropriate actions based on the health history and physical examination findings of the patient's condition. Try to record interventions as you perform them or soon afterward. Otherwise, you may forget to record important information. Note the time of each intervention to avoid the appearance that you took too long to intervene after assessing a significant finding.

Document the patient's response. Just because you have documented an intervention does not mean that your patient benefited from it. To indicate the effectiveness of an intervention, describe the patient's response (whether positive or negative). Be sure to evaluate the patient's emotional and physical responses.

Record referrals. Your documentation should indicate whether additional resources, such as home care, are needed, as well as any referrals you make to secure those resources. Record, too, your meetings with staff members from other disciplines who are involved in the patient's care. Also document the outcomes of discharge planning.

A patient's progress during your care and after discharge may depend on how well he understands his condition, treatment plan, and home care. When you document your teaching, clearly indicate your evaluation of the patient's understanding of the instructions you have provided. If you think that the patient needs additional instructions, note this so that other health care team members can cover that topic in their teaching.

HOW DOCUMENTATION HELPS YOU EVALUATE THE PLAN OF CARE

All the information you obtain from the health history and physical examination along with the nursing interventions and the patient's response to those interventions contribute to the plan of care. Thorough documentation helps you evaluate the plan and revise it as needed.

DOCUMENTING PRIORITY HEALTH PROBLEMS

Document initial information related to the patient's priority health problems. Follow up with documentation of ongoing health history and physical examination findings of parameters related to these problems. For example, if the patient has heart failure, you need to document ongoing findings related to the heart, lungs, peripheral pulses, and fluid balance.

Essential documentation for common priority health problems is presented in the sections that follow (see *Common Priority Health Problems*). Documentation of each problem is divided into the categories of *what the patient tells you, what you assess,* and *what you do and teach.*

COMMON PRIORITY HEALTH PROBLEMS

When documenting patient care, you will focus on what the patient tells you, what you assess, and what you do and teach. To help guide you through specific situations you may encounter in your daily practice, refer to the information that explains what to document when your patient experiences the following:
- Loss of a peripheral pulse
- Chest pain
- Myocardial infarction (MI)
- Heart failure
- Pneumonia

- Asthma attack
- Pulmonary embolism
- Pulmonary edema
- Pulmonary tuberculosis (TB)
- Severe pain
- Confusion
- Seizure
- Cerebrovascular accident (CVA)
- Hypoglycemia
- Hyperglycemia
- Pressure ulcer
- Surgery

WHEN YOUR PATIENT LOSES A PERIPHERAL PULSE

Loss of a peripheral pulse may signal interruption of circulation (a potentially life-threatening event). If your assessment reveals this finding, you will need to act rapidly. Besides reviewing your patient's medical history, you must quickly evaluate current health status. You will also need to notify the physician and record your findings accurately to ensure prompt, effective treatment.

DOCUMENT WHAT THE PATIENT TELLS YOU

Record an abbreviated version of the patient's medical history, especially noting a previous diagnosis of peripheral vascular disease, diabetes mellitus, heart disease, arterial occlusive disease, or other disorders that may predispose the patient to an arterial occlusion. If the patient reports chronic skin ulcers, injury, trauma, surgery, or wounds in the affected area, record that information. Pinpoint the exact location of the affected area, record the duration of the problem, and detail treatments the patient has received for the condition.

Next, document reports of pain, weakness, numbness, tingling, and decreased sensation in the arm or leg that has lost the pulse. Determine if the patient's symptoms are relieved by rest, and note this in the medical record. Also document other symptoms, even if they seem unrelated to the absent pulse. Because decreased circulation in an arm or leg may reflect a systemic problem, you will need to check for and document signs and symptoms of reduced cardiac output, such as hypotension, decreased level of consciousness (LOC), and chest pain.

DOCUMENT WHAT YOU ASSESS

Although signs and symptoms vary with the cause of the absent peripheral pulse, you can expect the following abnormal findings in the affected arm or leg:
- Weakness
- Pain
- Numbness
- Tingling

- Discolored nail beds or skin
- Edema
- Sluggish capillary refill
- Cool skin

Make sure you describe the affected arm or leg in detail, including its circumference, skin temperature and appearance, nail bed color, briskness of capillary refill, and the patient's ability to move the arm or leg.

Next, compare the affected arm or leg with the opposite one, and record your findings to help determine the circulatory status of the pulseless arm or leg. Measure the circumference of both arms or legs at two or more places (see *Documenting Your Measurements*).

DOCUMENTING YOUR MEASUREMENTS

If your patient loses the peripheral pulse, the circumference of the involved arm or leg may change. Change in circumference may indicate whether the underlying condition is improving or worsening. To ensure accurate assessment over time, always measure the arm or leg at exactly the same location each time and thoroughly document the location you are using.

When possible, mark the patient's skin at the top and bottom edges of the measuring tape. If you are using such skin markings as a guide, note this in your documentation. For instance, you might write, "Right leg circumference: 30 inches midthigh, 20 inches midcalf, measured using skin markings."

If you cannot mark the patient's skin, refer to an easy-to-find landmark to indicate where you took the measurement. For a thigh measurement, you might use the bend of the knee, as the following example shows: "Placed bottom edge of measuring tape on right anterior thigh, 6 inches above bend of knee."

You can also use a preprinted diagram to document measurement sites or to indicate skin abnormalities. To record a wound's location, for example, you can indicate its color and size in the margin. If the patient has multiple areas of skin breakdown, assign a number or letter to each area and then reference the areas in the narrative section of your note. For instance, you

may write, "Cultures taken from right leg wound A." You can also indicate changes in skin color or temperature on the human outline.

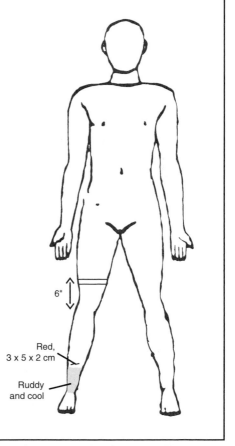

From Mosby: *Surefire documentation: how, what, and when nurses need to document,* St Louis, 1999, Mosby.

Then, using a Doppler device if possible, auscultate for a pulse in the arm or leg. Record the presence or absence of a bruit. If you see an open area or a break in the skin, document its location, size, and color and carefully describe the lesion's edges. Also document the amount, color, and odor of drainage.

Next, record information that might help determine the cause of the pulse loss. To do this, measure the apical pulse and determine if a pulse deficit exists; assess LOC; measure blood pressure; evaluate urine output; and note dyspnea, chest or back pain, abdominal pain or distention, and nausea or vomiting. These assessments may help identify the cause of the lost pulse, such as shock, hemorrhage, or aneurysm.

DOCUMENT WHAT YOU DO AND TEACH

As you intervene during the patient's acute illness and recovery, use the information below to guide your documentation and tailor the written plan of care to the patient's needs. Your documentation should also include the teaching you provide to help your patient prevent the underlying condition from recurring. Be sure to include the following, as needed:

- Ongoing monitoring of the affected arm or leg, along with vital signs
- Removal of a constricting item, such as a bandage
- Drugs and intravenous (IV) therapy
- Proper positioning
- Active or passive range-of-motion (ROM) exercises
- Antiembolism stockings
- Disease process
- Diagnostic tests
- Interventional procedures
- Precautions and follow-up tests for anticoagulation
- Activity
- Proper positioning of the arm or leg
- Avoidance of constrictive clothing, leg crossing, and staying in one position for prolonged periods
- Smoking cessation
- Proper nutrition
- Signs and symptoms to report
- Wound and skin care
- Scheduled follow-up visits

WHEN YOUR PATIENT HAS CHEST PAIN

Because chest pain may indicate a myocardial infarction (MI) or another potentially fatal condition, always take this symptom seriously. Act quickly to perform a focused assessment and intervene promptly as indicated. Remember, documentation of your assessment findings must convey the essential information the health care team needs to guide treatment, especially when your patient's life is in danger.

DOCUMENT WHAT THE PATIENT TELLS YOU

When documenting your patient's chest pain, record his exact description of this symptom, placing quotes around the patient's words. Ask the patient to rate pain severity on a scale of 0 to 10, with 0 representing *no pain* and 10 representing *the worst pain imaginable.*

Then have the patient point to the exact pain location and document his response. Ask if the pain radiates to other parts of the body, such as the jaws, shoulders, arms, or back. Document accompanying symptoms the patient reports, such as shortness of breath and nausea. Whenever possible, record the patient's own words, not your interpretation of them.

Next, document the pain's duration. Ask when the pain started and whether it is steady or intermittent. Determine if the patient has had chest pain before. If the patient has, ask him to compare the current pain with that in previous episodes. Carefully document this response.

Ask whether any factor (e.g., activity, stress, exposure to cold), triggered the chest pain. Find out if anything makes it better (e.g., rest, nitroglycerin) or worse (e.g., breathing deeply). Assess and document the patient's emotional status, noting, for instance, if he is anxious or reports a feeling of impending doom.

Health history. Document pertinent health history information, such as a history of heart disease, hypertension, or hypercholesterolemia. Note other risk factors for heart disease, such as a family history of heart disease, advanced age, history of smoking, diabetes mellitus, obesity, and a sedentary or stressful lifestyle. Document the use of estrogen or oral contraceptives. In addition, record chronic diseases, hospitalizations, procedures, and surgeries the patient reports.

Obtain a drug history, recording the names, doses, and administration times and routes for all drugs the patient uses. Record the time and amount of the last dose of each. Document drug and other allergies the patient reports.

DOCUMENT WHAT YOU ASSESS

Measure the patient's vital signs, especially noting tachycardia or bradycardia, an increased respiratory rate, and abnormally high or low blood pressure. Record your auscultation of heart sounds, including the presence of extra heart sounds or murmurs. If you hear abnormal sounds, note the stethoscope location, such as the fifth intercostal space, midclavicular line. Document whether the patient's heart rate is regular or irregular.

Then document patient actions (e.g., guarding, holding the chest) and behaviors (e.g., anxiety, restlessness) that suggest the patient is in pain. Note changes in mental status, too, such as decreased LOC, disorientation, and confusion.

Next, evaluate the patient's respiratory rate and pattern. Then record information regarding dyspnea, the patient's use of accessory breathing muscles, and any jugular vein distention. Obtain and document the patient's pulse oximetry reading. Then assess his skin, recording such abnormalities as coolness, clamminess, pallor, and cyanosis.

Arrange for the patient to undergo a baseline 12-lead electrocardiogram (ECG). Then review it with the physician to detect abnormal rhythms and other changes. Place a copy of the tracing at the bedside for quick comparison during future ECG evaluations.

DOCUMENT WHAT YOU DO AND TEACH

As you intervene during the patient's acute illness and recovery, expect to implement and document general interventions, as well as interventions specific to the underlying condition. As always, document your interventions and the patient's responses. Also, tailor the teaching plan to your patient's condition and treatment. Be sure to include the following, as needed:

- Diagnostic tests
- Fluid intake and output
- Oxygen therapy
- Continuous cardiac monitoring
- Drug and IV therapy
- Activity
- Emotional support
- Transfer to the intensive care unit (ICU)
- Hemodynamic monitoring
- Heart anatomy and physiology
- Disease process
- Interventional treatments
- Signs and symptoms to report
- Actions to take when chest pain occurs
- Cardiac risk factor reduction
- Nutrition
- Activity
- Resources for further information and support

WHEN YOUR PATIENT HAS A MYOCARDIAL INFARCTION

When caring for a patient who is experiencing an MI, accurate documentation can be as critical as rapid response. Your documentation can help ensure effective emergency treatment. It also helps tailor the plan of care to the patient's specific needs.

DOCUMENT WHAT THE PATIENT TELLS YOU

In this emergency you probably will not have time to gather and document a complete health history. However, once the crisis has passed, be sure to question the patient or a family member, or check medical records to obtain pertinent information.

To begin, determine if the patient has a history of atherosclerosis, coronary artery disease, or hyperlipoproteinemia. If so, record the date the condition was diagnosed and its treatment, including drugs, activity guidelines, and dietary restrictions. If the patient smokes cigarettes or did so in the past, record the number of packs smoked per day and the number of years the patient has smoked.

If the patient reports a history of hypertension and knows his most recent systolic and diastolic readings, document these readings to provide a baseline for comparison with current values. Record whether the patient complies with the hypertension treatment plan.

Find out if the patient has a history of diabetes mellitus. If so, record the date of diagnosis and the details of his treatment plan, including the type and dose of the oral antidiabetic drug or insulin taken. To help determine the effectiveness of diabetes treatment, document how often the patient monitors his blood glucose level at home, which methods he uses, and his most recent blood glucose level.

Then record the patient's reported activity level, including the types of activity and exercise performed and the number of days per week the patient exercises. If the patient describes a sedentary lifestyle, record this fact. Document the patient's weight and recent history of weight loss or gain.

If the patient has a family history of heart disease, note which family members are affected.

If the patient reports a previous MI, record the date and any complications. To aid your assessment of previous MI treatments and the patient's response, review the past medical record and document pertinent findings.

Next, document recent reports of crushing, substernal chest pain that radiates to the left arm, jaw, neck, or shoulder blades. Ask the patient to rate the pain's severity on a scale of 0 to 10, with 0 representing *no pain* and 10 representing *the worst pain imaginable.* Document this response, along with the time the pain started and factors that seem to improve or worsen it.

Ask if the patient recently had symptoms that typically precede or accompany an MI: indigestion or heartburn; more frequent angina attacks; feelings of impending doom; increased fatigue; and episodes of nausea, vomiting, or shortness of breath. Document this response fully. Discuss with the physician significant information you gather during the health history interview.

DOCUMENT WHAT YOU ASSESS

Although signs and symptoms of MI vary among patients, you should assess for and document the following expected abnormal findings:

- Anxiety
- Restlessness
- Dyspnea
- Tachypnea
- Diaphoresis
- Jugular vein distention
- Cool, mottled skin
- Diminished peripheral pulses
- S_4 or S_3 (abnormal heart sounds)
- Paradoxical splitting of S_2
- Systolic murmur
- Pericardial friction rub
- Low-grade fever

- Tachycardia and hypertension (with an anterior MI)
- Bradycardia and hypotension (with an inferior MI)

DOCUMENT WHAT YOU DO AND TEACH

As you intervene during the patient's acute illness and recovery, document care and teaching related to the following topics:

- Diagnostic tests
- Fluid intake and output
- Oxygen therapy
- Continuous cardiac monitoring
- Drug and IV therapy
- Activity
- Emotional support
- Transfer to the ICU
- Hemodynamic monitoring
- Heart anatomy and physiology
- Disease process
- Interventional treatments
- Signs and symptoms for the patient to report
- Actions to take when chest pain occurs
- Cardiac risk factor reduction
- Nutrition
- Smoking cessation
- Cardiac rehabilitation
- Resources for further information and support

WHEN YOUR PATIENT HAS HEART FAILURE

Successful management of heart failure focuses on three essential goals: (1) maintaining fluid balance, (2) controlling symptoms, and (3) recognizing warning signs of complications. Thorough documentation helps the health care team determine effective interventions and create a long-range treatment plan for your patient.

DOCUMENT WHAT THE PATIENT TELLS YOU

When obtaining your patient's health history, assess for and document signs, symptoms, and risk factors that could contribute to heart failure. If the patient has a history of heart failure, collect information about any past treatments received, noting their effectiveness.

Ask the patient to relate his medical history, especially heart or circulatory diseases. Along with this information, record the date of each diagnosis and treatment received.

Document past or present signs and symptoms of heart failure the patient describes, and note whether the patient has new or worsening symptoms. In particular, ask about shortness of breath, edema, cough, tachycardia, chest pain, orthopnea, and fatigue. Record this response in detail.

As necessary, ask the patient to elaborate on his symptoms. For example, if the patient says he gets tired from walking shorter and shorter distances, ask him how far he can walk now before tiring compared with how far he could walk previously. Your documentation might read, "Patient states that up to 1 week ago he could walk up to one block before feeling slightly short of breath. Now he becomes short of breath after walking about 10 feet."

Next, elicit and record information about the patient's diet and recent dietary changes. Document your assessment of the patient's sodium, fat, and cholesterol intake, as well as his understanding of how an improper diet can contribute to heart disease. Note whether the patient has gained or lost weight recently and whether he weighs himself at the same time each day.

Ask about urination patterns, and document recent changes in urine output and frequency of urination. Also inquire about the patient's daily fluid intake and document this answer.

If the patient reports a history of hypertension, document this along with the most recent blood pressure reading, if known. Record the names and doses of drugs the patient is using and his perception of the reason for using each one. In addition, document whether the patient complies with the prescribed drug regimen. Using the patient's own words, record exactly how he uses the drugs. Finally, document recent changes in the amount of daily activity, and determine if the patient has been under new or unusual stress.

DOCUMENT WHAT YOU ASSESS

Perform and document a thorough physical assessment to establish a baseline. As treatment progresses, your documentation will help the health care team track the patient's condition.

Vital signs. Record the patient's pulse, respiratory rate, and blood pressure every 4 hours (more often if they are unstable). Document whom you notified and how you intervened for abnormal values and changes, especially tachycardia, tachypnea, and hypotension. When measuring vital signs, also document daily weights (a valuable indicator of fluid gain or loss for a patient with heart failure).

Respiratory system. Auscultate the patient's lungs every 1 to 2 hours. Document adventitious breath sounds and changes from the previous assessment—especially increased congestion and decreased air movement. Notify the physician of changes indicative of a worsening condition, and document that you did so.

Then evaluate for and record the use of accessory breathing muscles and signs and symptoms of decreased perfusion and hypoxia. Document the time dyspnea occurs and precipitating factors. Ask the patient if anything has improved the dyspnea in the past, and record his answer.

Cardiovascular system. Check for jugular vein distention. When documenting this finding, include the degree of distention. Document your assessment of heart sounds every 1 to 2 hours. Be sure to record abnormal sounds, especially S_3 or a prominent systolic murmur, which may indicate fluid overload.

Tissue perfusion. Next, record indicators of decreased tissue perfusion, especially pallor, diaphoresis, and cool, clammy skin. Also note confusion and decreased LOC, which may signal decreased cardiac output.

Fluid balance. Assess for and document signs and symptoms of fluid overload. If the patient has edema, note its location and whether it is pitting or nonpitting. Record the degree of pitting, if present. Document changes from the previous assessment.

DOCUMENT WHAT YOU DO AND TEACH

As you intervene to manage the patient's heart failure, document exactly what you did, when you did it, and the patient's response. This helps you identify effective interventions and refine your plan of care as needed. In addition, document all teaching you provide, along with measurable indicators of the patient's understanding. Be sure your interventions, teaching, and documentation include the following topics:

• IV insertion
• Drug and IV therapy
• Oxygen therapy
• Cardiac and hemodynamic monitoring
• Heart anatomy, physiology, and disease process
• Fluid intake and output
• Daily weight
• Nutrition, including dietary or fluid restrictions and referral to a dietitian
• Signs and symptoms to report
• Activity limitations
• Diagnostic tests
• Home monitoring, such as blood pressure measurement and Holter monitoring

WHEN YOUR PATIENT HAS PNEUMONIA

Documentation for a patient with pneumonia can help him avoid complications, promote progress toward self-care, and prevent recurrences. During the health history interview and physical examination, stay alert for risk factors or other conditions that make the patient vulnerable to the disease.

DOCUMENT WHAT THE PATIENT TELLS YOU

Ask the patient to describe his symptoms and document them using his own words. Record the time of symptom onset, noting whether it was sudden or gradual. Ask about and record associated symptoms, such as fever, chills, cough, sputum production, weakness, fatigue, pain, and anorexia.

Risk factors. To further identify risk factors for pneumonia, note the patient's age and ask about a history of recent hospitalizations, surgery, chronic conditions, cardiopulmonary disease, immunosuppressive therapy, decreased LOC, and past bouts of pneumonia. Be sure to record complaints of difficulty eating, chewing, or swallowing, which predispose the patient to developing aspiration pneumonia. Document whether the patient has received a pneumococcal vaccine. If so, note the administration date.

Finally, record the patient's report of allergies to drugs, foods, chemicals, and environmental elements, such as dust, pollen, and pets.

Pain. Document chest pain, headache, or other pain your patient reports. Using the patient's own words, record the pain's characteristics, including intensity and duration. Note factors that the patient says make the pain better (e.g., splinting the chest while coughing, applying heat) or worse (e.g., coughing, breathing deeply).

DOCUMENT WHAT YOU ASSESS

Assess and record the patient's vital sign measurements every 4 hours or more often if he is unstable. If you detect a fever, tachycardia, tachypnea, or hypotension, document the finding, notify the physician, and document your notification. Record all laboratory test results you obtain, such as arterial blood gas (ABG) levels.

Respiratory status. Record the respiratory rate and rhythm. Then auscultate for breath sounds, and document abnormalities, such as diminished breath sounds, wheezes, or crackles. Next, record percussion findings, such as areas of dullness, which may indicate consolidation. Also record other findings, including dyspnea, nasal flaring, use of accessory breathing muscles, and abnormal breathing patterns.

If the patient has a cough, document its frequency and its effectiveness in clearing secretions. If the cough is productive, describe the amount of sputum produced, frequency of sputum production, as well as sputum color, odor, and other characteristics.

Oxygenation. Record physical findings that reflect the patient's oxygenation, such as nail bed color and respiratory effort. Record pulse oximetry readings at the time of your initial assessment. Then obtain and document oximetry readings whenever the patient's condition changes or as required by the physician or facility policy. If the patient is receiving supplemental oxygen, note the amount of oxygen being administered at the time of the oximetry reading, along with the oxygen flow rate and delivery device. Do the same when recording ABG levels. Always record and report significant levels or important changes from previous ABG levels.

Next, document the patient's skin color, turgor, and temperature, as well as capillary refill. Particularly note diaphoresis, pallor, and cyanosis, which may signal decreased oxygenation.

Finally, document your patient's LOC. Stay especially alert for confusion or disorientation—a sign of hypoxia or hypercapnia—and report this immediately.

DOCUMENT WHAT YOU DO AND TEACH

Record your interventions and teaching as you initiate them. This helps show that you provided timely and appropriate care, which may prove legally significant if the patient's care becomes an issue for litigation. Be sure to include the following, as needed:

• Frequent monitoring
• Oxygen therapy
• Pulse oximetry
• Fluid intake and output
• Drug and IV therapy
• Diagnostic tests
• Promoting coughing and deep breathing; performing chest physiotherapy and suctioning
• Nutrition
• Activity
• Disease process
• Infection prevention
• Signs and symptoms for the patient to report
• Recommended preventive vaccines
• Hydration
• Resources for further information and support

WHEN YOUR PATIENT HAS AN ASTHMA ATTACK

Potentially life threatening, an acute asthma attack calls for prompt, accurate assessment and expert intervention, as well as complete documentation of these actions. To avoid future asthma attacks and help maintain an optimal activity level, the patient also needs effective teaching. Thorough documentation of assessment, interventions, and teaching directs the plan of care during the acute episode. It can also help safeguard long-term health.

DOCUMENT WHAT THE PATIENT TELLS YOU

Even after stabilizing a patient with an acute asthma attack, difficulty breathing and speaking may prevent him from supplying information. If the patient can nod or shake the head, ask essential yes-or-no questions and record his responses. If a family member or friend accompanies the patient, obtain information from that person.

Then check the patient's medical record for data about a history of asthma or other respiratory problems, current drug use, and allergies. Be sure to note whether the patient uses oxygen, a nebulizer, or an inhaler at home, and document whether he is taking a steroid to treat asthma. If he is, record the dose and the date the patient started taking it. Also find out if the patient takes peak-flow measurements at home. Ask about and document the best measurement.

Next, record data about the current asthma attack, including its onset, duration, and accompanying symptoms. Ask the patient or his companion how often the patient experiences asthma attacks and whether the current episode differs from previous attacks. Carefully document the answers. Then identify and record recent exposure to irritants, such as smoke, allergens, and chemicals. Ask about symptoms of recent respiratory tract infections, such as fever and productive cough. In addition, document the treatments that have helped terminate previous asthma attacks.

DOCUMENT WHAT YOU ASSESS

Record your findings from a rapid assessment. Describe the following expected abnormal findings, if present, and any others you detect:

- Wheezing and dyspnea
- Diminished or absent breath sounds
- Difficulty speaking or performing activities (from dyspnea)
- Tachypnea
- Use of accessory breathing muscles
- Productive cough
- Tachycardia
- Hypotension
- Anxiety and diaphoresis
- Signs of decreased oxygenation, such as cyanosis
- Change in LOC

Record pulse oximetry readings, ABG levels, and peak-flow measurements if available.

DOCUMENT WHAT YOU DO AND TEACH

To prevent the asthma attack from progressing, intervene rapidly and record your actions as you take them. Expect to implement and document some or all of the following interventions and teaching points:

- Oxygen administration
- Pulse oximetry
- Nebulizer or inhaler administration
- Drug and IV therapy
- Diagnostic tests
- Upright positioning
- Breathing and relaxation techniques
- Energy conservation
- Emotional support
- Respiratory system anatomy and physiology
- Disease process
- Peak-flow measurements
- What to do if peak-flow measurements worsen or if an acute asthma attack occurs
- Use of a prescribed metered-dose inhaler, dry powder inhaler, or nebulizer
- Care of an inhaler and other respiratory equipment used at home
- Signs and symptoms to report
- Hygiene and infection prevention
- Allergen avoidance
- Breathing techniques
- Identifying and avoiding precipitating factors
- Pacing activities with rest
- Dietary and fluid recommendations
- Stress management and relaxation techniques
- Resources for further information and support

WHEN YOUR PATIENT HAS A PULMONARY EMBOLISM

Without prompt assessment and treatment, pulmonary embolism can lead to serious complications and, possibly, death. If you believe the patient has experienced a pulmonary embolism, notify the physician at once and take emergency steps to safeguard the patient's life. Then, as soon as possible, document the findings that led you to consider pulmonary embolism.

When the patient's condition allows, review the history for factors that predispose the patient to this disorder. Then perform a thorough physical examination, focusing on respiratory status and oxygenation. To show efficient nursing care and ensure clear communication with the rest of the health care team, document your interventions as you initiate them, along with the patient's response.

DOCUMENT WHAT THE PATIENT TELLS YOU

Record predisposing factors that the patient reports, such as a history of recent surgery, MI, heart failure, atrial fibrillation, venous insufficiency, thrombophlebitis, polycythemia vera, chronic illness, trauma, and immobilization after a fracture. Add other risk factors that you note, such as smoking, advanced age, and obesity. For a female patient, note recent pregnancy, childbirth, oral contraceptive use, and estrogen replacement therapy.

If the patient reports chest pain, ask him to describe it in detail and record the answer in his own words. Include its precise location and time of onset. Record the patient's rating of pain severity on a scale of 0 to 10, with 0 representing *no pain* and 10 representing *the worst pain imaginable.* Ask about and record factors that the patient says make the pain worse (e.g., breathing deeply, coughing) or better (e.g., lying still, splinting the chest while coughing). If the patient reports shortness of breath, document when this symptom was first noticed. Also assess and record the patient's anxiety level and if he reports a sense of impending doom.

DOCUMENT WHAT YOU ASSESS

Focus assessment and documentation on the patient's respiratory status and oxygenation. If you believe that a blood disorder has contributed to the pulmonary embolism, check the most recent hemoglobin, erythrocyte, and thrombocyte values. Document that you notified the physician of abnormal values, along with the notification time and the physician's orders. In addition, if you think the patient has deep vein thrombosis (DVT) that has embolized to the pulmonary vasculature, check the calves for evidence of erythema and edema. Note if the patient reports calf pain on dorsiflexion of the foot (Homans' sign), but refrain from performing the maneuver because of the risk of dislodging a clot.

Respiratory system. Document your assessment of the patient's respiratory status every 1 to 2 hours or as appropriate. Include respiratory rate and rhythm, chest expansion characteristics (e.g., asymmetry), as well as any hyperpnea, dyspnea, shallow breathing, or accessory muscle use.

Record the time of breath sound auscultation, noting such abnormalities as diminished breath sounds, wheezes, crackles, and friction rub. Document whether the patient has a cough. If the cough is productive, describe the amount of sputum produced and its characteristics.

DOCUMENT WHAT YOU DO AND TEACH

Act quickly to help the patient with a pulmonary embolism maintain adequate oxygenation and gas exchange. Try to document each intervention as you perform it, and then record the patient's response to your care and the teaching you provide. Be sure to cover the following areas:

- Oxygen therapy
- Vital sign measurements and pulse oximetry readings
- Drug and IV therapy
- Proper positioning
- Energy conservation
- Comfort measures
- Emotional support and anxiety relief
- Respiratory system anatomy and physiology
- Disease process
- Signs and symptoms of respiratory insufficiency
- Dietary restrictions
- Bleeding precautions
- Signs and symptoms to report
- Diagnostic tests
- Antiembolism stockings

WHEN YOUR PATIENT HAS PULMONARY EDEMA

Accurate documentation helps identify the cause of pulmonary edema and guides the health care team toward the most effective treatment. Pulmonary edema can rapidly progress to respiratory failure. By focusing your documentation on the key points described here, you can help your patient avert this acute emergency.

DOCUMENT WHAT THE PATIENT TELLS YOU

As necessary, gather information from the patient, family members, and existing medical records. In particular, document reports of chest pain. Using the patient's own words, record the pain's exact location, time of onset, duration, severity (on a scale of 0 to 10, with 0 representing *no pain* and 10 representing *the worst pain imaginable*), exacerbating factors (e.g., taking a deep breath), and alleviating factors (e.g., sitting upright).

Also check for and record preexisting cardiac or respiratory conditions that can precipitate pulmonary edema, past episodes of heart failure or acute respiratory distress syndrome, and a history of other predisposing factors, such as kidney or liver disease. Then record the names of drugs the patient reports taking and the allergies he describes.

DOCUMENT WHAT YOU ASSESS

During the acute crisis, record the patient's vital sign measurements frequently and obtain his weight daily. In addition, thoroughly document the crucial findings described here.

Respiratory system and oxygenation. Document your frequent auscultation of the patient's breath sounds, including adventitious sounds (e.g., crackles, wheezes). Note dyspnea, labored breathing, and use of accessory breathing muscles. Also document whether the patient has a cough. If the patient does have a cough, check for sputum production and describe the amount, color, and odor of the sputum, as well as other characteristics.

Then record significant skin findings, such as diaphoresis, abnormal temperature, clamminess, and cyanosis. Look for and document signs and symptoms of hypoxia, such as anxiety and restlessness. If the patient becomes short of breath during activity, record this fact. Indicate how much activity he can tolerate before becoming short of breath and how long it takes for his to recover a normal breathing pattern after rest. Also note if he has difficulty lying flat.

Finally, check for peripheral edema. Document its location, note any pitting, and record the degree of the pitting.

Cardiovascular system. Because pulmonary edema stresses the heart, document signs and symptoms of cardiac compromise. Record auscultation of heart sounds, noting decreased or abnormal sounds, such as an S_3. Document the quality of the pulse, which may be bounding in pulmonary edema. Also document that you assessed for jugular vein distention.

DOCUMENT WHAT YOU DO AND TEACH

Record your interventions as soon as possible after you implement them and be sure to document everything you teach. Keep these topics in mind as you intervene and teach:

- Airway, breathing, and circulation maintenance
- Oxygen therapy
- Continuous cardiac monitoring
- Pulse oximetry
- Diagnostic testing
- Drug and IV therapy
- Emotional support and anxiety relief
- Proper positioning
- Fluid balance
- Fluid intake and output
- Hemodynamic monitoring
- Heart and respiratory system anatomy and physiology
- Disease process
- Dietary and fluid restrictions
- Treatment procedures
- Oxygen and energy conservation techniques
- Signs and symptoms for the patient to report

WHEN YOUR PATIENT HAS PULMONARY TUBERCULOSIS

Documenting care for a patient with pulmonary tuberculosis (TB) can have far-reaching effects. Besides helping to ensure that the patient receives proper care, it can prevent the disease from being transmitted to others. By assessing and recording the patient's history, lifestyle, past treatments, and knowledge of TB and its transmission, you can evaluate risk for developing active disease and infecting others. Your interventions and teaching plan can then address these risks.

DOCUMENT WHAT THE PATIENT TELLS YOU

When obtaining the patient's medical history, be sure to elicit and record information about past pulmonary or infectious diseases and other respiratory conditions. If he has undergone a tuberculin skin test (intradermal injection of purified protein derivative [PPD]), record the test date and result. If the PPD reaction was positive, document other tests the patient has undergone, such as chest radiographs and sputum tests, and their results. Find out if the patient has been treated for TB before. If so, determine the dates and duration of treatment, names of all prescribed drugs, and the patient's compliance with treatment.

Then record current or recent symptoms your patient reports, including chronic cough, fever, chills, night sweats, bloody or purulent sputum, chest pain, weight loss, malaise, and anorexia.

Risk factors. Elicit and document your patient's risk factors for TB, such as a family history of the disease. Describe living arrangements, especially if the patient lives in an institution, community residence, nursing home, or shelter. Note whether the patient has spent time in prison, in a shelter, in the military, or as a homeless person. Record other risk factors, such as a history of alcoholism, IV drug use, and positive human immunodeficiency virus (HIV) status.

Document other risk factors you uncover, such as advanced age, a job in health care or day care, recent travel outside the country, or a condition that increases the risk of TB (e.g., malnutrition, chemotherapy, steroid or immunosuppressive therapy, chronic renal failure, other chronic disease, recent loss of more than 10% of body weight).

DOCUMENT WHAT YOU ASSESS

A patient who tests positive on a TB skin test does not necessarily have active TB. Your assessment can help determine the diagnosis and guide the interventions.

When performing and documenting a complete nursing assessment, focus on the following expected abnormal findings:
- Cough
- Fever
- Hemoptysis or purulent sputum
- Adventitious breath sounds
- Dyspnea
- Hoarseness
- Tachycardia
- Poor nutritional status

DOCUMENT WHAT YOU DO AND TEACH

Your teaching, the patient's understanding, and documentation of your interventions are crucial in preventing pulmonary TB transmission. Make sure that your interventions, teaching, and documentation include the following topics:

- Isolation procedures, including a double-door isolation room with negative-pressure ventilation
- Reporting to the local health authority and hospital infection control department
- Prevention of disease transmission
- Drug and IV therapy
- Oxygen therapy
- Pulse oximetry
- Assistance with positioning, turning, coughing, and deep breathing
- Suctioning, including proper care and disposal of suction equipment
- Diagnostic tests
- Drug compliance
- Nutrition
- Hygiene and infection prevention, including hand washing
- Proper disposal of sputum and tissues
- Follow-up testing
- Signs and symptoms for the patient to report
- Testing of family members and close contacts

WHEN YOUR PATIENT HAS SEVERE PAIN

For a patient in severe pain, developing the plan of care hinges on careful assessment, appropriate interventions, and thorough evaluation of the patient's response. Documentation plays an important role in tailoring the plan to your patient's needs. It also communicates vital information to other health care team members so that they can devise an effective pain management plan.

DOCUMENT WHAT THE PATIENT TELLS YOU

Obtain and record a thorough health history from the patient. Include all possible sources of pain, such as chronic diseases, illnesses, and surgeries. Record the patient's description of the circumstances when the pain first arose. Then elicit details about the pain, including the following:

- Onset
- Location and radiation
- Duration
- Nature (e.g., sharp, dull, stabbing)
- Severity rated on a 0 to 10 scale, with 0 representing *no pain* and 10 representing *the worst pain imaginable*
- Exacerbating factors
- Relieving factors

Ask the patient if the pain prevents him from performing certain motions or activities, interferes with activities of daily living, or decreases the quality of life. Also record any patient comments regarding usual activity levels, sleep patterns, and appetite.

Next, document the patient's use of analgesics, including over-the-counter preparations. Quoting the patient directly, record his perception of whether these drugs are effective or cause adverse effects.

Then ask the patient to describe his use of alcohol and street drugs. Also find out if the patient uses nonprescription drugs or other substances to control pain. Finally, ask about allergies to drugs and other substances. Document all responses carefully.

DOCUMENT WHAT YOU ASSESS

Record your findings from a thorough assessment. To avoid exacerbating the pain, be gentle when palpating, percussing, or auscultating the painful area.

First, document how well the patient can move the painful area, noting whether movement increases the pain. Describe weaknesses or functional limitations caused by the pain, and record diaphoresis or cool, clammy skin. In addition, record the patient's verbal response to pain, such as crying or shouting, and any nonverbal signs of pain, such as facial grimacing or guarding the painful area.

Next, measure and document the patient's vital signs. With severe pain, expect tachycardia, tachypnea, and hypertension. Assess whether the pain or analgesics have affected the patient's LOC or distorted his time perception. For instance, if the patient states, "My family left 1 hour ago," and you saw them leave 15 minutes earlier, then document this alteration in time perception. Finally, record what you observe about the patient's appetite.

DOCUMENT WHAT YOU DO AND TEACH

To evaluate the effectiveness of interventions and teaching, assess and record the patient's pain characteristics before and after each intervention, as well as his understanding of educational measures. As you document, be sure to cover the following general areas:

- Drug administration
- Comfort measures
- Balance between activity and rest
- External pain-relief measures, such as transcutaneous electrical nerve stimulation
- Emotional support
- Use of drugs for breakthrough pain, as indicated
- Use of patient-controlled analgesia
- Effective pain control strategies, such as positioning, distraction, relaxation, guided imagery, and external measures
- Signs and symptoms to report
- Activity and rest guidelines
- Factors that exacerbate pain
- Realistic expectations
- Ways to promote proper sleep patterns
- Avoidance of alcohol and substance abuse

- Stress management
- Importance of follow-up care and complying with treatment
- Resources for further information and support

WHEN YOUR PATIENT IS CONFUSED

When documenting care for a confused patient, you must show that you assessed for physiologic causes of the confusion, evaluated the patient's behavior carefully, and checked for exacerbating factors. You also must indicate that you took measures to help orient the patient and ensure his safety.

DOCUMENT WHAT THE PATIENT TELLS YOU

If your confused patient is not a reliable information source, try to obtain data about health history and current condition from family members, friends, and medical records. Check all three sources closely for clues to the cause of the confusion. Note information about chronic illnesses, hospitalizations, and surgeries, as well as a history of neurologic problems, cerebrovascular accident (CVA), or transient ischemic attacks.

To discover if an adverse drug effect, drug interaction, or inappropriate dose is causing the patient's confusion, record the names of all drugs the patient uses, along with their doses and administration times and routes.

Next, determine and record the patient's alcohol consumption pattern. Document information about his living situation, including the names of people who normally are with the patient during the day and at night, as well as the names of social contacts and other sources of support.

To help evaluate the patient's sleep pattern, find out if he is exposed to natural light during the day. Such exposure aids time orientation and affects circadian rhythms. Disruption of circadian rhythms may reduce sleep, possibly causing confusion. Document how much sleep the patient usually gets, and describe use of sedatives or other measures to promote sleep.

Also ask about sensory deficits, such as decreased visual acuity, hearing, and sensation. Describe corrective devices the patient uses, such as eyeglasses or a hearing aid, and record the patient's perception of the effectiveness of these devices.

DOCUMENT WHAT YOU ASSESS

Because confusion can take many behavioral forms and stem from various physical causes, you will need to perform and document a complete patient assessment. Include the following information.

Onset and symptoms. If you notice that your patient becomes confused at certain times of day, document the behaviors, symptoms, and activities that occur at these times. Note whether the confusion has a gradual or sudden onset, and record the names, doses, and administration times of drugs received that day.

Determine if the patient experiences weakness when confused. Assess for and document bilateral handgrip and arm and leg strength. Note difficulty with coordinating fine and gross movements, and document speech abnormalities, such as garbled speech, word searching, aphasia, and difficulty articulating words. Also describe whether the patient is alert or lethargic. If he falls asleep frequently, record how long he can stay awake at one time and how easily you can arouse him from sleep.

Cognitive functions. Record your assessment of the patient's orientation to time, place, situation, and person. Using direct quotes, document the patient's answers to questions you ask when evaluating reality orientation. When recording the ability to understand what others say, use measurable behaviors. Do not simply rely on the patient's statement that he understands. For instance, document whether the patient can repeat instructions, follow commands appropriately, and demonstrate procedures taught to him.

Also record your assessment of the patient's short-term, midrange, and long-term memory. Start by asking the patient to repeat several words, then ask what he did yesterday, and, finally, question the patient about events that occurred many years ago.

Note whether the patient can focus on one activity for an extended period of time. In addition, note whether statements made by the patient are appropriate or inappropriate. Record inappropriate statements in the patient's own words, and be sure to include a description of the circumstances. To make sure you did not misinterpret anything, ask the patient to explain his statement and record this explanation.

If your patient exhibits abnormal behaviors or makes statements that suggest he is hallucinating, describe the specific behaviors and record the patient's statements in his exact words. In addition, document the patient's emotional status, noting anxiety, irritability, or depression. If the patient's behavior suggests he may harm himself or others, document this behavior and the measures you take to ensure safety, such as providing one-to-one supervision.

Sensory deficits. Document visual, hearing, or other sensory deficits you detect. Record exactly what the patient says and what you observe. For instance, you may write, "Patient states his hearing is adequate when wearing a hearing aid. Patient did not respond to his name when it was spoken in a normal volume from 2 feet away while he was wearing the hearing aid."

DOCUMENT WHAT YOU DO AND TEACH

Document interventions you take to keep your patient safe, decrease his confusion, and address its cause. Thorough documentation helps detect factors that worsen or ease confusion. Teaching a confused patient and his family helps ensure safe, appropriate care while the patient is hospitalized and after discharge. If the patient is so confused that you question whether he is capable of consenting to treatment, notify the physician (see *Is Your Patient Competent?*).

IS YOUR PATIENT COMPETENT?

Legally, every adult is considered competent unless a judge finds otherwise in a formal hearing. A confused patient may be legally competent but unable to consent to treatment or otherwise participate in the treatment plan. If the patient cannot understand the nature of the treatment, he is considered clinically incompetent (or incapacitated).

Determining clinical competency

In most facilities the attending physician decides whether a patient is clinically competent. Nursing documentation of the patient's physical and psychosocial responses to therapy may play a major role in the physician's decision. To determine clinical competency, the physician typically evaluates whether the patient can do the following:
- Make definitive decisions
- Understand the information provided
- Engage in rational decision making and appreciate the possible outcomes of each option
- Make a reasonable decision about treatment

Murky legal waters

If the patient falls short in any of the previously mentioned areas, the physician usually tries to obtain consent from the patient's closest relative or appointed health care decision maker. If the patient is legally competent, obtaining the consent of a surrogate may lead to a legal action for battery, based on unauthorized touching of the patient.

To clarify the issue, lawmakers are addressing the family's surrogate decision-making power. Typically, they favor granting such power if the family acts in good faith. Therefore obtaining a surrogate's consent generally is considered safer than relying solely on the consent of a clinically incompetent patient.

Documenting care

If you care for a clinically incompetent patient, obtain the names of all family members and identify the closest relative, family-appointed spokesperson, or surrogate decision maker to contact about treatment decisions. In addition, document conversations you have with these people. Record their names and telephone numbers in the medical record and your nursing documentation.

Depending on the cause of the patient's confusion, you may need to document the following interventions and teaching points:
- Frequent observation and orientation
- Safety measures
- Management of stimulation
- Sensory and communication needs
- Drug therapy
- Laboratory test results
- Potential hazards of taking nonprescription or herbal preparations without consulting the physician
- Importance of avoiding potential substances of abuse, such as alcohol
- Signs and symptoms for the caregiver and/or family to report
- Ways for the caregiver and/or family to monitor the patient's condition
- Follow-up tests

- Nutrition
- Importance of daily social contact and routine social activities
- Appropriate stimuli, such as a newspaper, radio, clock, calendar, and television
- Avoidance of drastic changes, such as rearrangement of furniture
- Keeping the home clean and clutter free
- Effective ways to manage agitation and irritability
- Resources for further information and support

WHEN YOUR PATIENT HAS A SEIZURE

Typically, a seizure is self-limited and poses no immediate threat to the patient's life. However, during a seizure, a patient may fall or aspirate gastric contents into the lungs. In addition, status epilepticus (a series of uninterrupted seizures) may cause permanent brain damage or even death unless halted promptly by the administration of diazepam, phenobarbital, or another anticonvulsant agent. Your assessment and in-depth documentation of the patient's status and the actions taken to keep him safe can prove important to diagnosis and treatment. For instance, your detailed record of the patient's condition before, during, and after the seizure can help determine the seizure type and, possibly, its cause.

DOCUMENT WHAT THE PATIENT TELLS YOU

Ask your patient if he has experienced a seizure before, and determine if he has had other neurologic problems. Document the patient's responses; then record a history of diseases and conditions that increase the risk of seizures, such as hypoglycemia, head trauma, and alcohol or drug use.

If the patient has a history of seizures, document the date of the initial diagnosis and the current treatment plan, including prescribed drugs. Record the names, doses, and administration frequency of anticonvulsant agents he is taking, along with the time and amount of the last dose. If the patient reports a history of alcohol or drug use, document the substance, the time of last use, and the amount taken. Next, explore factors associated with previous seizures, such as lack of sleep or emotional distress, and document these facts in the patient's medical record. In addition, record any nonspecific symptoms the patient may have experienced just before a seizure, such as headaches, mood changes, lethargy, muscle spasms, or jerking. Be sure to note the symptom's timing relative to the seizure. If the patient says he usually has an aura before a seizure, document the description of the aura in the patient's exact words. For instance, the patient may describe a pungent smell, an unusual taste, nausea, indigestion, a rising or sinking feeling in his stomach, or a visual disturbance, such as seeing flashing lights.

DOCUMENT WHAT YOU ASSESS

Besides offering valuable clues to the seizure type and its cause, accurate documentation of your patient's condition and behavior just before, during, and after the seizure provides baseline information that can help the health care team detect changes in his status. If you did not witness the seizure, try to obtain information from someone who did.

Begin your documentation by describing events that preceded the seizure, such as an aura, outcry, or other behavior. Also record the following information:
- Time the seizure began
- Time it ended
- Length of clonic and tonic phases, if present
- LOC before, during, and after the seizure
- Neurologic status
- Pupil responses and arm and leg strength after the seizure
- Specific body parts affected by the seizure
- Vital signs during the seizure (if they can be assessed without harming the patient)
- Vital signs after the seizure
- Respiratory status, noting cyanosis and other signs of inadequate oxygenation
- Urinary or bowel incontinence

The patient may receive care before the seizure ends, such as drugs to halt the seizure and position changes to prevent injury. Record these interventions. In addition, document the name, dose, and administration time and route of the anticonvulsant agent given, and note its effectiveness in resolving the seizure.

Assessment after the seizure. After the seizure ends, examine the patient for injuries sustained during the seizure and assess his overall condition. Document your findings thoroughly. Depending on the seizure type and severity, the patient may display various behaviors immediately after the seizure. Besides documenting his LOC, check for and record other signs and symptoms that occur. Expected findings after a seizure include the following:
- Confusion
- Emotional lability
- Lethargy
- Fatigue
- Increased sensitivity to bright lights and noise
- Amnesia related to the seizure

Continue to observe and document the patient's condition until he returns to baseline status.

DOCUMENT WHAT YOU DO AND TEACH
To promote continuity of care throughout your patient's stay, record the interventions and teaching you perform to maintain safety before, during, and after the seizure. Include the following items:
- Maintenance of the bed in a low position, near the nurses' station
- Raised and padded side rails
- Call button within easy reach
- An emergency airway, supplemental oxygen, and suction equipment at the bedside
- Resuscitation equipment and an emergency drug tray nearby

- Patient instruction to report an aura immediately
- Patient positioning to one side to maintain an open airway and prevent aspiration
- Removal of potentially dangerous objects from the area
- Physician notification
- Staying at the patient's side until the seizure ends, avoiding restraining the patient
- Drug and IV therapy
- Reorientation, reassurance, and reassessment of patient frequently (See *How Often Should You Reassess Your Patient?*)

HOW OFTEN SHOULD YOU REASSESS YOUR PATIENT?

The Joint Commission (formerly The Joint Commission on Accreditation of Healthcare Organizations [JCAHO]) has developed the following recommendations for patient reassessment. Keep in mind that these recommendations represent the minimum requirements. Your patient may need more frequent reassessment.

Patient	When to Reassess
Same-day surgery patient	On return from postanesthesia unit and immediately before discharge
Stable patient in medical-surgical unit	Every 24 hours
Patient with decreasing neurologic status	Every 15 minutes
Patient in labor	Every 15 minutes
Patient with active gastrointestinal (GI) bleeding	Continuously, on a one-to-one basis
Suicidal patient	Continuously, on a one-to-one basis
Patient in rehabilitation	Every 1 to 2 weeks
Long-term care patient	Monthly

- Diagnostic testing
- Regular dental care to treat trauma to the teeth, gums, and mouth
- Measures to help prevent seizures
- Medical alert identification
- Information about driver's license status
- Resources for further information and support

WHEN YOUR PATIENT HAS A CEREBROVASCULAR ACCIDENT

A patient who experiences a CVA or brain attack may be in immediate danger of airway obstruction and further brain damage. To help ensure prompt treatment and develop an effective nursing plan of care, you must document this condition thoroughly and record the responses to rapid interventions. Your documentation provides a crucial record of events throughout the course of the patient's illness.

Not all patients who have had a CVA require similar care. The history and assessment findings you will document and the interventions you will perform depend on the brain area affected and the cause of the CVA. The most common causes include thrombosis, embolus, and intracerebral hemorrhage. Although diagnostic tests help identify the precipitating condition, timely and effective management hinges on precise nursing observation and documentation.

DOCUMENT WHAT THE PATIENT TELLS YOU

During the health history interview, obtain information about the patient's medical history and symptoms just before and during the CVA. If your patient cannot communicate, interview family members and check medical records for relevant information.

Medical history. Document a history of hypertension, cerebral aneurysm, or a bleeding disorder because these conditions can cause intracerebral hemorrhage. Also record a history of rheumatic heart disease, endocarditis, posttraumatic valvular disease, open-heart surgery, and atrial fibrillation and other arrhythmias (these conditions suggest cerebral embolism as the cause of CVA). You should ask if the patient has a history of peripheral vascular disease, hyperlipidemia, heart disease, diabetes mellitus, transient ischemic attacks, and trauma. Record the information you obtain.

Next, document the names and doses of prescription and over-the-counter drugs the patient has been taking. If the patient is taking an antihypertensive or anticoagulant agent, find out when it was last taken and in what dose. Record the answer.

Your patient's lifestyle may provide clues to the cause of his CVA. Documenting this information also promotes more effective rehabilitation planning. Gather as much data as possible about the patient's smoking history, dietary sodium and fat intake, daily activity level, and drug history.

Symptoms. Record information about the patient's condition during the days and hours that led up to the CVA. Ask family members if the patient cannot tell you himself. For example, document reports of headache, weakness, dizziness, confusion, memory disturbances, mood swings, tingling, numbness, poor muscle coordination, visual impairment (e.g., double vision), facial drooping, difficulty swallowing or talking, stiff neck, seizures, bowel or bladder incontinence, and bounding pulse.

DOCUMENT WHAT YOU ASSESS

Besides aiding diagnosis and treatment, the data you collect and document during your physical assessment help ensure continuity of care by providing a baseline for later comparison. When documenting your assessment, focus especially on the patient's respiratory, neurologic, and cardiovascular systems.

Respiratory system. Quickly check your patient for a patent airway, and then take steps to maintain it. Measure respiratory rate, pattern, and effort; evaluate skin color; and review pulse oximetry or ABG analysis results. Immediately notify the physician of abnormalities or changes in the patient's status. Then document your findings and your notification of the physician, including the time of notification.

Neurologic system. Accurate documentation of neurologic status can help care-givers track the patient's progress or deterioration. Record your frequent assessments of his LOC. Remember, though, to document only specific and objective data, not interpretations of your findings (see *Recording the Level of Consciousness: Objectivity Counts*).

RECORDING THE LEVEL OF CONSCIOUSNESS: OBJECTIVITY COUNTS

When documenting your patient's level of consciousness (LOC), include only specific, objective observations, not vague terms that one reader may interpret differently than another. For instance, if the patient is sitting up in bed talking with visitors, record this fact in detail. Do not state merely that he is *alert*. If he is unresponsive with no reflexes, describe him that way rather than simply writing *comatose*. For more hints, review the following documentation:

Do Write	Do Not Write
Awake and aware of the environment and interacting with visitors.	Alert
Oriented to his name, place, and today's date, including the year.	Appears to know where he is
Sleeps when not stimulated. He is easily aroused by verbal stimulation, then is oriented to his name, place, and today's date.	Lethargic
Aroused with difficulty. Requires physical versus verbal stimulation.	Obtunded
Nonsensical verbal responses.	
Aroused only with painful stimuli. No verbal response.	Stuporous
Reflex activity only with painful stimulation. Cannot be aroused.	Semicomatose
No response or reflex reactions.	Comatose

Because hemiplegia is a common sign of CVA, assess for and document weakness, numbness, and tingling in the arms or legs. Report these problems to the physician promptly. Also check for and record facial drooping, loss of voluntary movement, changes in reflexes, and speech difficulties. When documenting these findings, describe the specific areas of the body affected and the severity of the abnormality.

Next, evaluate for aphasia (defective language function). Remember that aphasia may be receptive, expressive, or mixed. To detect receptive aphasia (inability to understand language), assess the patient's ability to follow simple commands. To detect expressive aphasia (inability to express or form words), ask the patient to identify an object or a person. Document your findings, which may suggest that the patient has a specific type of aphasia or mixed aphasia (both types).

Cardiovascular system and other findings. Evaluate and document your patient's cardiovascular system. Measure and record blood pressure; typically, a CVA increases blood pressure, requiring frequent monitoring and an antihypertensive agent. If you administer an antihypertensive drug, document its effectiveness. Be sure to notify the physician if you detect a drop in blood pressure, which may promote brain tissue ischemia or death or indicate continued life-threatening bleeding. Document your notification, including its time, the physician's orders, and your actions.

Monitor and document the patient's blood glucose level, which may increase as a result of steroid therapy used to reduce cerebral edema caused by the CVA. Record your findings.

DOCUMENT WHAT YOU DO AND TEACH

Document all actions you take to maintain the patient's respiratory status and vital signs, to curb further cerebral ischemia and infarction, to prevent injury, to prevent or manage CVA complications, and to help the patient communicate needs. Also provide teaching to your patient and his family. Be sure to cover the following general areas:

- Diagnostic tests
- Drug and IV therapy
- Artificial airway, if needed
- Positioning to maintain a patent airway
- Pulse oximetry
- Oxygen therapy
- Suctioning as needed
- Endotracheal intubation and mechanical ventilation, if needed
- Nothing by mouth (NPO) status, until swallowing ability is established
- Fluid intake and output
- Assistance with personal hygiene
- Skin protection measures
- Administration of gastric feedings, if ordered
- Raised side rails and nearby placement of the call button
- Toileting schedule and bowel program
- Turning the patient frequently and using pressure relief devices, such as a special mattress and heel protectors
- Passive ROM exercises
- Antiembolism stockings
- Footboards, slings, splints, and braces
- Help with communication
- Referrals to a speech, occupational, or physical therapist
- Disease process
- Ways to reduce risk factors for CVA recurrence
- Signs and symptoms to be reported
- Safety measures and devices to use at home, such as a shower chair
- Adaptive measures to use when performing activities of daily living
- Use of ambulatory aids, if needed
- Home exercise program
- Telephone numbers for home health agencies
- Resources for further information and support

WHEN YOUR PATIENT HAS HYPOGLYCEMIA

Defined as a low blood glucose level, hypoglycemia can lead to coma, irreversible brain damage, and death unless treated promptly and effectively. The condition occurs primarily in type 1 diabetic patients who do not eat enough food, who self-administer too much insulin, or who engage in unusual exertion. Other causes of hypoglycemia include cancer of the stomach, liver, or lung; adrenal gland hypofunction; malnutrition; liver dysfunction; alcoholism; and strenuous exercise.

To establish a foundation for the plan of care, focus your documentation on the patient's history of diabetes mellitus or other disorders, recent food and fluid intake, activity level, recent infections or emotional stress, and alcohol use. Be sure to document all physical assessment findings, laboratory test results, nursing interventions, and patient responses to interventions.

DOCUMENT WHAT THE PATIENT TELLS YOU

Most diabetic patients experience warning symptoms of hypoglycemia. Ask your patient to describe how he has been feeling for the past few hours, and record the patient's response in his own words. If the patient noticed warning signs, try to determine (and then document) exactly when they began and how they progressed. Expect to document the following symptoms:
- Nervousness or shakiness
- Dizziness or feeling faint
- Numbness or tingling in the hands and feet
- Weakness
- Diaphoresis
- Hunger or nausea
- Headache
- Palpitations
- Double vision

If the patient reports such symptoms, ask if he has had them before. If so, find out if the patient knows what caused them. Record any responses in the patient's exact words.

DOCUMENT WHAT YOU ASSESS

Although the patient's symptoms are important, you will also need to document objective signs of hypoglycemia. If you witnessed the hypoglycemic episode, record your observation of the following:
- Tremors
- Personality changes, such as aggressiveness, stubbornness, negativity, or depression
- Decreased LOC, such as confusion, difficulty speaking, delirium, seizures, or loss of consciousness
- Poor coordination
- Cold, clammy skin
- Increased heart rate or a slow, bounding pulse
- Increased respiratory rate

DOCUMENT WHAT YOU DO AND TEACH

Hypoglycemia can rapidly progress to neurologic compromise, so you will need to intervene immediately and notify the physician. After verifying hypoglycemia, vary interventions in accordance with the patient's LOC. Remember to take these general actions and to teach the following key points to prevent recurrence of hypoglycemia:

- Finger-stick glucose levels, using a portable blood glucose meter
- Administration of 15 g of a simple oral carbohydrate (e.g., juice, candy, dextrose, honey) if your patient is conscious and can swallow
- Administration of an IV carbohydrate (e.g., dextrose) or subcutaneous, intramuscular, or IV glucagon, if your patient is unresponsive and cannot swallow
- IV access
- Cause of hypoglycemia
- Importance of maintaining a normal blood glucose level
- Signs and symptoms to recognize and actions to take
- Safety measures
- Importance of carrying an oral carbohydrate at all times
- Importance of eating regular meals and snacks, plus what to do if the patient is sick and unable to eat (sick-day rules)
- Importance of wearing medical alert identification
- Importance of having regular medical checkups

WHEN YOUR PATIENT HAS HYPERGLYCEMIA

Defined as a high blood glucose level, hyperglycemia seldom poses an immediate threat until the glucose level exceeds 240 mg/dl. With extreme blood glucose level elevation, the patient's condition may rapidly progress to ketoacidosis, a potentially fatal metabolic disorder.

Although commonly caused by diabetes mellitus, hyperglycemia also may stem from Cushing's syndrome, physical stress (e.g., trauma, burns, surgery), and certain drugs (including corticosteroids and thiazide diuretics). In a diabetic patient, common causes of hyperglycemia include insufficient insulin dose, dietary noncompliance, infection, and gastrointestinal (GI) illness.

To provide a basis for the nursing plan of care and the interdisciplinary treatment plan, first determine if your patient has been diagnosed with diabetes. Then explore and document other aspects of the patient's health history, including recent food intake, infections, and physical injury.

DOCUMENT WHAT THE PATIENT TELLS YOU

Ask the patient how he has been feeling over the past few days, and record the response in the patient's exact words. The following are symptoms of hyperglycemia:

- Weakness
- Unusual thirst
- Frequent urination
- Anorexia
- Vomiting

- Drowsiness
- Abdominal pain
- Headache

Then find out if the patient has had hyperglycemia previously. If so, record the symptoms experienced at that time.

DOCUMENT WHAT YOU ASSESS

Next, perform a physical examination. Expect to assess and document the following signs and symptoms of hyperglycemia:

- Flushed cheeks
- Dry skin and mouth
- Acetone (sweet) breath odor
- Kussmaul's respirations (fast, deep, labored breathing), especially if the blood glucose level exceeds 500 mg/dl
- Weak, rapid pulse
- Low blood pressure
- Restlessness
- Decreased LOC (possibly unresponsiveness)
- Electrolyte abnormalities, particularly potassium imbalance
- Glucose and ketones in the urine
- Signs of infection, such as a fever, increased pulse rate, or hot, dry skin that is flushed

DOCUMENT WHAT YOU DO AND TEACH

Besides documenting your rapid interventions, record the patient's responses to these general interventions to show that you took appropriate actions to reverse hyperglycemia and that the patient knows how to prevent further hyperglycemia:

- Insulin administration
- Glucose monitoring
- Fluid and electrolyte balance
- Pathophysiology of the disorder
- Mechanisms of hyperglycemia and ketoacidosis
- Prescribed drugs, including their names, doses, administration times and routes, adverse effects, and storage
- Insulin administration, if indicated
- Signs and symptoms of hypoglycemia and hyperglycemia; actions to take if these conditions occur
- Use of a blood glucose monitor
- Importance of regular blood glucose monitoring
- Effect of diet, infection, stress, and exercise on the glucose level
- Dietary restrictions
- Foot care
- Importance of seeing the physician regularly and having regular eye examinations
- Resources for further information and support

WHEN YOUR PATIENT HAS A PRESSURE ULCER

A pressure ulcer is an ulceration of the skin and underlying tissue. It results from prolonged pressure, primarily on a bony prominence, and reflects ischemia and tissue hypoxia. A pressure ulcer may take a long time to heal and demands meticulous care by all health care providers.

When documenting your nursing care, include the patient's risk factors for developing a pressure ulcer, your assessment findings and interventions, and the patient's response. This information helps the health care team evaluate the treatment regimen's effectiveness as healing progresses.

DOCUMENT WHAT THE PATIENT TELLS YOU

To determine when the pressure ulcer developed and to detect contributing health care problems, obtain and document a thorough history from your patient and family members. Ask them to describe any changes in the ulcer's size, appearance, drainage, and odor. Document their descriptions accurately.

Then record the patient's complete medical history. Especially note risk factors for pressure ulcers, such as diabetes mellitus, peripheral vascular disease, immunosuppression, smoking, and delayed healing. Collect and document data about the patient's dietary habits to determine whether nutritional needs are being met. Determine if the patient has a history of incontinence, and document this information. Finally, ask about and record the patient's usual daily routine, including his activity level. If the patient is bedridden, ask which positions he most often maintains.

DOCUMENT WHAT YOU ASSESS

When documenting your initial assessment, be as specific as you can, especially when describing the pressure ulcer's size, stage, appearance, drainage, and odor. Remember, your record provides a baseline for evaluating healing and gauging treatment effectiveness.

Wound stage. Assess the stage of the pressure ulcer according to this guide:
• *Stage I.* Skin redness is unrelieved by removal of the pressure source.
• *Stage II.* Skin is chafed, cracked, blistered, or peeling, but the damage is superficial.
• *Stage III.* The full thickness of the skin and, possibly, subcutaneous (fatty) tissue is lost. Drainage, eschar, and necrotic tissue may be present.
• *Stage IV.* A deep, craterlike ulcer shows destruction of the full thickness of the skin and deeper tissues. Muscle and bone may be exposed and damaged.
• *Unable to stage.* Area covered with necrotic tissue; unable to stage precisely.
You may document wound appearance in a narrative format or by drawing a picture of the wound and labeling it appropriately. When describing wound characteristics, include the following features:
• Precise location
• Diameter in centimeters
• Depth in centimeters

- Amount, color, and location of granulation tissue (moist, pink tissue that represents new growth)
- Amount, color, and location of eschar (black or gray, scablike, crusty tissue covering the wound)
- Amount, color, and location of necrotic tissue (dry, black tissue that represents tissue death)
- Amount and description of drainage
- Description of odor
- Length and location of any undermining (cavity beneath the wound opening) or tunneling
- Color and temperature of the surrounding skin

Describe the amounts of granulation tissue, eschar, and necrotic tissue in percentages of total wound tissue. For instance, if granulation tissue accounts for about half of the pressure sore, record this as 50% granulation.

Nutritional and hydration status. Adequate nutrition and fluid intake are crucial for pressure ulcer healing. To assess your patient's nutritional and hydration status, evaluate and document the skin's general appearance and turgor. Also record the results of serum albumin and total protein assays.

DOCUMENT WHAT YOU DO AND TEACH

Your interventions for a patient with a pressure ulcer should focus on promoting healing and preventing further skin breakdown. Record each action you take and your patient's response. Also document interdisciplinary and collaborative consultations and interventions (see *Taking the Team Approach to Wound Care*).

TAKING THE TEAM APPROACH TO WOUND CARE

When developing a holistic plan of care for a patient with a pressure ulcer, expect to consult these health care team members. Document all pertinent communication with team members.

Dietitian	For strategies on optimizing the patient's nutrition
Occupational therapist	For advice on frequent repositioning to maximize pressure relief
Wound/ostomy practitioner	To help assess the wound, form a plan of care, and evaluate the wound care regimen's effectiveness
Medical social worker	For referrals and resource information to ensure continuity of care after discharge
Plastic surgeon	To surgically repair, débride, and close certain wounds

---

Your documentation for careful interventions and teaching should include the following areas:
- Wound care
- Pressure reduction
- Frequent turning and repositioning

- Good hygiene
- Overhead trapeze to assist in repositioning
- Pathophysiology of pressure ulcers
- Wound care regimen
- Signs and symptoms to report
- Importance of good hygiene and skin care
- Nutrition and fluid requirements to promote healing
- Use of pressure reduction or pressure relief devices
- Importance of frequent repositioning

WHEN YOUR PATIENT HAS SURGERY

With more same-day surgeries being performed and shorter hospital stays for major surgery, you may find it a challenge to gather and document all the necessary patient information in the time allotted. Yet, no matter how briefly you care for a patient, you must document all the care you provide. Besides serving as the basis for evaluating the plan of care, your documentation reflects the standard of care provided. This can prove important if the patient later sues you, other health care team members, or your health care facility.

DOCUMENT WHAT THE PATIENT TELLS YOU

Before surgery, document the patient's medical history. Ask the patient to describe previous health problems, the treatments received for them, and the effectiveness of those treatments. Then document the information about previous surgeries and other medical procedures. Find out if the patient has experienced an allergic reaction to a food, drug, anesthetic agent, contrast medium, or dye. If the patient has never been anesthetized, ask if anyone in his family has experienced a reaction to an anesthetic agent.

Determine if the patient has had a problem with bleeding, such as easy bruising, blood in the urine or stool, or difficulty stopping a cut from bleeding. Also document the use of warfarin or nonsteroidal antiinflammatory agents. These factors indicate that the patient may have bleeding problems during and after surgery.

Next, have the patient tell you what he knows about the scheduled procedure, and document his response. If the patient will go home shortly after surgery, record the type of transportation to be used and the name of the person accompanying the patient home. Also document whether someone will be at home when the patient arrives or if he will be alone that night.

Next, ask the patient when he last ate or drank and what drugs (if any) were taken that day. Record the patient's reply in his own words. Then question the patient about any recent symptoms, especially if they seem unrelated to the reason for the upcoming surgery. In particular, document shortness of breath, chest pain, nausea, anxiety, and urinary difficulties.

Record the date of the patient's last bowel movement, and indicate whether he moves his bowels regularly. Also document the patient's usual activity level and daily routine, which may be disrupted during the recovery period.

Ask the patient if he has ever smoked. When documenting the answer, include the number of cigarettes smoked per day (currently and in the past).

In addition, find out if the patient regularly drinks alcohol or uses recreational drugs, and record the response. Document the patient's use of hearing aids, eyeglasses, and dentures. Finally, record the name of the patient's primary care physician.

During the postoperative period. After the patient returns from surgery, record reports of discomfort and other problems. Ask the patient to rate the pain's severity on a scale of 0 to 10, with 0 representing *no pain* and 10 representing *the worst pain imaginable.* Document this answer. In addition, record the following complaints:
• Urinary urgency with inability to void
• Shortness of breath
• Chest pain
• Nausea
• Leg pain or cramping
• Anxiety or fear

DOCUMENT WHAT YOU ASSESS

Perform a physical examination before and after surgery, and document your findings.

Preoperative findings. Remember that your preoperative examination provides a baseline for later assessments. Notify the physician of abnormal findings, such as the following:
• Hypertension or hypotension
• Tachycardia or bradycardia
• Fever
• Abnormal breath sounds
• Irregular heart rate
• Abdominal firmness or distention
• Cold or discolored arms or legs

Postoperative findings. Document your postoperative physical examination findings, and then compare them with preoperative findings. Measure and record the patient's vital signs every 5 to 15 minutes for the first hour after surgery and then hourly. Auscultate the lungs, noting the rate, rhythm, and depth of respirations; document these data carefully. Then palpate peripheral pulses, recording the strength of each pulse. Document any reported pain on ankle dorsiflexion.

Next, record the amount of urine in the drainage bag, if present. Use this measurement as a baseline when assessing urine output over the next several hours. Then auscultate and palpate the patient's abdomen, recording abdominal tone and the type of bowel sounds.

Document the appearance of the dressing and the area around the incision, including the amount and color of drainage and skin discoloration. Assess the insertion site for tubes, drains, and catheters, and record their appearance.

Review the patient's latest blood chemistry and hematology results. Notify the physician of abnormal values, and document that you did so.

DOCUMENT WHAT YOU DO AND TEACH

Document all interventions you performed before and after surgery. In your preoperative documentation, include the steps you took to prepare the patient for surgery, including teaching. Document perioperative care accordingly (see *Documenting Perioperative Care*).

DOCUMENTING PERIOPERATIVE CARE

Before your patient is transferred from the postanesthesia care unit to the surgery suite, review your documentation to make sure it addresses all important aspects of his medical and recent history, the surgery he has just undergone, his postanesthesia care, and his current condition.

Medical and recent history
When documenting history information, be sure to include the following:
- The patient's medical and surgical history
- Events leading to current surgery
- Complications related to previous surgery or anesthesia (Document this prominently at the front of the section.)
- Drug or food allergies
- Current drugs
- Tobacco use

Surgery
Surgery documentation should cover the following:
- Type of procedure performed
- Time surgery began and ended
- Type of anesthesia used
- Duration of anesthesia
- Range of patient's vital signs during surgery
- Name, dose, administration time and route of each drug administered
- Fluid intake, output, and loss
- Use of devices to stop blood flow to a particular area, such as a tourniquet
- Type and location of drains, tubes, implants, and dressings left in place
- Patient's tolerance of the procedure
- Surgical complications

Postanesthesia period
During the postanesthesia period, you may document vital signs, assessment findings, and interventions on a postanesthesia flow sheet. No matter where you record the information, your documentation of the patient's postanesthesia course should include the following:
- Vital signs
- Level of consciousness (LOC)
- Skin color
- Name, dose, administration time and route of each analgesic or other drug given

DOCUMENTING PERIOPERATIVE CARE—cont'd

- Patient's respiratory status, including the time of endotracheal tube removal, use of supplemental oxygen (if ordered), and arterial blood gas (ABG) levels or pulse oximetry readings
- Unusual events or complications, such as vomiting, hypothermia, arrhythmias, swollen tongue, or postspinal headache
- Interventions used to treat unusual events or complications documented earlier

Current condition
At the end of your postanesthesia documentation, document the patient's current condition. If the patient is being discharged to home (as with same-day surgery), be sure to document other pertinent findings, such as whether or not the patient can eat, walk, and urinate, as well as your patient's understanding of discharge instructions. In addition, be sure to include the following:
- Vital signs
- LOC
- Interventions that will continue in the surgical unit

In your postoperative notes, record that you implemented all postoperative orders and helped the patient return to a baseline level of functioning. Make sure you cover the following areas in your documentation:
- Completion of preoperative checklist
- NPO status
- Signed consent form
- Correct identification band
- Removal of personal clothing, jewelry, and prosthetics, such as dentures and contact lenses
- Taping of wedding ring, if permitted
- Itemized list of valuables
- Postanesthesia care unit transfer information
- Fluid intake and output
- Diagnostic testing
- Coughing and deep-breathing exercises
- Splinting of incision
- Pain control
- Drug and IV therapy
- Antiembolism stockings
- Leg and foot exercises
- Emotional support to the patient and family
- Instructions for resuming previous drugs at home
- Recommended activity level
- Dietary recommendations or restrictions
- Care of the incision and remaining drains
- Signs and symptoms to be reported
- Dates and times of follow-up medical appointments

INDEX

A

Abbreviated assessment, 23
Abdominal aorta, 226
Abdominal aortic aneurysm, 179–181
Abdominal distention, 256–259
  assessment of, 256–257
  asymmetrical, 256
  causes of, 257–259
  percussion of, 238–239, 246
Abdominal pain, 249–256
  acute, 250
  assessment of, 249–253
  peritonitis, 249, 253
Abdominal region
  anatomy of, 226
  assessment of, 16
  auscultation of, 235, 237
  bimanual palpation, 242
  bowel sounds, 236–237, 246, 256–257
  chief complaints of, 245–273
    cholecystitis. *See* Cholecystitis
    constipation, 248–249, 260–261
    diarrhea, 261–266
    distention. *See* Abdominal
      distention
    erectile dysfunction, 272
    fecal incontinence, 259
    hematuria, 268
    menstrual abnormalities, 268–270
    nausea and vomiting, 246–249
    penile discharge or lesions,
      270–272
    rectal bleeding, 272–273
    urinary frequency, 266–267
    urinary incontinence, 259–260
    urination difficulty or pain,
      267–268
    vaginal discharge or lesions,
      270–272
  contraction of muscles, 241
  examination of, 231–232, 244, 311–312
  female genitalia
    age-related changes, 243
    anatomy of, 229–231, 233
    palpation of, 243–244
  fluid shifts in, 234
  friction rubs, 236, 237

Abdominal region (*Continued*)
  inguinal lymph nodes, 240
  inspection of, 232–234
    abnormal findings, 234
    normal findings, 233–234
    patient positioning for, 232
  male genitalia
    anatomy of, 231, 233
    palpation of, 243
  mass in, 241–242
  palpation of, 16, 239
  percussion of, 237, 239
  peritoneal inflammation, 242–243
  pregnancy-related changes, 35
  quadrants, 236–238
  vascular sounds, 236
Abducens nerve, 72, 93*t*
Abrasions, corneal, 108
Absent heart sounds, 161, 170
Abuse
  history-taking, 9–10
  by hostile patients, 27–28
Achilles reflex, 286–288
Acoustic nerve, 72, 93*t*
Acoustic neuroma, 130
Acromion process, 131–132
Actinic keratoses, 203–204
Actinic lentigines, 58
Actinic purpura, 58
Acute abdominal pain, 250
Acute angle-closure glaucoma,
  115–116, 120
Acute arterial occlusion, 301–302
Acute bacterial conjunctivitis, 114
Acute keratitis, 116
Acute labyrinthitis, 130
Acute otitis externa, 120–121, 126
Acute otitis media, 126–127
Acute vision loss, 119
Adie's pupil, 109
Adrenal glands, 226
Advanced open-angle glaucoma, 120
Adventitious breath sounds, 166
Aerophagia, 258–259
Age-related macular degeneration, 120
Aggravating factors, 5
Aging. *See also* Older adults
  blood pressure affected by, 44–45

ENGLISH-SPANISH TRANSLATIONS

ENGLISH	ESPAÑOL	PRONUNCIATION
Parts of the Body	**Las Partes del Cuerpo**	**las PAR-tays dehl KWAIR-poh**
Head and Neck	La cabeza y el cuello	la kah-BAY-sah ee el KWAY-yoh
Skull	el cráneo	CRAH-nay-oh
Forehead	la frente	FRAYN-tay
Temple	la sién	see-EN
Eye	el ojo	OH-hoh
Nose	la nariz	nah-REES
Ear	a oreja/el oído	h-RAY-hah/oh-WEE-do
Throat	la garganta	gar-GAHN-tah
Mouth	la boca	BOH-kah
Tongue	la lengua	LAYN-gwah
Teeth	los dientes	dee-AYN-tays
Cheek	la mejilla	may-HEE-yah
Chin	la barbilla	bar-BEE-yah
Skin	la piel	pee-EHL
Hair	el pelo	PAY-loh
Arm and Hand	**Brazo y mano**	**BRAH-soh ee MAH-noh**
Bones	los huesos	WAY-sohs
Fingers	los dedos	DAY-dohs
Thumb	el pulgar	pool-GAHR
Shoulder	el hombro	OHM-broh
Wrist	la muñeca	moo-NYAY-kah
Elbow	el codo	KOH-doh
Muscles	los músculos	MOOS-koo-lohs
Leg and Foot	**Pierna y pie**	**pee-AIR-nah ee pee-AY**
Pelvis	la pelvis	PEHL-bees
Thigh	el muslo	MOOS-loh
Knee	la rodilla	roh-DEE-yah
Ankle	el tobillo	toh-BEE-yoh
Toes	los dedos (del pie)	DAY-dohs (del pee-AY)
Chest	**Pecho**	**PAY-choh**
Rib	la costilla	kohs-TEE-yah
Heart	el corazón	koh-rah-SOHN
Chest/breast	el pecho/seno/busto	PAY-choh/SAY-noh/BOOS-toh
Waist	la cintura	seen-TOO-rah
Abdomen	**Abdomen**	**ahb-DOH-mayn**
Stomach	el estómago	ays-TOH-mah-goh
Liver	el hígado	EE-gah-doh
Spleen	el bazo	BAH-so
Gallbladder	la vesícula biliar	bay-SEE-koo-lah bee-LEE-ahr
Appendix	la apéndice	ah-PAYN-dee-say
Rectum	el recto	RAYK-toh
Groin	la ingle	EEN-glay
Back	**La espalda**	**la ays-PAHL-dah**
Lung	el pulmón	pool-MOHN
Spine	la espina dorsal	ays-PEE-nah DOHR-sahl
Kidney	el riñón	ree-NYOHN
Hip	la cadera	kah-DAIR-ah
Buttock	la nalga	NAHL-gah
Anus	el ano	AH-noh